Diabetes Remission

Editor

BETUL A. HATIPOGLU

ENDOCRINOLOGY AND METABOLISM CLINICS OF NORTH AMERICA

www.endo.theclinics.com

Consulting Editor
ADRIANA G. IOACHIMESCU

March 2023 • Volume 52 • Number 1

ELSEVIER

1600 John F. Kennedy Boulevard • Suite 1800 • Philadelphia, Pennsylvania, 19103-2899

http://www.theclinics.com

ENDOCRINOLOGY AND METABOLISM CLINICS OF NORTH AMERICA Volume 52, Number 1
March 2023 ISSN 0889-8529, ISBN 13: 978-0-323-96058-8

Editor: Taylor Hayes
Developmental Editor: Jessica Cañaberal

Endocrinology and Metabolism Clinics of North America (ISSN 0889-8529) is published quarterly by Elsevier
Inc., 360 Park Avenue South, New York, NY 10010-1710. Months of issue are March, June, September, and
December. Periodicals postage paid at New York, NY and additional mailing offices. Subscription prices are
USD 406.00 per year for US individuals, USD 907.00 per year for US institutions, USD 100.00 per year for US
students and residents, USD 481.00 per year for Canadian individuals, USD 1121.00 per year for Canadian institutions, USD 527.00 per year for international individuals, USD 1121.00 per year for international institutions,
USD 100.00 per year for Canadian students/residents, and USD 245.00 per year for international students/res-
idents. To receive student/resident rate, orders must be accompanied by name of affiliated institution, date of
term, and the signature of program/residency coordinator on institution letterhead. Orders will be billed at individual rate until proof of status is received. Foreign air speed delivery is included in all *Clinics* subscription prices.
All prices are subject to change without notice. **POSTMASTER:** Send address changes to *Endocrinology and
Metabolism Clinics of North America*, Elsevier Health Sciences Division, Subscription Customer Service, 3251
Riverport Lane, Maryland Heights, MO 63043. **Customer Service: Telephone: 1-800-654-2452** (U.S. and Canada); **1-314-447-8871** (outside U.S. and Canada). **Fax: 1-314-447-8029. E-mail: journalscustomerservice-u-
sa@elsevier.com (for print support); journalsonlinesupport-usa@elsevier.com (for online support).**

Reprints. For copies of 100 or more, of articles in this publication, please contact the Commercial Rights
Department, Elsevier Inc., 360 Park Avenue South, New York, NY 10010-1710; phone: +1-212-633-3874;
fax: +1-212-633-3820; E-mail: reprints@elsevier.com.

Endocrinology and Metabolism Clinics of North America is covered in *MEDLINE/PubMed (Index Medicus),
EMBASE/Excerpta Medica, Current Contents/Clinical Medicine, Current Contents/Life Sciences, Science
Citation Index, ISI/BIOMED, BIOSIS,* and *Chemical Abstracts.*

Contributors

CONSULTING EDITOR

ADRIANA G. IOACHIMESCU, MD, PHD, FACE
Associate Professor of Medicine and Neurosurgery Co-Director, The Emory Pituitary Center Emory University School of Medicine, Atlanta, Georgia, USA

EDITOR

BETUL A. HATIPOGLU, MD
Professor of Medicine, Case Western Reserve University School of Medicine, Vice Chair, UH System Clinical Affairs, Department of Medicine, Medical Director, Diabetes and Obesity Center, Mary B. Lee Chair in Adult Endocrinology, University Hospitals Cleveland Medical Center, Cleveland, Ohio, USA

AUTHORS

VANCE L. ALBAUGH, MD, PhD
Metamor Institute, Integrative Physiology and Molecular Medicine Laboratory, Pennington Biomedical Research Center, Louisiana State University, Baton Rouge, Louisiana, USA

DIMA ALFAKARA, MD
Endocrinology Fellow, Department of Endocrinology, University Hospitals of Cleveland, Cleveland, Ohio, USA

SADEER AL-KINDI, MD
Assistant Professor of Medicine, Harrington Heart and Vascular Institute, University Hospitals Cleveland Medical Center, Case Western Reserve University School of Medicine, Cleveland, Ohio, USA

CHRISTOPHER AXELROD, MS
Integrative Physiology and Molecular Medicine Laboratory, Pennington Biomedical Research Center, Louisiana State University, Baton Rouge, Louisiana, USA

ASHOK BALASUBRAMANYAM, MD
Professor of Medicine, Rutherford Professor of Diabetes Research, Division of Diabetes, Endocrinology, and Metabolism, Baylor College of Medicine, Houston, Texas, USA

KATHRYN P. BELMONT, BS
Integrative Physiology and Molecular Medicine Laboratory, Pennington Biomedical Research Center, Louisiana State University, Baton Rouge, Louisiana, USA

JULIA BLANCHETTE, PhD, RN
Nurse Scientist, Division of Endocrinology, University Hospitals Cleveland Medical Center, Center for Diabetes and Obesity, Cleveland, Ohio, USA

TANICIA DALEY, MD
Division of Pediatric Endocrinology, Children's Healthcare of Atlanta, Emory University School of Medicine, Atlanta, Georgia, USA

JOSE J, ECHEGARAY, MD
Assistant Professor, University Hospitals Eye Institute/Department of Ophthalmology and Visual Sciences, Case Western Reserve University, Vitreoretinal Diseases and Surgery, Ocular Immunology and Uveitis, University Hospitals, Cleveland, Ohio, USA

CRAIG B. FREY, DPM, AACFAS
Staff, University Hospitals Podiatric Medicine and Surgery, Director, University Hospitals Advanced Limb Salvage and Reconstruction, Fellowship Director, Residency Director, Cleveland, Ohio, USA

REVITAL GORODESKI BASKIN, MD
Department of Endocrinology, Obesity Program Director, Diabetes and Obesity Center, University Hospitals of Cleveland, Cleveland, Ohio, USA

NOUR HAMMAD, MD
Division of Nephrology and Hypertension, University Hospitals Cleveland Medical Center, Louis Stokes Cleveland VA Medical Center, Cleveland, Ohio, USA

ZUBAIDAH NOR HANIPAH, MD
Metamor Institute, Pennington Biomedical Research Center, Louisiana State University, Baton Rouge, Louisiana, USA; Department of Surgery, Faculty of Medicine and Health Sciences, University Putra Malaysia, Selangor, Malaysia

SHUAI HAO, MD
Division of Pediatric Endocrinology, Children's Healthcare of Atlanta, Emory University School of Medicine, Atlanta, Georgia, USA

MOHAMED HASSANEIN, MD
Division of Nephrology, University of Mississippi Medical Center, Jackson, Mississippi, USA

BETUL A. HATIPOGLU, MD
Professor of Medicine, Case Western Reserve University School of Medicine, Vice Chair, UH System Clinical Affairs, Department of Medicine, Medical Director, Diabetes and Obesity Center, Mary B. Lee Chair in Adult Endocrinology, University Hospitals Cleveland Medical Center, Cleveland, Ohio, USA

SCOTT ISAACS, MD, FACP, FACE
Adjunct Associate Professor of Medicine, Emory University School of Medicine, Medical Director, Atlanta Endocrine Associates, Atlanta, Georgia, USA

NUPUR KIKANI, MD
Assistant Professor of Medicine, Department of Endocrine Neoplasia and Hormonal Disorders, The University of Texas MD Anderson Cancer Center, Houston, Texas, USA

CHRISTIAN KIM, MD
University Hospitals Eye Institute/Department of Ophthalmology and Visual Sciences, Case Western Reserve University, Cleveland, Ohio, USA

JOHN P. KIRWAN, PhD
Integrative Physiology and Molecular Medicine Laboratory, Pennington Biomedical Research Center, Louisiana State University, Baton Rouge, Louisiana, USA

SHREE KURUP, MD, FACP
Professor, University Hospitals Eye Institute/Department of Ophthalmology and Visual Sciences, Case Western Reserve University, Vitreoretinal Diseases and Surgery, Ocular Immunology and Uveitis, University Hospitals, Cleveland, Ohio, USA

ISSAM MOTAIREK, MD
Harrington Heart and Vascular Institute, University Hospitals Cleveland Medical Center, Case Western Reserve University School of Medicine, Cleveland, Ohio, USA

RICHARD PARK, DPM
Resident, University Hospitals Podiatric Medicine and Surgery, Cleveland, Ohio, USA

SAMANTHA PAUL, MD
University Hospitals Eye Institute/Department of Ophthalmology and Visual Sciences, Case Western Reserve University, Cleveland, Ohio, USA

MAHBOOB RAHMAN, MD
Louis Stokes Cleveland VA Medical Center, Division of Nephrology and Hypertension, University Hospitals Cleveland Medical Center, Case Western Reserve University, Cleveland, Ohio, USA

RACHEL ROBINSON, DPM
Attending, University Hospitals Podiatric Medicine and Surgery, Cleveland, Ohio, USA

FRANCESCO RUBINO, MD
Department of Diabetes, Bariatric and Metabolic Surgery, King's College Hospital, Denmark Hill, London, United Kingdom

PHILIP R. SCHAUER, MD
Professor of Metabolic Surgery, Metamor Institute, Pennington Biomedical Research Center of Louisiana State University, Baton Rouge, Louisiana, USA

WARREN SOBOL, MD
Associate Professor, University Hospitals Eye Institute/Department of Ophthalmology and Visual Sciences, Case Western Reserve University, Vitreoretinal Diseases and Surgery, Ocular Immunology and Uveitis, University Hospitals, Cleveland, Ohio, USA

MOHAMED KAMEL SOLIMAN, MD
Department of Ophthalmology, Assiut University Hospitals, Assiut, Egypt; Case Western Reserve University, Vitreoretinal Diseases and Surgery, Ocular Immunology and Uveitis, Department of Ophthalmology, University Hospitals, Cleveland, Ohio, USA

GUILLERMO E. UMPIERREZ, MD
Division of Endocrinology, Metabolism and Lipids, Emory University School of Medicine, Atlanta, Georgia, USA

PRIYATHAMA VELLANKI, MD
Division of Endocrinology, Metabolism and Lipids, Emory University School of Medicine, Atlanta, Georgia, USA

ANURADHA VISWANATHAN, MBBS
Section for Pediatric Endocrinology, Cleveland Clinic Children's, Cleveland, Ohio, USA

JAMIE R. WOOD, MD
University Hospitals Rainbow Babies and Children's Hospital, Case Western Reserve University, Cleveland, Ohio, USA

COURTNEY YODER, DPM
Attending, University Hospitals Podiatric Medicine and Surgery, Cleveland, Ohio, USA

Contents

Rekindling Hope for Remission: Current Impact of Diabetes for Our World's Future Health and Economy   1

Betul A. Hatipoglu

> The individual and societal burdens of living with a chronic disease are a global issue. Diabetes directly increases health care costs to manage the disease and the associated complications and indirectly increases the economic burden through long-term complications that hinder the productivity of humans worldwide. Thus, it is crucial to have accurate information on diabetes-related costs and the geographic and global economic impact when planning interventions and future strategies. Health care systems must work with government agencies to plan national-level pre diabetes and diabetes strategies and policies. Public health services must focus on diabetes screening prevention and remission.

Root Cause for Metabolic Syndrome and Type 2 Diabetes: Can Lifestyle and Nutrition Be the Answer for Remission   13

Revital Gorodeski Baskin and Dima Alfakara

> Obesity and its association with metabolic syndrome are implicated in many disease states. Research has focused on the role of diet and lifestyle modifications in the evolution of prediabetes to diabetes seeking ways to intervene and improve outcomes. Proven nutritional include leaner proteins, an abundance of vegetables, extra-virgin olive oil, and controlled portioning of carbs and starches. The transition from a sedentary state to an exercise routine of moderate intensity has shown efficacy in lowering metabolic risks. The synergy of dietary and physical activity modifications are the building blocks for lifestyle modifications examined in this review as a means of preventing obesity-related diabetes.

Intervention with Therapeutic Agents, Understanding the Path to Remission in Type 2 Diabetes: Part 1   27

Shuai Hao, Guillermo E. Umpierrez, Tanicia Daley, and Priyathama Vellanki

> Type 2 diabetes is characterized by progressive decline in pancreatic β-cell function. Studies in adult subjects with newly diagnosed type 2 diabetes have reported that intensive insulin therapy followed by various antihyperglycemic medications can delay β-cell decline. However, this improvement is lost after cessation of therapy. In contrast, youth with type 2 diabetes experience a more rapid loss in β-cell function compared

with adults and have loss of β-cell function despite being on insulin and other antihyperglycemic medications. In part one of this two-part review, we discuss studies aiming to achieve diabetes remission with insulin and oral antidiabetic medications.

Type 2 diabetes is characterized by progressive decline in pancreatic β-cell function. Newer agents, such as glucagon-like peptide-1 receptor agonist (GLP-1RA) and dual incretin agonists, can augment β-cell function and delay the need for additional antihyperglycemics. However, the effect on β-cell function ceases after stopping the medications. When combined with intensive lifestyle modifications, higher doses of GLP-1RA than those used for diabetes treatment can be used to induce weight loss. More research is needed on whether the weight loss achieved with GLP1-RA can be sustained after stopping medication and in turn can sustain diabetes remission.

Bariatric surgery improves glucose homeostasis and glycemic control in patients with type 2 diabetes. Over the past 20 years, a breadth of studies has been conducted in humans and rodents aimed to identify the regulatory nodes responsible for surgical remission of type 2 diabetes. The review herein discusses central mechanisms of type 2 diabetes remission associated with weight loss and surgical modification of the gastrointestinal tract.

Long-term remission of type 2 diabetes following lifestyle intervention or pharmacotherapy, even in patients with mild disease, is rare. Long-term remission following metabolic surgery however, is common and occurs in 23% to 98% depending on disease severity and type of surgery. Remission after surgery is associated with excellent glycemic control without reliance on pharmacotherapy, improvements in quality of life, and major reductions in microvascular and macrovascular complications. For patients with type 2 diabetes, early intervention with metabolic surgery, when beta cell function still remains intact, provides the greatest probability of long-term remission as high as 90% or more.

The prevalence of diabetic retinopathy is steadily increasing as the population of patients with diabetes grows. In the past decade, the development of anti-VEGF agents has dramatically changed the treatment landscape for diabetic retinopathy and diabetic macular edema (DME). Newer agents in development aim to reduce the treatment burden of diabetic retinopathy.

Diabetic Kidney Care Redefined with a New Way into Remission

Nour Hammad, Mohamed Hassanein, and Mahboob Rahman

> Diabetic kidney disease has been a leading cause for end-stage kidney disease. Traditional methods to slow progression include tight glycemic control, blood pressure control, and use of renin–angiotensin axis inhibitors. Finerenone and sodium glucose co-transporters have shown proven benefit in diabetic kidney disease regression recently. Other potential targets for slowing the decline in diabetic kidney disease are transforming growth factor beta, endothelin antagonist, protein kinase C inhibitors, advanced glycation end product inhibition, Janus kinase-signal transducer and activator of transcription pathway inhibition, phosphodiesterase 3 or 5 inhibitors, and Rho kinase inhibitor. These targets are at various trial phases and so far, show promising results.

Nagging Pain and Foot Ulcers Can be Treated into Remission

Craig B. Frey, Richard Park, Rachel Robinson, and Courtney Yoder

> Lower extremity ulcerations are very common in patients with diabetes. These wounds lead to amputation in a surprisingly large percentage of patients with diabetes. The mortality rate following amputation in a patient with diabetes is alarmingly high. Preventive treatment is pivotal to avoid the numerous complications associated with diabetic ulcerations. However, at the onset of ulceration, early treatment under the supervision and guidance of a specialist can result in remission. Diabetic peripheral neuropathy is also a life-altering and debilitating disease. Although some patients experience numbness, some experience pain that can be sharp, shooting, and tingling. Although treatment is challenging and often requires medication, newer modalities, such as stimulation and physical therapy, have shown promise in reversing the devastating effects of peripheral neuropathy.

Ameliorating Cardiovascular Risk in Patients with Type 2 Diabetes

Issam Motairek and Sadeer Al-Kindi

> Patients with type 2 diabetes (T2D) are at an increased risk of cardiovascular disease (CVD), which constitutes the most common cause of morbidity and mortality in these patients. Intensive CVD risk factor control can ameliorate the elevated CVD associated with T2D. In this review, we provide an overview of CVD risk factor control, including traditional (blood pressure, glycemia, lipid, thrombosis, and lifestyle modifications) and nontraditional (social and environmental determinants of health) in patients with T2D, including evidence on management and outcomes.

Nonalcoholic Fatty Liver Disease

Scott Isaacs

> Management of nonalcoholic fatty liver disease (NAFLD) is crucial for type 2 diabetes (T2D) remission because they are linked through the common pathophysiology of insulin resistance and lipotoxicity. One in three patients with T2D has nonalcoholic steatohepatitis leading to fibrosis, cirrhosis, and hepatocellular carcinoma. Noninvasive testing with imaging and/or serum biomarkers can assess the risk for advanced liver disease. A liver biopsy is

only necessary in select patients where there is diagnostic doubt. Treatments for NAFLD parallel T2D remission strategies focusing on weight loss and managing comorbid conditions through lifestyle modification, antiobesity medications, and/or bariatric surgery, and T2D medications with proven efficacy.

Heterogeneous forms of Ketosis-prone diabetes (KPD) are characterized by patients who present with diabetic ketoacidosis (DKA) but lack the typical features and biomarkers of autoimmune T1D. The A-β+ subgroup of KPD provides unique insight into the concept of "remission" since these patients have substantial preservation of beta-cell function permitting the discontinuation of insulin therapy, despite initial presentation with DKA. Measurements of C-peptide levels are essential to predict remission and guide potential insulin withdrawal. Further studies into predictors of remission and relapse can help us guide patients with A-β+ KPD toward remission and develop targeted treatments for this form of atypical diabetes.

Type 1 diabetes is a chronic autoimmune disorder that results in destruction of insulin-producing cells in the pancreas. The autoimmune process is thought to be waxing and waning resulting in variable endogenous insulin secretion ability. An example of this is the honeymoon phase or partial remission phase of type 1 diabetes, during which optimal control of blood glucoses can be maintained with significantly reduced exogenous insulin, and occasionally exogenous insulin can be temporarily discontinued altogether. Understanding this phase is important because even fairly small amounts of endogenous insulin secretion is associated with reduced risk of severe hypoglycemia and microvascular complications.

To date, people living with type 1 diabetes depend on external subcutaneous insulin while waiting for a cure, or a feasible method to preserve, replace, and generate fully functioning β cells that secrete appropriate insulin in response to glucose. Current work includes evaluating renewable sources of β cells, transplantation methods without immunosuppressives, and methods to preserve β-cell function. Such methods include β-cell encapsulation, scaffolding, immune modulation, gene editing, and disease-modifying therapies. The purpose of this article is to review the progress and describe β-cell therapies over the past 5 years.

ENDOCRINOLOGY AND METABOLISM CLINICS OF NORTH AMERICA

SERIES OF RELATED INTEREST

Medical Clinics
https://www.medical.theclinics.com
Primary Care: Clinics in Office Practice
https://www.primarycare.theclinics.com/

VISIT THE CLINICS ONLINE!
Access your subscription at:
www.theclinics.com

Foreword

Diabetes Remission

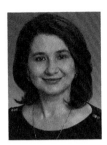

Adriana G. Ioachimescu,
MD, PhD, FACE
Consulting Editor

The "Diabetes Remission" issue of the *Endocrinology and Metabolism Clinics of North America* presents our current understanding of the mechanisms and implications of attaining significantly improved glycemia in patients who no longer require pharmacologic treatment. The guest editor is Dr Betul Hatipoglu, Professor of Medicine at Case Western Reserve University School of Medicine. Dr Hatipoglu has done extensive work in the field of diabetes and pancreatic islet cell transplantation.

Diabetes remission is a relatively new concept that reflects the advances in diabetes management. In 2021, experts defined it as achieving an improvement of HbA_{1c} to 6.5% or less for at least 3 months and in absence of pharmacotherapy. This concept is multifaceted, with socioeconomic, educational, and pharmacologic implications. The underlying pathogenetic links depend on the diabetes type and treatment modalities. The authors discuss the effectiveness of various modalities that can result in type 2 diabetes remission, including lifestyle interventions, bariatric surgery, and medications. Also included in our issue is an update on the islet cell transplantation for patients with type 1 diabetes. Diabetes complications should be monitored in patients who attain the favorable outcome of near-normal glycemia. Our issue includes discussions about nephropathy, retinopathy, neuropathy, and foot ulcers.

Achieving remission is a worthwhile task that requires multidisciplinary collaboration between endocrinologists, internists, diabetes educators, surgeons, and other team members. The teamwork entails a long-term approach to care, so that, it is hoped, remission is maintained. The methodology is patient-centric, dependent on diabetes type, complications, and various other individual factors that may impact the disease course.

I hope you will find this issue of the *Endocrinology and Metabolism Clinics of North America* a great resource for your practice. I would like to thank Dr Hatipoglu, our guest editor, and the authors for their valuable contributions. As with every issue of the

Endocrinol Metab Clin N Am 52 (2023) xiii–xiv
https://doi.org/10.1016/j.ecl.2022.11.001
0889-8529/23/© 2022 Published by Elsevier Inc.

endo.theclinics.com

Endocrinology and Metabolism Clinics of North America, I am grateful to the Elsevier editorial staff for their continuous support.

Adriana G. Ioachimescu, MD, PhD
The Emory Pituitary Center
Emory University School of Medicine
1365 B Clifton Road, NorthEast B6209
Atlanta, GA 30322, USA

E-mail address:
aioachi@emory.edu

Preface

Time to Rethink Diabetes Care

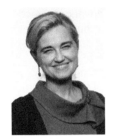

Betul A. Hatipoglu, MD
Editor

The American Diabetes Association and an international group of experts published a consensus report in August 2021 proposing an "HbA_{1c} <6.5% (48 mmol/mol) that occurs spontaneously or after an intervention and persists for at least 3 months after stopping glucose-lowering pharmacotherapy" as the definition of remission.[1] Diabetes remission is an encouraging diagnosis for type 2 diabetes (T2D). Several articles in this issue of *Endocrinology and Metabolism Clinics of North America* examine interventions demonstrating some effectiveness for diabetes remission, such as bariatric surgery, low-calorie diets, and carbohydrate restriction, among others.

Endocrinologists and others who clinically manage diabetes now have a diagnostic criterion for remission, and caregivers can offer hope when counseling some people living with T2D. Interventions may achieve glycemic control for some patients for a prolonged period. However, diabetes is currently a nationwide epidemic. The percentage of patients with an HbA_{1c} >9% is increasing despite more than 40 new treatment options approved since 2005 and improved technologies. We need a fresh look at diabetes care programs to find what is working and what needs improvement.

At the root of the issue is the current care model for diabetes. Fewer than 6500 adult endocrinologists care for patients in the United States.[2] This is an alarmingly small number given the estimated 34.1 million adults, 18 years or older, living with diabetes in 2018.[3] Diabetes care by an endocrinologist is associated with lower morbidities and health care costs, and fewer readmissions.[4] The approximate ratio is 46,000 patients per endocrinologist, which is an impossible need to meet with the expected further decline in full-time adult endocrinologists in the United States through 2025.[5] It is time to rethink our care models.

To meet the rising demand for endocrine care will require inclusive team-based care for diabetes management. Within the last year, we launched this team-based model at University Hospitals, Cleveland to organize diabetes care to be patient-centric, to better utilize resources, to support primary care, and to maximize value. This model

Endocrinol Metab Clin N Am 52 (2023) xv–xvii
https://doi.org/10.1016/j.ecl.2022.09.001
0889-8529/23/© 2022 Published by Elsevier Inc.

endo.theclinics.com

employs a multidisciplinary team approach without the classic patient interaction by the entire team. The model seeks to increase capacity to see more patients more quickly by the most appropriate provider, and to improve diabetes management and care across the continuum. Our diabetes care team operates in the outpatient setting of our health system, connecting the experience and wisdom of the endocrinologist to disciplines more readily available to see patients with T2D. Team members include an endocrinologist, diabetes educator, nutrition services, advanced practice providers, and others as needed, such as a PharmD, social worker, nurse navigator, and when needed, consultations from psychiatry, nephrology, and cardiology interacting with primary care.

The diabetes care team engages primary care physicians through meetings, building a relationship as a diabetes resource and endocrinology referral service. Primary care providers discuss their difficult diabetes patients with the team, and the team recommends care interventions based on the patient's needs, serving as a coach more than a consultant. Each patient referral is assigned to the appropriate team member who quickly implements the intervention.

As with any chronic disease, including diabetes, it takes a team approach to connect all the services to help the patient manage their disease. If we can catch T2D and intervene early in the disease course and encourage substantial weight loss and lifestyle changes, there is greater potential to restore β-cell function and achieve remission.[6]

Of course, sustainability of a coaching rather than a consulting team-based diabetes care model is only possible if billing and reimbursement in the United States recognize and value the work. This will require a paradigm shift from the classic physician reimbursement and specialist care to a team supported by endocrinology leadership, from caring for advanced and complications of the disease to prevention and remission. The future of our population health heavily depends on today's vision.

Betul A. Hatipoglu, MD
Case Western Reserve University
School of Medicine
Department of Medicine
Diabetes & Obesity Center
University Hospital Cleveland Medical Center
11100 Euclid Avenue
Cleveland, OH 44106, USA

E-mail address:
Betul.Hatipoglu@UHhospitals.org

REFERENCES

1. Riddle MC, Cefalu WT, Evans PH, et al. Consensus report: definition and interpretation of remission in type 2 diabetes. Diabetes Care 2021;44(10):2438–44.

2. Romeo GR, Hirsch IB, Lash RW, et al. Trends in the endocrinology fellowship recruitment: reasons for concern and possible interventions. J Clin Endocrinol Metab 2020;105(6):1701–6.

3. Centers for Disease Control and Prevention. National Diabetes Statistics Report, 2020. Centers for Disease Control and Prevention, U.S. Dept of Health and Human Services. 2020. Available at: https://www.cdc.gov/diabetes/data/statistics-report/index.html?CDC_AA_refVal=https%3A%2F%2Fwww.cdc.gov%2Fdiabetes%2Fdata%2Fstatistics%2Fstatistics-report.html. Accessed June 15, 2021.

4. Lash RW. Endocrinology: growing need, but shrinking workforce. Medscape; 2017. Available at: https://www.medscape.com/viewarticle/881849. Accessed June 23, 2021.
5. Vigersky RA, Fish L, Hogan P, et al. The clinical endocrinology workforce: current status and future projections of supply and demand. J Clin Endocrinol Metab 2014;99(9):3112–21.
6. White MG, Shaw JAM, Taylor R. Type 2 diabetes: the pathologic basis of reversible β-cell dysfunction. Diabetes Care 2016;39(11):2080–8.

Rekindling Hope for Remission

Current Impact of Diabetes for Our World's Future Health and Economy

Betul A. Hatipoglu, MD

KEYWORDS

- Diabetes • Remission • Global economic burden • Social determinants of health
- World health • Prediabetes • Direct and indirect costs

KEY POINTS

- The global economic burden of diabetes for medical costs is predicted to be $1028 billion by 2030 and $1054 billion by 2045.
- North America, East Asia, and the Pacific are projected to contribute the most to the global gross domestic product for diabetes, whereas Latin America and the Caribbean will likely face the highest regional gross domestic product.
- Health care systems must work with their government agencies to plan national pre-diabetes and diabetes strategies.
- Public health services need to focus on diabetes screening prevention and remission and encourage patients with chronic disease to use health care services.
- Diabetes is a health, economic, and psychosocial burden on individuals with diabetes and all three must be part of chronic health care.

INTRODUCTION

The individual and societal burdens of living with a chronic disease have never been as prominent a global issue as in the 21st century. The United Nations has acknowledged that diabetes is a major global health challenge.[1] Diabetes prevalence has been increasing worldwide over the last several decades, yet it accelerated at an unimaginable rate during the COVID-19 pandemic[2] (**Fig. 1**).[3] Back in 2000, the International Diabetes Federation (IDF) stressed the impact of diabetes on the world's economy in the first *Diabetes Atlas*.[4] By around 2015, diabetes was already the 15th most common cause of shortened life expectancy in the world,[5] especially among

Case Western Reserve University, School of Medicine, Department of Medicine University Hospitals Cleveland Medical Center, Department of Medicine, Adult Endocrinology, 11100 Euclid Avenue, Cleveland, OH 44106, USA
E-mail address: bxh258@case.edu

Endocrinol Metab Clin N Am 52 (2023) 1–12
https://doi.org/10.1016/j.ecl.2022.06.006
endo.theclinics.com

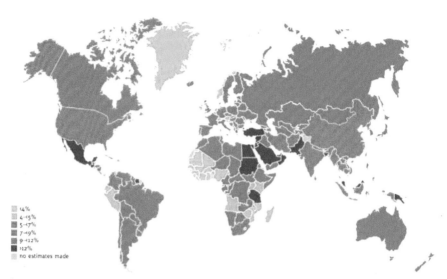

Fig. 1. Estimated age-adjusted comparative prevalence of diabetes in adults (20–79 years) in 2021. (*From* International Diabetes Federation. IDF Diabetes Atlas, 10th edition. Brussels, Belgium: International Diabetes Federation, 2021. http://www.diabetesatlas.org.)

socioeconomically disadvantaged and high-risk populations.[6] Diabetes not only directly increases health care costs to manage the disease and the associated acute and chronic complications, it also indirectly, and perhaps on a larger scale, increases the economic burden through long-term complications that hinder the productivity of humans worldwide.[7,8]

Given the global burden of diabetes, we need to further evaluate the impact on population health and the economy to make fair and equal decisions for resource utilization and distribution. A particular emphasis must be on prevention and diabetes remission.[9] To plan interventions and future strategies, it is crucial for organizations such as the World Health Organization (WHO) to have access to accurate information on diabetes-related costs and the economic impact by geographic region and on a global scale. Traditionally, health care providers have not received education on the business models accompanying the science. Therefore, shifting our vision by including the costs of a disease, such as diabetes, for both direct medical care and lost productivity (indirect costs) and its contribution to our global economy can better inform how we treat the disease and the person, and perhaps identify the most urgently needed areas.[10]

This article intends to focus your attention on the importance of working toward diabetes remission and the impact it can have on an individual, societal, and global level. Together we will examine the impact in different regions of the world, with the objective of justifying why we need resources, business planning, and government awareness of these expenses to achieve a healthier, happier world.

DIABETES IMPACT BY REGION

Although analyzing the impact of diabetes worldwide is quite challenging and studies scarce, one study took the 2015 data and projected the global economic effects of diabetes by 2030.[11] This study, of course, could not foresee the unexpected effect of COVID-19 on diabetes.[2] For their calculations, Bommer and colleagues[10] obtained prevalence and mortality data for 184 countries from the IDF *Diabetes Atlas,* including details from regions of sub-Saharan Africa, East Asia, the Pacific, Europe, Central Asia, Latin America, the Caribbean, the Middle East, North Africa, North America, and South Asia.[3] The authors estimate that the economic burden of diabetes in 2030 will exceed 2015 levels by 88%, jumping from 1.5% to 2.2% of the global gross domestic product (GDP). The results are astonishing and provoke true urgency, in which the IDF estimates health expenditures for diabetes of $1028 billion by 2030 and $1054 billion by 2045 (**Fig. 2**). Stratifying different regions into economic scenarios regarding the global economic burden, North America, East Asia, and the Pacific are projected to contribute the most to the global GDP, whereas Latin America and the Caribbean will likely face the highest burden for local GDP.[11]

EUROPEAN UNION

Pohlmann and colleagues[12] reviewed three large health care systems in the European Union using publicly available data from France,[13] Germany,[14] and Italy.[15] This review primarily focused on type 2 diabetes (T2D), identified cost sources, and suggested unit costs to support health economist research. In France, the total economic burden for T2D was based on 5% of their total health expenditures and was estimated to be EUR

At a glance	2021	2030	2045
Total world population	7.9 billion	8.6 billion	9.5 billion
Adult population (20–79 y)	5.1 billion	5.7 billion	6.4 billion
Diabetes (20–79 y)			
Prevalence[i]	10.5%	11.3%	12.2%
Number of people with diabetes	536.6 million	642.7 million	783.2 million
Number of deaths due to diabetes	6.7 million	–	–
Total health expenditure due to diabetes[ii] (2021 USD)	USD 966 billion	USD 1,028 billion	USD 1,054 billion
Hyperglycaemia in pregnancy (20–49 y)			
Proportion of live births affected[iii]	16.7%	–	–
Number of live births affected	21.1 million	–	–
Impaired glucose tolerance (20–79 y)			
Prevalence[i]	10.6%	11.0%	11.4%
Number of people with impaired glucose tolerance	541.0 million	622.7 million	730.3 million
Impaired fasting glucose (20–79 y)			
Prevalence[i]	6.2%	6.5%	6.9%
Number of people with impaired glucose tolerance	319.0 million	369.7 million	440.8 million
Type 1 diabetes (0–19 y)			
Number of children and adolescents with type 1 diabetes	1.2 million	–	–
Number of newly diagnosed cases each year	184,100	–	–

i Prevalence is standardised to each national population for the respective year
ii Health expenditure for people with diabetes is assumed to be on average two-fold higher than people without diabetes
iii Prevalence is standardised to world population for the respective year

Fig. 2. Estimated total number of adults (20–79 years) with diabetes in 2021, 2030, and 2045. (*From* International Diabetes Federation. IDF Diabetes Atlas, 10th edition. Brussels, Belgium: International Diabetes Federation, 2021. http://www.diabetesatlas.org.)

8.5 billion in 2013.[16] In Germany, T2D-related costs were 10% of health insurance expenses (2009–2010), resulting in an estimated EUR 16.1 billion.[17] In Italy, the probabilistic estimated direct cost was near EUR 9.6 billion, and indirect costs resulting from early retirement and loss of workforce was an additional EUR 10.7 billion in 2012.[18] The authors concluded that diabetes-related complications, including renal, neuropathic and ophthalmologic complications,[19–21] and adverse events, in particular hypoglycemia,[22] are the most important cost drivers in these three countries.[12]

COUNTRIES OF ASIA

China has witnessed a dramatic increase in the prevalence of diabetes, from 2.5% in 1994 to 11.6% in 2010.[23] Perhaps, more concerning in China is the 15.5% of adults estimated to have prediabetes.[24] Given their limited effort to prevent, manage, and treat diabetes, the economic burden and attributed complications are expected to rise. They are first in the top 10 listing of countries or territories relative to the prevalence of diabetes (**Table 1**). Further complicating the impact is the estimated 76.4% of patients with diabetes who have at least one complication.[25] The authors observed a health expenditure increase from $0.25 billion in 1993 (0.07% of the GDP) to $8.65 billion in 2008 (0.21% of the GDP).[25] Diet, decreasing levels of physical activity, and obesity, like the rest of the world, have contributed to the rapid increase of diabetes in China.[26]

In India, diabetes prevalence among urban adults was 12% in 2000 compared to 18.6% in South India in 2006.[27] In Asia, women have a 2- to 3-fold higher risk of gestational diabetes, causing an epidemic of young-onset diabetes. Additionally, a history of gestational diabetes affects the metabolic health of the child. The combination of gestational diabetes, in utero nutritional imbalance, childhood obesity, and

Table 1

Top 10 countries or territories for number of adults (20–79 years) with diabetes in 2021 and 2045

	2021			2045	
Ranks	Country or Territory	Number of People with Diabetes (Millions)	Ranks	Country or Territory	Number of People with Diabetes (Millions)
1	China	140.9	1	China	174.4
2	India	74.2	2	India	124.9
3	Pakistan	33.0	3	Pakistan	62.2
4	United States of America	32.2	4	United States of America	36.3
5	Indonesia	19.5	5	Indonesia	28.6
6	Brazil	15.7	6	Brazil	23.2
7	Mexico	14.1	7	Bangladesh	22.3
8	Bangladesh	13.1	8	Mexico	21.2
9	Japan	11.0	9	Egypt	20.0
10	Egypt	10.9	10	Turkey	13.4

(*From* International Diabetes Federation. IDF Diabetes Atlas, 10th edition. Brussels, Belgium: International Diabetes Federation, 2021. http://www.diabetesatlas.org.)

overnutrition in adulthood fuels the epidemic in Asian countries.[28] Thus, prevention and control of diabetes should be a top public health priority among Asian populations.[27]

Studies in some Asian countries also suggest that exposure to toxins, such as persistent organic pollutants, is associated with metabolic syndrome and diabetes.[29,30] For example, research on chronic arsenic exposure in Taiwan and Bangladesh revealed a strong association with diabetes risk.[31]

MIDDLE EAST AND NORTH AFRICA

The Middle East and North Africa (MENA) region on the IDF 2021 atlas has the highest percentage (24.5%) of diabetes-related deaths among people 20–79 years of age.[3] Additionally, the MENA region has the highest regional prevalence at 16.2%. A study by Haghravan and colleagues[32] reviewed diabetes prevention and control programs from 12 Middle Eastern countries. In Iran, 17 medical universities piloted a national diabetes prevention and control program from 1999 to 2001, and The National Diabetes Service Framework was established in 2016 to achieve goals set by the WHO for 2025. Turkey addressed the prevention and control of cardiovascular disease and diabetes through a National Tobacco Control Program in 2007 and food and physical activity initiatives. In Tunisia, a consensus on diabetes prevention was proposed by the public and private sectors. Saudi Arabia started a national program to improve awareness and education about diabetes. Many other countries in the region such as Jordan, Kuwait, The United Arab Emirates, Qatar, and Bahrain developed comprehensive national strategies consistent with global strategic objectives for diabetes, childhood obesity, smoking, exercise, and diet.

AFRICA

The greatest increase in diabetes prevalence is expected to occur in Africa, although, unfortunately, endemic infections have received more attention. Currently, diabetes-related health care cost information is sparse, but available data confirm similar global trends. For example, estimated expenditures in Nigeria are $1.071 billion annually, in Cameroon direct medical costs are $148/mo/individual, and in Sudan are $175/y for medications and ambulatory care only.[33] One challenge in Africa is that patients and families pay most of their expenses, and rising health care costs will be catastrophic for individuals.[33]

JAPAN

In Japan, where the quality of diabetes treatment is higher than in many other regions in the world, the economic burden of diabetes is still serious. Japan is ahead of most countries, proactively implementing intervention trials for prediabetes to prevent overt diabetes and attributed complications.[34]

LATIN AMERICA

Unfortunately, the rapid growth of diabetes in middle-income countries is widening the gap in global health disparities. Diabetes is an overall public health problem in Latin America. The estimated economic burden in Mexico in 2011 was $7.7 billion, of which $3.4 billion was direct and $4.3 indirect costs.[35] Arrendondo and colleagues[36] reported a 26% increase in the economic burden from epidemiological changes in diabetes in Mexico from 2014 to 2016, and a comparative analysis with six other selected Latin American countries found similar epidemiological trends. These countries illustrate potentially disastrous health disparities, generating further economic burden, once more emphasizing the need to redesign the current approach to disease care. It is important to shift the focus toward prevention and remission-oriented models to meet expected challenges from diseases such as diabetes.[35]

NORTH AMERICA

According to the Centers for Disease Control and Prevention (CDC), more than 34.2 million Americans have diabetes, and around 88 million, or 1 out of 3, adults have prediabetes.[37] When the global economic burden of increasing diabetes prevalence was examined under a unified framework, Bommer and colleagues[10] identified patterns of diabetes-related costs and determined research needs in low-income regions. Indirect costs, including diabetes-associated morbidity and premature mortality, accounted for 34.7% of the total global burden, but the share and composition of these costs varied widely across countries. As diabetes prevalence increased in the world, the United States ranked 4th (**Table 1**) and contributed to the largest share of global costs, and was the region with the highest percentage of GDP.

In 2019, the IDF estimated global health expenditures for diabetes to be $760 billion and projected it to increase to $845 billion by 2045.[38] Disparities between high-, middle-, and low-income countries were large, with estimated expenditures 300 times higher in high-income compared to low-income countries. The United States ($294.6 billion) had the highest expenditures. Patients in the 60–69-year age group had the highest diabetes-related costs annually ($177.7 billion), followed by the 50–59-year ($173.0 billion) and 70–79-year ($171.5 billion) groups. Expenditures were slightly higher for women compared to men.

An even more generous $327 billion was estimated when the cost of diagnosed diabetes in 2017 was calculated, including $237 billion in direct medical costs and $90 billion in reduced productivity.[8,39] In the United States, 1 in 4 health care dollars is spent to care for people with diabetes, and half of that is directly for diabetes care. Indirect costs include loss of workdays ($3.3 billion) and diminished productivity at work ($26.9 billion), reduced productivity if not employed ($2.3 billion), diabetes-related disability causing unemployment ($37.5 billion), and 277,000 premature deaths attributed to diabetes as a result of workforce loss ($19.9 billion).[8,39]

In the United States, 53% of total direct costs in 2012 solely treated diabetic complications.[40] Diabetic complications are mostly preventable, and if not, can potentially be delayed. Diabetes-related chronic kidney disease, for example, has been linked to a 49% increase in annual health care expenditures in the United States.[41] One of the most devastating, costly diabetic complications, however, is diabetic foot disease from neurological or vascular damage, or both, resulting in 5.4 times higher costs.[42] Macrovascular complications, such as cardiovascular disease and congestive heart failure, not only remain the number one cause of mortality, despite advances in therapy, but incur higher health care costs compared to cases without diabetes.[43]

A study nearly 3 decades ago calculated the direct costs of illness and factors affecting these costs among Medicaid-insured patients who were ≤65 years old.[44] The services comprising total direct costs were hospitalization (29.2%), prescription medicines (28.2%), outpatient care (21.3%), and physician encounters (14.3%). Factors significantly linked to cost and a person's use of health care were the numbers of comorbidities and of different physicians who were visited, insulin dependence in T2D, and complications, particularly renal dysfunction. Patients who successfully controlled their diabetes with diet and exercise had lower health care costs and use, emphasizing the importance of prevention/remission through lifestyle modification.

FUTURE STRATEGIES FOR THE DIABETES PANDEMIC

Screening is an urgent priority noted on the world map for undiagnosed diabetes (**Fig. 3**). A systematic review of the economic benefits of screening programs implemented in different countries for T2D and prediabetes found screening was more cost-effective than no screening in 62% (8 of 13) of studies, with targeted or opportunistic screening more economical than universal.[45]

Ali and colleagues[46] synthesized findings from Natural Experiments for Translation in Diabetes studies, which assessed diabetes health programs or policies implemented by the community, government, or other nonresearchers. Provider-focused interventions (eg, education and electronic screening decision support), and patient reminders and decreased copayments improved glucose screening and testing. Patient-focused lifestyle modification programs had modest to low success. Low-intensity strategies (eg, well coaching) saw small decreases in weight, whereas high-intensity diabetes prevention programs achieved moderate enrollment, weight loss, and short term slightly lower health expenditures. Health plans that used incentives increased medication adherence, whereas those that mandated moves to high-deductible plans increased delays in accessing health care for acute complications (eg, cellulitis). Lower-income patients were especially prone to delaying care, causing increased rates and acuity of emergency department visits for diabetic complications and other severe conditions.

In the United States, the CDC widely promotes a prediabetes awareness campaign that connects people to an evidence-based lifestyle change program to prevent T2D.[37] Researchers in Ireland have simulated the potential economic and health impact if a nationwide prevention program were implemented and reduced the

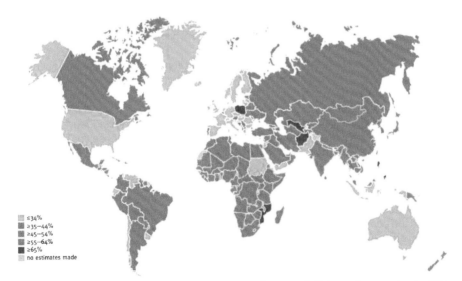

≤34%
≥35–44%
≥45–54%
≥55–64%
≥65%
no estimates made

Fig. 3. Proportion of adults (20–79 years) with undiagnosed diabetes by country in 2021. (*From* International Diabetes Federation. IDF Diabetes Atlas, 10th edition. Brussels, Belgium: International Diabetes Federation, 2021. http://www.diabetesatlas.org.)

incidence of diabetes.[47] Based on a projected increase of 198,000 more people with T2D by 2036, they estimated that prevention could hypothetically reduce T2D cases between 2000 (0.5%) and 19,000 (4.6%) by 2036. Thus, identifying prediabetes and implementing prevention programs are worth pursuing.

Knowing that patients often need help learning to manage their diabetes and other health problems, we need self-management tools and interventions to build patients' skills and confidence. When quality improvement interventions recommended by the American Diabetes Association were examined, such as patient self-management support, team approach, patient education, and other support, the mean decline in HbA_{1c} was 0.5% (0.3–0.6).[48] Teljeur and colleagues[49] reviewed cost and cost-effectiveness studies of self-management interventions. Evidence suggests that education self-management programs are cost-effective or superior to usual care, and telemedicine-type interventions are possibly cost-effective.[50] Whereas some pharmacist-led and behavioral interventions were reviewed, the evidence was promising but insufficient to come to any conclusions.[51]

Economic simulation modeling for T2D is an important tool for epidemiologists, policymakers, clinicians, and other stakeholders.[52] However, modeling needs to address diabetes progression in racial and ethnic minorities and incorporate health equity in health economic analyses. Thus, redesigning programs to effectively combat the barriers and gaps in implementation for populations with the most need should be an urgent public health priority.

Diabetes care is as much a social issue as a clinical disease and requires an infrastructure that addresses both social and medical needs.[53] Eight grantees in the Bridging the Gap: Reducing Disparities in Diabetes Care initiative are implementing strategies to address both needs, providing social support services, connecting health care and community organizations, and initiating information technology and protocols to identify high-risk patients and make referrals.[53] Psychosocial factors are important contributors to the disease burden. For instance, coping with the disease and diabetes fatigue can affect a person's overall mental health. It can also be difficult to navigate the health system and interact with multidisciplinary teams, and ongoing psychosocial challenges can reduce the patient's health-related quality of life. When planning interventions, we need to include psychosocial support tools and teach patients chronic disease management skills.[54]

Sustaining these interventions will require upfront funding and alternative payment models to support and incentivize these efforts. Innovations in financing that support medical and social determinants of health for patients with diabetes are starting to emerge.[55] New value-based payment approaches that reward the quality of care delivered are being used in the public and private sectors, replacing fee-for-service models that solely reimburse for volume. Evidence suggests that these financing innovations are funding integrated care teams that can address the medical and social needs of patients with diabetes.

Social determinants of health are also linked to our environment and the prevention of diabetes is closely tied to environmental factors. We see a growing interest in the impact of health care and human activities on the environment and the close interaction with the economy. For example, adding insulin to oral agents for patients with T2D over the past 30 years has added an extra 1057 kg of CO_2 emissions/patient in the United Kingdom.[56] Endocrine-disrupting chemicals (EDCs) affect many parts of our endocrine system, contributing to the development of metabolic disorders by disrupting peroxisome proliferator-activated receptors, estrogen receptors, and thyroid hormone receptors, among other metabolic signaling pathways. Current evidence suggests a relationship between prenatal exposure to bisphenol A (BPA) and childhood obesity, and exposure to perfluoroalkyl and polyfluroalkyl substances and phthalates in adulthood with gestational diabetes, impaired glucose tolerance, obesity, and T2D.[57]

Many US medical societies have made EDCs and their effect on metabolism and diabetes a top priority and are actively working with government agencies to minimize their impact on our health.[57]

SUMMARY

Health care systems need to work with their government agencies to plan prediabetes and diabetes strategies and policies at a national level. Moreover, public health services need to focus on diabetes screening prevention and remission, as well as delay-related complications by encouraging patients with chronic diseases, such as diabetes and hypertension, to use health care services. Health care agencies must redesign their consultative services and use a team care approach with referrals to secondary/tertiary care when needed and heavily consider psychosocial determinants of health as part of chronic health care. Environmental health is important for human health and EDCs should be a top priority for environmental agencies. Within the large universal health care system, the impact of one system on another could not have been better realized than during our experience with the COVID-19 pandemic.

Of course, diabetes prevention is our first strategy against this disease. Yet, knowing that 1 out of 2 people in the world is an undiagnosed diabetic, remission of diabetes rekindles our hope as we battle increasing prevalence across the world.

DISCLOSURE

The author has nothing to disclose.

ACKNOWLEDGMENT

The work was partially funded by the Mary B. Lee Chair in Adult Endocrinology awarded to Dr. Hatipoglu.

REFERENCES

1. United Nations General Assembly. General Assembly adopts resolution stressing cooperation for universal economic development as it acts on over 40 second committee reports. Resolution adopted by the Sixty-first General Assembly, GA/10564 Plenary, 83rd Meeting on 20 December 2006: World Diabetes Day Resolution No. A/RES/61/2252007. Available at: https://www.un.org/press/en/2006/ga10564.doc.htm. Accessed July 16, 2022.
2. Mulder H, Fall T. The COVID-19 pandemic may be receding but the diabetes pandemic rages on. Diabetologia 2022;65(6):915–6.
3. International Diabetes Federation. IDF diabtes atlas. 10th edition. Brussels: International Diabetes Federation; 2021. Available at: https://www.diabetesatlas.org. Accessed May 22, 2022.
4. Williams R. The costs of diabetes. 1st edition. Brussels, Belgium: International Diabetes Federation; 2000. p. 225–31.
5. Wang H, Naghavi M, Allen C, et al. Global, regional, and national life expectancy, all-cause mortality, and cause-specific mortality for 249 causes of death, 1980–2015: a systematic analysis for the Global Burden of Disease Study 2015. Lancet 2016;388(10053):1459–544.

6. Spencer Bonilla G, Rodriguez-Gutierrez R, Montori VM. What we don't talk about when we talk about preventing type 2 diabetes-addressing socioeconomic disadvantage. JAMA Intern Med 2016;176(8):1053–4.
7. Williams R, Van Gaal L, Lucioni C, et al. Assessing the impact of complications on the costs of Type II diabetes. Diabetologia 2002;45(7):S13–7.
8. American Diabetes Association. Economic costs of diabetes in the US in 2017. Diabetes Care 2018;41(5):917–28.
9. Riddle MC, Cefalu WT, Evans PH, et al. Consensus report: definition and interpretation of remission in type 2 diabetes. Diabetes Care 2021;44(10):2438–44.
10. Bommer C, Heesemann E, Sagalova V, et al. The global economic burden of diabetes in adults aged 20-79 years: a cost-of-illness study. Lancet Diabetes Endocrinol 2017;5(6):423–30.
11. Bommer C, Sagalova V, Heesemann E, et al. Global economic burden of diabetes in adults: projections from 2015 to 2030. Diabetes Care 2018;41(5):963–70.
12. Pohlmann J, Norrbacka K, Boye KS, et al. Costs and where to find them: identifying unit costs for health economic evaluations of diabetes in France, Germany and Italy. Eur J Health Econ 2020;21(8):1179–96.
13. Chevreul K, Durand-Zaleski I, Bahrami SB, et al. France: Health system review. Health Syst Transit 2010;12(6):1–291, xxi-xxii.
14. Busse R, Blumel M. Germany: Health system review. Health Syst Transit 2014; 16(2):1–296, xxi.
15. Ferre F, de Belvis AG, Valerio L, et al. Italy: health system review. Health Syst Transit 2014;16(4):1–168.
16. Charbonnel B, Simon D, Dallongeville J, et al. Direct medical costs of type 2 diabetes in france: an insurance claims database analysis. Pharmacoecon Open 2018;2(2):209–19.
17. Jacobs E, Hoyer A, Brinks R, et al. Healthcare costs of Type 2 diabetes in Germany. Diabet Med 2017;34(6):855–61.
18. Marcellusi A, Viti R, Mecozzi A, et al. The direct and indirect cost of diabetes in Italy: a prevalence probabilistic approach. Eur J Health Econ 2016;17(2):139–47.
19. Turchetti G, Bellelli S, Amato M, et al. The social cost of chronic kidney disease in Italy. Eur J Health Econ 2017;18(7):847–58.
20. Kahm K, Laxy M, Schneider U, et al. Health care costs associated with incident complications in patients with type 2 diabetes in Germany. Diabetes Care 2018; 41(5):971–8.
21. Bongiovanni I, Couillerot-Peyrondet AL, Sambuc C, et al. [Cost-effectiveness analysis of various strategies of end-stage renal disease patients' care in France]. Nephrol Ther 2016;12(2):104–15.
22. Veronese G, Marchesini G, Forlani G, et al. Costs associated with emergency care and hospitalization for severe hypoglycemia. Nutr Metab Cardiovasc Dis 2016;26(4):345–51.
23. Mao W, Yip CW, Chen W. Complications of diabetes in China: health system and economic implications. BMC Public Health 2019;19(1):269.
24. Yang W, Lu J, Weng J, et al. Prevalence of diabetes among men and women in China. N Engl J Med 2010;362(12):1090–101.
25. Hu H, Sawhney M, Shi L, et al. A systematic review of the direct economic burden of type 2 diabetes in China. Diabetes Ther 2015;6(1):7–16.
26. Yang G, Kong L, Zhao W, et al. Emergence of chronic non-communicable diseases in China. Lancet 2008;372(9650):1697–705.
27. Chan JC, Malik V, Jia W, et al. Diabetes in Asia: epidemiology, risk factors, and pathophysiology. JAMA 2009;301(20):2129–40.

28. Yajnik CS. Nutrient-mediated teratogenesis and fuel-mediated teratogenesis: two pathways of intrauterine programming of diabetes. Int J Gynaecol Obstet 2009; 104(Suppl 1):S27–31.

29. Fujiyoshi PT, Michalek JE, Matsumura F. Molecular epidemiologic evidence for diabetogenic effects of dioxin exposure in U.S. Air Force veterans of the Vietnam war. Environ Health Perspect 2006;114(11):1677–83.

30. Lee DH, Steffes MW, Jacobs DR Jr. Can persistent organic pollutants explain the association between serum gamma-glutamyltransferase and type 2 diabetes? Diabetologia 2008;51(3):402–7.

31. Chen CJ, Wang SL, Chiou JM, et al. Arsenic and diabetes and hypertension in human populations: a review. Toxicol Appl Pharmacol 2007;222(3):298–304.

32. Haghravan S, Mohammadi-Nasrabadi F, Rafraf M. A critical review of national diabetes prevention and control programs in 12 countries in Middle East. Diabetes Metab Syndr 2021;15(1):439–45.

33. Mapa-Tassou C, Katte JC, Mba Maadjhou C, et al. Economic impact of diabetes in Africa. Curr Diab Rep 2019;19(2):5.

34. Urakami T, Kuwabara R, Yoshida K. Economic impact of diabetes in Japan. Curr Diab Rep 2019;19(1):2.

35. Arredondo A, Reyes G. Health disparities from economic burden of diabetes in middle-income countries: evidence from Mexico. PLoS One 2013;8(7):e68443.

36. Arredondo A, Azar A, Recaman AL. Diabetes, a global public health challenge with a high epidemiological and economic burden on health systems in Latin America. Glob Public Health 2018;13(7):780–7.

37. Centers for Disease Control and Prevention. National diabetes prevention program. centers for disease control and prevention. 2021. Available at: https://www.cdc.gov/diabetes/prevention/index.html. Accessed May 22, 2022.

38. Williams R, Karuranga S, Malanda B, et al. Global and regional estimates and projections of diabetes-related health expenditure: Results from the International Diabetes Federation Diabetes Atlas, 9th edition. Diabetes Res Clin Pract 2020; 162:108072.

39. Centers for Disease Control and Prevention. Type 2 diabetes. centers for disease control and prevention. 2021. Available at: https://www.cdc.gov/diabetes/basics/type2.html. Accessed May 10, 2022.

40. Zhuo X, Zhang P, Hoerger TJ. Lifetime direct medical costs of treating type 2 diabetes and diabetic complications. Am J Prev Med 2013;45(3):253–61.

41. Coresh J, Astor BC, Greene T, et al. Prevalence of chronic kidney disease and decreased kidney function in the adult US population: Third National Health and Nutrition Examination Survey. Am J Kidney Dis 2003;41(1):1–12.

42. Armstrong DG, Swerdlow MA, Armstrong AA, et al. Five year mortality and direct costs of care for people with diabetic foot complications are comparable to cancer. J Foot Ankle Res 2020;13(1):16.

43. Li R, Bilik D, Brown MB, et al. Medical costs associated with type 2 diabetes complications and comorbidities. Am J Manag Care 2013;19(5):421–30.

44. Guo JJ, Gibson JT, Gropper DM, et al. Empiric investigation on direct costs-of-illness and healthcare utilization of Medicaid patients with diabetes mellitus. Am J Manag Care 1998;4(10):1433–46.

45. Einarson TR, Bereza BG, Acs A, et al. Systematic literature review of the health economic implications of early detection by screening populations at risk for type 2 diabetes. Curr Med Res Opin 2017;33(2):331–58.

46. Ali MK, Wharam F, Kenrik Duru O, et al. Advancing health policy and program research in diabetes: findings from the Natural Experiments for Translation in Diabetes (NEXT-D) Network. Curr Diab Rep 2018;18(12):146.

47. Pierse T, O'Neill S, Dinneen SF, et al. A simulation study of the economic and health impact of a diabetes prevention programme in Ireland. Diabet Med 2021;38(6):e14540.

48. Nuckols TK, Keeler E, Anderson LJ, et al. Economic evaluation of quality improvement interventions designed to improve glycemic control in diabetes: a systematic review and weighted regression analysis. Diabetes Care 2018;41(5):985–93.

49. Teljeur C, Moran PS, Walshe S, et al. Economic evaluation of chronic disease self-management for people with diabetes: a systematic review. Diabet Med 2017; 34(8):1040–9.

50. Lee JY, Lee SWH. Telemedicine cost-effectiveness for diabetes management: a systematic review. Diabetes Technol Ther 2018;20(7):492–500.

51. Cohen LB, Taveira TH, Wu WC, et al. Pharmacist-led telehealth disease management program for patients with diabetes and depression. J Telemed Telecare 2020;26(5):294–302.

52. Dadwani RS, Laiteerapong N. Economic simulation modeling in type 2 diabetes. Curr Diab Rep 2020;20(7):24.

53. Gunter KE, Peek ME, Tanumihardjo JP, et al. Population health innovations and payment to address social needs among patients and communities with diabetes. Milbank Q 2021;99(4):928–73.

54. O'Brien CL, Ski CF, Thompson DR, et al. The Mental Health in Diabetes Service (MINDS) to enhance psychosocial health: study protocol for a randomized controlled trial. Trials 2016;17(1):444.

55. Saulsberry L, Peek M. Financing diabetes care in the U.S. health system: payment innovations for addressing the medical and social determinants of health. Curr Diab Rep 2019;19(11):136.

56. Marsh K, Ganz M, Nortoft E, et al. Incorporating environmental outcomes into a health economic model. Int J Technol Assess Health Care 2016;32(6):400–6.

57. Kahn LG, Philippat C, Nakayama SF, et al. Endocrine-disrupting chemicals: implications for human health. Lancet Diabetes Endocrinol 2020;8(8):703–18.

Root Cause for Metabolic Syndrome and Type 2 Diabetes

Can Lifestyle and Nutrition Be the Answer for Remission

Revital Gorodeski Baskin, MD[a],*, Dima Alfakara, MD[b]

KEYWORDS

- Metabolic syndrome • Lifestyle modifications • Ketogenic diet • Mediterranean diet
- Intermittent fasting • Moderate-intensity exercises • Band exercises

KEY POINTS

- The metabolic syndrome is a risk factor for the development of type 2 diabetes and cardiovascular disease.
- Nutritional changes with the goal of weight loss have been shown to augment the natural progression of the metabolic syndrome.
- Physical activity, especially of moderate intensity, has additional therapeutic benefits in lowering these metabolic risks.

Metabolic syndrome is a known precursor for many disease states. Decades of research have specifically investigated how obesity contributes to insulin resistance, hyperinsulinemia, pancreatic β-cell dysfunction, and consequent type 2 diabetes mellitus (T2DM). Lifestyle and behavioral changes are integral in the prevention of this process. Can a physiologic cascade be modulated and even halted with something as simple as weight loss? The hypothesis is logical, but losing weight is not a simple proposition and may not be the only solution. The early phases of metabolic syndrome can be significantly modified through nutritional changes, with a focus on dietary caloric restriction and physical activity (PA).

Himsworth[1] described two subtypes of diabetes: the insulin-sensitive type and the insulin-insensitive type. He believed an unknown factor existed that sensitized the

[a] Department of Endocrinology, Diabetes and Obesity Center, University Hospitals of Cleveland, 11100 Euclid Avenue, Cleveland, OH 44106, USA; [b] Department of Endocrinology, University Hospitals of Cleveland, 11100 Euclid Avenue, Cleveland, OH 44106, USA
* Corresponding author.
E-mail address: rgorodeski@gmail.com

Endocrinol Metab Clin N Am 52 (2023) 13–25
https://doi.org/10.1016/j.ecl.2022.10.007
0889-8529/23/© 2022 Elsevier Inc. All rights reserved.

body and its organs to insulin, and that this factor was either lacking or being restricted in those with insulin-insensitive diabetes. Dr Gerald Reaven proposed in his 1988 American Diabetes Association Banting Award Lecture that "although this concept may seem outlandish at first blush," insulin resistance is the underlying cause of T2DM and importantly for coronary artery disease (independent of diabetes).[2] He described "Syndrome X" as hyperinsulinemia, impaired glucose tolerance (IGT), hypertension, decreased high-density lipoprotein cholesterol (HDL-C), and hypertriglyceridemia. Dr Reavan was the first to propose the clustering of these risk factors for cardiovascular disease with insulin resistance at its center.[3,4] Syndrome X has since had various names, including "insulin resistance syndrome," "the deadly quartet," "hypertriglyceridemic waist," and "metabolic syndrome."[5]

The Centers for Disease Control and Prevention (CDC) reports a >35% increased prevalence of metabolic syndrome between 1988 and 2012.[6] This equated to greater than one-third of the adult population in the United States having an increased risk of T2DM and atherosclerotic cardiovascular disease in every sociodemographic group. The International Diabetes Federation estimates that by 2035, 10.1% (592 million cases) of the world population could have T2DM.[7] Ninety percent of T2DM cases have resulted from the combination of sedentary living and occupations, high fat, carbohydrate-rich, and processed diets, obesity, excessive alcohol intake, smoking, stress, and poor sleep habits.[8,9]

Once diagnosed, T2DM contributes to multi-organ dysfunction, leading to diabetic nephropathy, retinopathy, neuropathy, and a combination of macro and microvascular complications. T2DM and its associated hyperinsulinemic state are related to adipocyte dysfunction, cytokine activation, and destructive chronic inflammation.[10] In addition to the toll on individuals, billions of dollars spent annually on diabetes and related complications have caused a global economic burden. In the United States alone, the cost of diabetes increased by 26% from 2012 to 2017 due to clinic/hospital visits, medications, supplies, and indirect costs.[11]

Prediabetes is described as the precursor to T2DM and is thought to occur over many years to decades, with a slow and potentially reversible onset. It is believed that skeletal muscle insulin resistance is the primary pathophysiologic component that precedes β-cell dysfunction.[12]

Eventually, progressive β-cell function loss with worsening insulin resistance culminates in the recognizable clinical presentation of diabetes. Yet early intervention can prevent β-cell destruction. The interlude between genetics, epigenetics, and lifestyle decisions has contributed to the molecular and physiologic mechanism of T2DM development.[13] Prevention of prediabetes progressing to T2DM along with the strive toward diabetic remission has been the focus of medicine for decades.

PA plays a very important role in metabolic syndrome, and the progression of prediabetes to T2DM. High PA (vs low PA) has, in epidemiologic terms, suggested a ~30% reduction in the relative diabetes risk.[14] An inverse association has been noted between PA and the risk of T2DM, including vigorous activity, leisure-time activity, moderate activity, low-intensity activity, and walking.[15] Performing 30 min of moderate-to-vigorous intensity PA was associated with a 15% (7 to 255, $P < 0.001$) difference in insulin sensitivity, as defined in homeostasis model assessment insulin sensitivity calculation (HOMA-IS), an index of insulin sensitivity and specifically hepatic insulin resistance.[16] The benefit of regular PA has been an important component of lifestyle modification (LSM) recommendations in the management of the metabolic syndrome. Conversely, a sedentary lifestyle can accelerate the process.

Globally, a sedentary lifestyle is listed as the fourth highest risk factor for increased mortality.[17] Per an ongoing state-based telephone interview survey evaluation conducted by The CDC Behavioral Risk Factor Surveillance System (BRFSS) collects data from states and US territories and from 2017 to 2020 found a 25.3% overall prevalence of low-level PA for 52 jurisdictions.[18] In addition, they noted that 8.3% of deaths in the United States were associated with inadequate levels of PA in the 40 to 69 years and ≥70-year age groups.[19] The CDC has adopted PA guidelines for the general population, which includes 150 to 300 min of moderate-intensity aerobic exercise/week, 75 to 150 min of vigorous-intensity aerobic activity/week, or a combination of moderate- and vigorous-intensity activity of equivalent times/week.[20] Improvements in disease risk factors have been observed with the addition of exercise routines, dietary modifications, and weight loss. It is important to note that the role of exercise alone in preventing the progression of prediabetes to diabetes remains unclear. The intensity of exercise, duration per episode, and weekly frequency remain unclear and require additional research.

Lifestyle reforms have helped prevent T2DM. These include dietary interventions with primarily calorie-restricted diets and exercise. One of the first studies to evaluate this was conducted in Da Qing, China in 1986.[21] They enrolled 577 individuals with IGT, as defined by World Health Organization criteria, and randomized them to diet only, exercise only, diet plus exercise, or control. Patients were followed over a 6-year period and the incidence of diabetes was determined. The incidence of diabetes at 6 years per intervention was 43.8% (95% confidence interval [CI], 35.5–52.3) for diet, 41.1% (95% CI, 33.4–49.4) for exercise, and 46.0% (95% CI, 37.3–54.7) for diet plus exercise compared with 67.7% (95% CI, 59.8–75.2) for the control group, with a $P < 0.05$ (similar whether subjects were lean or overweight, body mass index [BMI] >25 kg/m^2). The investigators successfully showed a statistically significant diabetes incidence reduction with lifestyle interventions.

The Diabetes Prevention Program was one of the largest randomized clinical trials in the United States to evaluate the impact of lifestyle interventions in patients with impaired fasting glucose (IFG) and IGT.[22] The 3234 participants were randomized to placebo or metformin (MET) (850 mg twice/day) or to lifestyle interventions. The latter included recommendations to follow the Food Guide Pyramid and a diet similar to the National Cholesterol Education Program Sep 1 diet, to reduce their weight by a minimum of 7%, and to do moderate intensity exercise for ~150 min/week. Over the 2.8 years of follow-up, the trial showed a significant reduction in the incidence of diabetes of 58% (95% CI, 48% to 66%) in the lifestyle group, compared with 31% (95% CI, 17% to 43%) in the MET (vs placebo) group. In addition, per 100 person-years, the incidence of diabetes was 4.8, 7.8, and 11.0 in the lifestyle group, MET, and placebo groups, respectively. The risk of diabetes was reduced by 90% in participants that lost weight and achieved the required PA.[13]

The Finnish Diabetes Prevention Study enrolled 522 overweight patients (mean BMI 31) with IGT to either an intervention or a control group with a follow-up for a mean of 3.2 years.[23] The intervention group was advised to lower their fat intake to <30% of their energy consumption, increase intake of fiber, vegetables, whole grains, and low-fat dairy products, and start moderate exercise for a minimum of 30 min/day (both endurance and circuit-type resistance training). The trial showed a 58% reduction in diabetes ($P < 0.001$) and a net weight loss of 3.5 ± 5.5 kg in the intervention group and 0.8 ± 4.4 kg in the control group by the end of year 2 of the study ($P < 0.001$).

A study in Japan randomized 458 male participants with IGT to an intensive intervention lifestyle group or control group.[24] The control group was advised to maintain a BMI <24 kg/m^2 with diet and exercise. The intervention group was advised to maintain a BMI <22 kg/m^2 and were given quarterly lifestyle instructions during outpatient clinic visits. Over the 4 years of follow-up, the intervention group lost 2.8 kg, whereas the control group lost 0.39 kg ($P < 0.001$). Diabetes incidence was 3.0% in the intervention group and 9.3% in the control group. Although the weight loss was minimal, the impact on diabetes risk reduction was 67.4% ($P < 0.001$). As previously shown, even a 5% loss of body weight has been shown to improve insulin sensitivity by 30%.[13]

The Indian Diabetes Prevention Program was a prospective community-based study that randomized 531 patients of Asian Indian descent with IGT and a BMI of 25.8 ± 3.5 kg/m^2 to 1 of 4 groups and measured for progression to T2DM over a median of 30 months.[25] The groups included a control, LSM, MET, and LSM plus MET. The LSM group was advised to walk briskly for a minimum of 30 min daily, reduce refined carbohydrates, fats, total calories, and sugar consumption, and amplify fiber. Compared with the control group, the relative risk reduction of diabetes development with LSM was 28.5% (95% CI, 20.5–37.3; $P = 0.018$), with MET was 26.4% (95% CI, 19.1–35.1; $P = 0.029$), and with LSM + MET was 28.2% (95% CI, 20.3–37.0; $P = 0.022$). The lifestyle intervention was able to prevent diabetes and adding MET (500 mg/day) did not show an extra benefit. Each of the aforementioned studies highlights the benefits of LSMs in slowing the progression toward disease.

The Mediterranean diet has also been linked to health benefits including improvements in insulin resistance and insulin sensitivity, diabetes, glucagon-like peptide-1 activity, inflammation, oxidative stress, cardiovascular disease, atrial fibrillation, certain cancer types, lipid-lowering effects, platelet aggregation, gut-microbiota, cognition, Alzheimer's disease, among others.[26–28] The Mediterranean diet was originally based on the dietary pattern of the 22 countries bordering the Mediterranean Sea.[26] As these countries have undergone modernization, their traditional diets have changed, making it difficult to consistently define the components of the diet. Most agree that the Mediterranean diet consists of a wealth of non-starchy vegetables, fresh fruits, legumes, non-processed whole grain breads, nuts, seeds, extra-virgin olive oil, fish, poultry, and eggs, low consumption of red meat (once/week), low amounts of dairy products, butter, sugar drinks, and red wine.[26,27,29] An abundance of research has linked the Mediterranean diet to long-lasting improvement in prediabetes and diabetes management.

Many staples of the Mediterranean diet are foods that contain a variety of phytochemicals and polyphenols. Phytochemicals contribute an antioxidant effect and may help inhibit gut glucose absorption and aid with insulin sensitivity.[28] Flavonoids, which are present in a variety of plants, are polyphenols that have been studied relative to T2DM risk. Wedick and colleagues[30] studied non-diabetics from the Nurses' Health Study, Nurses' Health Study 2, and the Health Professionals Follow-Up Study, and noted a lower risk of T2DM with a higher consumption of the flavonoid subclasses of anthocyanins, specifically blueberries and apples/pears.

Extra-virgin olive oil is essential to the Mediterranean diet. Its health benefits for T2DM have been evaluated and are thought to be related to the high concentration of bioactive polyphenols and their anti-inflammatory and antioxidant properties.[31] In one study, 79 patients with T2DM were randomized to 500 mg of oral olive leaf extract daily or placebo.[32] Participants taking the extract showed significantly lower fasting plasma insulin levels and hemoglobin A1C (HbA1c). The investigators did not note a significant difference in the postprandial plasma insulin levels. The PREDIMED study was a parallel-group, randomized, primary cardiovascular prevention trial in Spain that evaluated 3541 patients with high cardiovascular risk but not diabetic.[33] Participants were randomized to either a Mediterranean diet supplemented with extra-virgin olive oil, Mediterranean diet supplemented with nuts, or control diet (advised on a low-fat

diet) and followed over a median of 4.1 years. The study showed a statistically significant 40% relative risk reduction (multivariate-adjusted hazard ratio [HR], 0.60; 95% CI
0.43 to 0.85) in diabetes in the Mediterranean diet group supplemented with extra-
virgin olive oil. As a demonstration of the benefits of the dietary intervention, the PRE-
DIMED study noted a diabetes risk reduction with dietary changes only, as they did not
include a PA or weight loss component in their study.

It is valuable to explore further how specific diets can impact glucose metabolism.
The "Western Diet" has traditionally been high in red meats, saturated fats, sweets,
refined grains, and processed foods.[34,35] In contrast, plant-based diets have been
characterized as high in vegetables, fruits, legumes, nuts, and seeds. Many benefits
have been described with a plant-based diet including possible prevention of diabetes. Tian and colleagues[36] reviewed the risk of T2DM with the consumption of protein (both animal and non-animal based). Their meta-analysis found a higher risk of
T2DM with the intake of total protein and animal protein. In females, plant protein
was associated with a lower T2DM risk, and specifically soy plant protein was associated with a lower risk as well. Red and processed meats were both associated
with a higher risk of T2DM. Finally, egg and fish were not associated with a decreased
diabetes risk. The next three studies further highlight the impact of a plant-based diet
on metabolic syndrome and its association with diabetes.

The Adventist Health Study-2 was a prospective study of 26,187 women and 15,200
men from the Adventist denomination without diabetes at baseline. Diabetes developed in 2.12% of non-vegetarians, 0.54% of vegans, 1.08% of lacto ovo vegetarians,
1.29% of pesco vegetarians, and 0.92% of semi-vegetarians.[35] Vegan patients had a
77% risk reduction in developing diabetes.[34]

The Rotterdam Study included 6798 participants from the Netherlands who had a
diet high in plant-based foods and low in animal products.[34] The median follow-up
was 5.7 and 7.3 years and showed 928/6798 cases of prediabetes and 642/6798
cases of T2DM. The higher the intake of plant-based food the lower the risk of insulin
resistance, prediabetes, and T2DM. When adjusting for BMI, this remained statistically
significant for insulin resistance ($B = -0.05$ [$-0.06;-0.04$]) and diabetes (HR = 0.87
[0.79; 0.99]).[37]

Staija and colleagues[38] included 4,102,369 person-years from three cohorts (Nurses'
Healthy Study, Nurses' Health Study 2, and Health Professionals Follow-Up Study), all
were free of chronic diseases. A plant-based diet index was evaluated and within that
there was a "healthful" index component. The sweets/desserts, fruit juices, sweetened
beverages, refined grains, and potatoes were the less healthy plant foods and received
reverse scores in the plant-based index. The data analysis showed a 34% lower risk of
developing diabetes in individuals who consumed high-quality plant-based food and
were most adherent to the "healthful" plant-based dietary index, independent of
BMI.[38,39] The study concluded that the shift away from less-healthy plant-based food
and animal protein is associated with a lower risk of T2DM development.

The low-carbohydrate ketogenic diet (LCKD) has recently been a focus of interest
and investigation. It is a more drastic approach to eating when contrasted with the
Mediterranean and plant-based diets. In the early twentieth century, ketogenic diets
were the principal treatment option for diabetes (at that time type 1 and T2DM were
not yet differentiated).[40] Before the introduction of insulin, from 1915 until 1922, diabetes experts Drs. Elliott P. Joslin and Frederick M. Allen encouraged a "starvation
diet" for their patients with diabetes.[41] This ketogenic diet was not meant to be a
cure but was meant to maximize the length of life. Although the extreme diet they
implemented contributed to hypoglycemia and even death among patients with
type 1 diabetes, it often benefited those with T2DM. In 1919, Dr Allen and his

associates co-authored *The Rockefeller Series*. The book described 76 patients with diabetes and included details of the strict dietary restrictions used as treatments for their disease as well as their clinical outcomes.[41] Dr Allen was optimistic about his approach to treatment, but did straightforwardly report that 43% of his patients died by 1917.[41]

Interestingly, around the same time, diabetes experts recommended ketosis for their patients. Dr Russel Wilder, who coined the term ketogenic diet, treated children with medication-refractory seizures with this diet, for which a physiologic mechanism of benefit is still unknown.[40,42] At that time, the ketosis diet was a 4:1 ratio of fat to carbohydrate plus protein consistency. In the years since, there have been variations in the ratio of the components, and most have targeted a carbohydrate intake of <20 to 30 g/day, limiting it to 5% to 10% of the total daily dietary requirement.[40]

The physiologic changes occurring during ketosis result from the dramatic deprivation of carbohydrates. As glycogen storage depletes, insulin secretion lowers, and lipolysis of fat in adipose tissue increases with consequent oxidation of free fatty acids and ketone body formation.[43] This state of nutritional ketosis leads to free fatty acids and ketone bodies being used as the energy and fuel source for all vital organs, most importantly, the brain.[42] Nutritional ketosis produces a blood ketone level of 0.5 to 3 mg/dL, a 5- to 10-fold lower level than the range that occurs in diabetic ketoacidosis. In addition, blood glucose levels and pH are maintained in the normal range in contrast to those in diabetic ketoacidosis.[43] Many believe that consuming a very LCKD likely leads to reduction in insulin levels and elevation in ketone bodies, and that together these lead to an appetite suppressant/anorexic effect, improved satiety, weight loss, and improvement in prediabetes and diabetes.[44,45] The following two studies illustrate a keto diet's impact on blood sugar.

Saslow and colleagues[46] conducted a parallel-group, randomized (1:1) trial, including 34 adults with a BMI >25 and an HbA1c of >6.0%. They randomized patients to a very LCKD or a moderate-carbohydrate, calorie-restricted, low fat diet. At 12 months, the ketogenic diet group showed an HbA1c reduction from 6.6% to 6.1%, whereas the moderate carbohydrate group showed a reduction from 6.9% to 5.7% ($P = 0.007$). In addition, the ketogenic diet group showed a greater weight loss and reduction in diabetes medication use.

Hussain and colleagues[47] recruited 363 participants from Kuwait medical center who were overweight (BMI >25 kg/m^2) with a fasting serum glucose >125 mg/dL. Participants were advised to choose between a low-calorie diet and an LCKD for a 24-week intervention trial. Results indicated that both groups had significant ($P < 0.0001$) improvements in BMI, body weight, and waist circumference by the 24th week, but the percentage lost was greater in the ketogenic group. Although blood sugar levels dropped in both groups, the ketogenic group had a significantly greater drop in blood glucose and HbA1c levels ($P < 0.0001$). The ketogenic group also showed a larger significant decrease in total cholesterol, low-density lipoprotein, and triglycerides and a significant increase in HDL-C ($P < 0.0001$). Though only 6 weeks long, this study did enroll a large group of participants and successfully showed the biochemical benefits of the ketognic diet.

Intermittent fasting (IF) is a dietary intervention that involves calorie restriction for a period of time for one or several days per week, or a prolonged overnight fast.[48] This dietary intervention has gained popularity, but has been implemented in varied ways with no clear unified guidelines. Most share the concept of the "feeding window" being short and the fasting time being long (16–24 h), and a "balanced and healthy" diet encouraged.[48] IF is further broken down to alternate-day fasting, time-restricted feeding, periodic prolonged fasting, intermittent calorie restriction, and religious fasting (eg, Ramadan).[49,50] These variable approaches to IF have made it difficult to compare findings in the literature, but there have been extensive reviews of the impact of IF on diabetes and weight loss.

Stockman and colleagues[49] noted that IF in animal studies was associated with improvements in both serum glucose and insulin. In human studies, there was a documented decrease in fasting insulin with no simultaneous drop in fasting glucose and, therefore, not a clear association with insulin sensitivity improvements.[49] Patterson and colleagues[50] reported that 11 of 16 intervention trials of IF regimens showed statistically significant weight loss. They noted a weight loss benefit with alternate-day fasting as well as glucose and insulin concentration reductions. However, the research did not consistently show superiority of alternate-day fasting for weight loss with calorie-restricted dietary plans. In a review by Barnosky and colleagues,[51] IF and alternate-day fasting (ADF) were compared with traditional calorie restriction diets. They showed that all three dietary approaches reduced body weight, in which calorie restriction was slightly more beneficial. The effect on diabetic risk parameters (fasting insulin, insulin sensitivity, and visceral fat mass) was comparable throughout all three dietary interventions.

Another area of study is PA. As discussed above, the link between physical inactivity and metabolic syndrome has been observed and studied in the literature. Lakka and colleagues[52] conducted a cross-sectional study of 1069 middle-aged men without diabetes, cardiovascular disease, or cancer to investigate the association of leisure-time PA and cardiorespiratory fitness on metabolic syndrome. Men who engaged in <3.6 h/week of any leisure-time PA were 64% more likely to have metabolic syndrome than those participating in >6.8 h/week of PA. Men with <1 h/week of at least moderate-intensity PA were 63% more likely to have metabolic syndrome than those with ≥3.0 h/week of such PA. They also assessed VO2max, which is a measure of endurance and accounts for the rate of oxygen consumption measured during exercise. The leisure-time PA group showed a lower VO2max, and this was correlated with a higher risk of metabolic syndrome.

Fowler and colleagues[53] conducted a cross-sectional study of 6,500 randomly selected US adults as part of the National Health and Nutrition Examination Survey to evaluate three objectives. First, they examined the relationship between insulin resistance (indexed using HOMA-IR) and PA (indexed by the total-MET-minutes per week). Second, they examined the influence of age, sex, race, smoking, and BMI on insulin sensitivity and PA. Third, they analyzed the impact of waist circumference on the association between insulin resistance and PA. As expected, results showed that as levels of weekly PA increased, mean HOMA-IR decreased significantly, after controlling for sex, age, race, BMI, and smoking (with a weakening of association in the latter two). Interestingly, the same relationship did not persist when adjusting for differences in waist circumference. More specifically, in adults in the small, medium, and large waist quartiles, there was no relationship between PA and insulin resistance (HOMA-IR). In contrast, in the largest quartile of waist/abdominal obesity (extra-large waists), there was a strong association showed between PA and HOMA-IR. This suggests that visceral and hepatic fat depots are of extra metabolic importance and when reduced through diet and exercise, show an improvement in diabetes risk.

Similar to the diets, not all exercises are equal. Although leisure exercise is better than none at all, it likely is not as metabolically beneficial as moderate to higher intensity exercise. Yoo and colleagues[54] conducted a cohort study of 280,194 Korean patients without diabetes and followed participants in clinic visits over a median duration of 4.13 years. Participants were divided into PA groups according to their self-reported level of intensity, including sedentary, mild PA, and health-enhancing PA.[54]

Their aim was to investigate the association between PA and HOMA-IR as an index of insulin resistance, and adjusted for waist circumference as a confounding factor. Independent of waist circumference, they found that increasing PA or maintaining health-enhancing PA was associated with a lower insulin resistance index ($P < 0.001$), improvement in HOMA-IR ($P < 0.001$), and a lower risk of HOMA-IR progression ($P < 0.001$). Of particular importance, even after the health-enhancing group decreased their PA level over time, the insulin resistance index was lower in that group when compared with the sedentary group ($P < 0.001$). The outcome of this study suggested a strong inverse relationship between PA and insulin resistance in non-diabetics. In addition, independent of BMI and waist circumference, they noted a lasting positive effect of the exercise even after its activity level decreased, though the duration of the improvement remains unknown. Moreover, it is unclear whether this applies to those with preexisting insulin resistance.

The importance of exercise intensity is further shown in the below study. Even with minimal weight loss, moderate-intensity walking can significantly improve the metabolic syndrome. Slentz and colleagues[55] conducted a 6-month parallel clinical trial on 195 adults with elevated fasting glucose and BMI in the overweight/obese range, but without diabetes, uncontrolled hypertension, or cardiovascular disease. Patients were randomized into four groups: low amount of exercise (equivalent to walking 8.6 miles/week) of moderate intensity, high amount of exercise (equivalent to 13.8 miles/week) of moderate intensity, high amount of exercise of vigorous-intensity, or diet plus moderate-intensity exercise (and an additional aim of a weight loss of 7%). They sought to evaluate the impact of these interventions on glucose homeostasis measures. Results showed that the diet plus exercise group experienced a statistically significant decrease in fasting glucose ($P < 0.001$) compared with the exercise-only groups. Fasting glucose was unchanged in the exercise-only groups. The diet plus exercise group [#4] and the high amount of moderate-intensity exercise group both had similar benefits regarding the glucose tolerance findings. Interestingly, the high amount of moderate-intensity exercise group had a significantly better outcome relative to glucose homeostasis compared with the vigorous-intensity exercise group, despite the fact that the former group showed only a modest weight loss of 2 kg (4.4 lbs). Slentz and colleagues suggested that moderate-intensity walking of ~13.8 miles per week (and minimal weight loss) may be nearly as effective as a combination of diet plus exercise (with a more pronounced weight loss) in preventing the progression of prediabetes to diabetes.

Looking again at the importance of higher intensity exercise, Tjonna and colleagues[56] conducted a randomized pilot trial evaluating the impact of high-intensity exercise compared with moderate-intensity exercise on metabolic syndrome risk factors, including insulin action, blood pressure, and endothelial function. Thirty-two patients with metabolic syndrome were randomized to aerobic interval training, continuous moderate exercise, or control for a 16-week trial. All groups spent about the same time exercising, but the intensity of the workouts varied among the groups. Both exercise groups showed improvement in body weight, waist circumference, and systolic and diastolic blood pressures ($P < 0.05$). The aerobic interval group showed a more significant effect on fasting glucose, insulin sensitivity, and β-cell function ($P < 0.05$), and a 25% increase in HDL-C ($P < 0.05$). At the end of 16 weeks, and in contrast to any of the control subjects, 46% in the aerobic interval group ($P < 0.05$) and 37% in the continuous moderate exercise group ($P = 0.23$; between-group difference, $P < 0.05$) were no longer considered to have metabolic syndrome. This study showed the impact of high-intensity exercise in reducing and even reversing risk factors for metabolic syndrome when compared with moderate-intensity exercise.

In our technologically savvy world, many rely on smartphones and smartwatches to monitor the number of steps achieved daily. This tracking mechanism can help increase activity level awareness in sedentary and active individuals and aid in goal modifications. Chiang and colleagues[57] randomized 32 sedentary college students in the obese category and nondiabetic to one of three groups for an 8-week intervention. The groups included a walking step (WSG), walking exercise (WEG), and control. The WSG was asked to reach 12,000 steps/weekday (Monday–Friday), the WEG combined the aforementioned step goal with walking exercises (30 min of continuous moderate-intensity, defined as 103 steps/min, brisk walking pace) 3 days per week, and controls were asked to maintain their usual lifestyle and diet. After the 8-week intervention, the WEG showed statistically significant improvements in the visceral fat area, HDL-C, fasting glucose, and triglycerides ($P < 0.05$). The WSG only showed significant improvements in HDL-C ($P < 0.05$). Chiang and colleagues speculated that the WEG met a moderate-intensity level of exercise, whereas the WSG likely did not. Therefore, the higher intensity exercise showed significant benefit for components of the metabolic syndrome, whereas the lower intensity exercise was less robustly beneficial. As tracking steps has become a popular venture for many, the ability to monitor the outcome of our PA interventions is more attainable and serves as a useful source of motivation.

It is important to note that not all individuals can or are able to participate in intensive interval training as their mode of exercise. Band exercises (use of elastic bands for resistance) are a reasonable option to consider because they are affordable, require no gym memberships or expensive equipment, and are easy to do while traveling. They provide both strength training and muscle toning benefits. Son and colleagues[58] evaluated the impact of resistance band exercise training on metabolic syndrome. Thirty-five sedentary postmenopausal Korean participants with abdominal obesity, hypertension, and metabolic syndrome, were randomized using a two-armed parallel design to a non-exercise control group or a resistance band exercise group for 12 weeks. The resistance band exercise program consisted of a supervised 60-min session three times/week, with a gradual increase in intensity over the 3-month study period. The resistance band exercise group showed a statistically significant improvement in both glucose and insulin levels, HOMA-IR, lipid levels, blood pressure, BMI, and body fat percentage ($P < 0.05$). In addition, lean body mass and HDL-C were noted to increase in the exercise group ($P < 0.05$). This form of PA may have therapeutic effects for metabolic syndrome. Given the ease of use of this mode of exercise, the results are highly encouraging even for those with limited means or access to a gym.

In conclusion, this review delved into a variety of LSMs, both dietary and PA, that have been studied to determine their impact on minimizing the risks of metabolic syndrome and its natural progression to cardiovascular disease. As Dr Gerald Reaven first introduced Syndrome X, now labeled metabolic syndrome, we have increasingly understood how the combination of IGT, hyperinsulinemia, uncontrolled blood pressure, and high LDL and triglycerides contribute to metabolic dysfunction. The Mediterranean diet, plant-based diet, and very LCKD have shown significant therapeutic benefits on prediabetes and diabetes. IF is more controversial as many studies have shown that calorie restriction is equally as beneficial in its metabolic consequences, and likely more sustainable over the long term. Exercise in different intensities and durations, has been a vital partner in this strive toward reducing cardiovascular risk. Interestingly, higher intensity exercise with even minimal weight loss has been significantly beneficial in delaying diabetes progression. Moderate-intensity walking and resistance band exercises have also shown statically beneficial results. Armed with this growing trove of information, we can confidently recommend LSMs as a vital therapy to our high-risk patients in their journey to reverse the metabolic syndrome, decrease cardiovascular risk, and improve their overall health.

CLINICS CARE POINTS

- Intermittent fasting, though showing some benefits, is not as effective as long-term calorie-restricted diets.
- Resistant bands can be highly effective for improving fitness when access to gyms is limited.

DISCLOSURE

The authors have nothing to disclose.

REFERENCES

1. Himsworth HP. Diabetes mellitus: its differentiation into insulin-sensitive and insulin-insensitive types. 1936. Int J Epidemiol 2013;42:1594–8.
2. Reaven GM. Banting lecture 1988. Role of insulin resistance in human disease. Diabetes 1988;37:1595–607.
3. Lemieux I, Despres JP. Metabolic Syndrome: Past, Present and Future. Nutrients 2020;12. https://doi.org/10.3390/nu12113501.
4. Fahed G, Aoun L, Bou Zerdan M, et al. Metabolic syndrome: updates on pathophysiology and management in 2021. Int J Mol Sci 2022;23. https://doi.org/10.3390/ijms23020786.
5. Rochlani Y, Pothineni NV, Kovelamudi S, et al. Metabolic syndrome: pathophysiology, management, and modulation by natural compounds. Ther Adv Cardiovasc Dis 2017;11:215–25.
6. Moore JX, Chaudhary N, Akinyemiju T. Metabolic syndrome prevalence by race/ethnicity and sex in the United States, National Health and nutrition examination survey, 1988-2012. Prev Chronic Dis 2017;14:E24.
7. International Diabetes Federation. IDF diabetes atlas (6th edition). 2013. Available at: wwwidforg/diabetesatlas. Accessed February 10, 2015.
8. Ezzati M, Riboli E. Behavioral and dietary risk factors for noncommunicable diseases. N Engl J Med 2013;369:954–64.
9. Chen L, Magliano DJ, Zimmet PZ. The worldwide epidemiology of type 2 diabetes mellitus–present and future perspectives. Nat Rev Endocrinol 2011;8:228–36.
10. Mirabelli M, Chiefari E, Arcidiacono B, et al. Mediterranean diet nutrients to turn the tide against insulin resistance and related diseases. Nutrients 2020;12. https://doi.org/10.3390/nu12041066.
11. American Diabetes A. Economic costs of diabetes in the U.S. in 2017. Diabetes Care 2018;41:917–28.
12. DeFronzo RA, Tripathy D. Skeletal muscle insulin resistance is the primary defect in type 2 diabetes. Diabetes Care 2009;32(Suppl 2):S157–63.
13. Khan RMM, Chua ZJY, Tan JC, et al. From pre-diabetes to diabetes: diagnosis, treatments and translational research. Medicina (Kaunas) 2019;55. https://doi.org/10.3390/medicina55090546.
14. Kolb H, Martin S. Environmental/lifestyle factors in the pathogenesis and prevention of type 2 diabetes. BMC Med 2017;15:131.

15. Aune D, Norat T, Leitzmann M, et al. Physical activity and the risk of type 2 diabetes: a systematic review and dose-response meta-analysis. Eur J Epidemiol 2015;30:529–42.
16. Yates T, Henson J, Edwardson C, et al. Objectively measured sedentary time and associations with insulin sensitivity: Importance of reallocating sedentary time to physical activity. Prev Med 2015;76:79–83.
17. World Health Organization. Global health risks: mortality and burden of disease attributable to selected major risks 2009. Geneva, Switzerland: WHO Press; 2009.
18. CDC. https://www.cdc.gov/physicalactivity/data/inactivity-prevalence-maps/indexhtml. Accessed January 2022.
19. Carlson SA, Adams EK, Yang Z, et al. Percentage of deaths associated with inadequate physical activity in the United States. Prev Chronic Dis 2018;15:E38.
20. Piercy KL, Troiano RP, Ballard RM, et al. The physical activity guidelines for americans. JAMA 2018;320:2020–8.
21. Pan XR, Li GW, Hu YH, et al. Effects of diet and exercise in preventing NIDDM in people with impaired glucose tolerance. The Da Qing IGT and Diabetes Study. Diabetes Care 1997;20:537–44.
22. Knowler WC, Barrett-Connor E, Fowler SE, et al, Diabetes Prevention Program Research G. Reduction in the incidence of type 2 diabetes with lifestyle intervention or metformin. N Engl J Med 2002;346:393–403.
23. Tuomilehto J, Lindstrom J, Eriksson JG, et al. Prevention of type 2 diabetes mellitus by changes in lifestyle among subjects with impaired glucose tolerance. N Engl J Med 2001;344:1343–50.
24. Kosaka K, Noda M, Kuzuya T. Prevention of type 2 diabetes by lifestyle intervention: a Japanese trial in IGT males. Diabetes Res Clin Pract 2005;67:152–62.
25. Ramachandran A, Snehalatha C, Mary S, et al, Indian Diabetes Prevention P. The Indian Diabetes Prevention Programme shows that lifestyle modification and metformin prevent type 2 diabetes in Asian Indian subjects with impaired glucose tolerance (IDPP-1). Diabetologia 2006;49:289–97.
26. Tosti V, Bertozzi B, Fontana L. Health benefits of the mediterranean diet: metabolic and molecular mechanisms. J Gerontol A Biol Sci Med Sci 2018;73:318–26.
27. Martin-Pelaez S, Fito M, Castaner O. Mediterranean diet effects on type 2 diabetes prevention, disease progression, and related mechanisms. Nutrients 2020;12. https://doi.org/10.3390/nu12082236.
28. Guasch-Ferre M, Merino J, Sun Q, et al. Dietary polyphenols, mediterranean diet, prediabetes, and type 2 diabetes: a narrative review of the evidence. Oxid Med Cell Longev 2017;2017:6723931.
29. Davis C, Bryan J, Hodgson J, et al. Definition of the mediterranean diet; a literature review. Nutrients 2015;7:9139–53.
30. Wedick NM, Pan A, Cassidy A, et al. Dietary flavonoid intakes and risk of type 2 diabetes in US men and women. Am J Clin Nutr 2012;95:925–33.
31. Santangelo C, Filesi C, Vari R, et al. Consumption of extra-virgin olive oil rich in phenolic compounds improves metabolic control in patients with type 2 diabetes mellitus: a possible involvement of reduced levels of circulating visfatin. J Endocrinol Invest 2016;39:1295–301.
32. Wainstein J, Ganz T, Boaz M, et al. Olive leaf extract as a hypoglycemic agent in both human diabetic subjects and in rats. J Med Food 2012;15:605–10.
33. Salas-Salvado J, Bullo M, Estruch R, et al. Prevention of diabetes with Mediterranean diets: a subgroup analysis of a randomized trial. Ann Intern Med 2014; 160:1–10.

34. Jardine MA, Kahleova H, Levin SM, et al. Perspective: Plant-Based Eating Pattern for Type 2 Diabetes Prevention and Treatment: Efficacy, Mechanisms, and Practical Considerations. Adv Nutr 2021;12:2045–55.

35. Tonstad S, Stewart K, Oda K, et al. Vegetarian diets and incidence of diabetes in the Adventist Health Study-2. Nutr Metab Cardiovasc Dis 2013;23:292–9.

36. Tian S, Xu Q, Jiang R, et al. Dietary protein consumption and the risk of type 2 diabetes: a systematic review and meta-analysis of cohort studies. Nutrients 2017;9. https://doi.org/10.3390/nu9090982.

37. Chen Z, Zuurmond MG, van der Schaft N, et al. Plant versus animal based diets and insulin resistance, prediabetes and type 2 diabetes: the Rotterdam Study. Eur J Epidemiol 2018;33:883–93.

38. Satija A, Bhupathiraju SN, Rimm EB, et al. Plant-based dietary patterns and incidence of type 2 diabetes in us men and women: results from three prospective cohort studies. PLoS Med 2016;13:e1002039.

39. McMacken M, Shah S. A plant-based diet for the prevention and treatment of type 2 diabetes. J Geriatr Cardiol 2017;14:342–54.

40. Choi YJ, Jeon SM, Shin S. Impact of a ketogenic diet on metabolic parameters in patients with obesity or overweight and with or without type 2 diabetes: a meta-analysis of randomized controlled trials. Nutrients 2020;12. https://doi.org/10.3390/nu12072005.

41. Mazur A. Why were "starvation diets" promoted for diabetes in the pre-insulin period? Nutr J 2011;10:23.

42. Batch JT, Lamsal SP, Adkins M, et al. Advantages and disadvantages of the ketogenic diet: a review article. Cureus 2020;12:e9639.

43. Gershuni VM, Yan SL, Medici V. Nutritional ketosis for weight management and reversal of metabolic syndrome. Curr Nutr Rep 2018;7:97–106.

44. Westman EC, Feinman RD, Mavropoulos JC, et al. Low-carbohydrate nutrition and metabolism. Am J Clin Nutr 2007;86:276–84.

45. Johnstone AM, Horgan GW, Murison SD, et al. Effects of a high-protein ketogenic diet on hunger, appetite, and weight loss in obese men feeding ad libitum. Am J Clin Nutr 2008;87:44–55.

46. Saslow LR, Daubenmier JJ, Moskowitz JT, et al. Twelve-month outcomes of a randomized trial of a moderate-carbohydrate versus very low-carbohydrate diet in overweight adults with type 2 diabetes mellitus or prediabetes. Nutr Diabetes 2017;7:304.

47. Hussain TA, Mathew TC, Dashti AA, et al. Effect of low-calorie versus low-carbohydrate ketogenic diet in type 2 diabetes. Nutrition 2012;28:1016–21.

48. Zubrzycki A, Cierpka-Kmiec K, Kmiec Z, et al. The role of low-calorie diets and intermittent fasting in the treatment of obesity and type-2 diabetes. J Physiol Pharmacol 2018;69.

49. Stockman MC, Thomas D, Burke J, et al. Intermittent fasting: is the wait worth the weight? Curr Obes Rep 2018;7:172–85.

50. Patterson RE, Sears DD. Metabolic effects of intermittent fasting. Annu Rev Nutr 2017;37:371–93.

51. Barnosky AR, Hoddy KK, Unterman TG, et al. Intermittent fasting vs daily calorie restriction for type 2 diabetes prevention: a review of human findings. Transl Res 2014;164:302–11.

52. Lakka TA, Laaksonen DE, Lakka HM, et al. Sedentary lifestyle, poor cardiorespiratory fitness, and the metabolic syndrome. Med Sci Sports Exerc 2003;35:1279–86.

53. Fowler JR, Tucker LA, Bailey BW, et al. Physical Activity and Insulin Resistance in 6,500 NHANES Adults: The Role of Abdominal Obesity. J Obes 2020;2020: 3848256.
54. Yoo TK, Oh BK, Lee MY, et al. Association between physical activity and insulin resistance using the homeostatic model assessment for insulin resistance independent of waist circumference. Sci Rep 2022;12:6002.
55. Slentz CA, Bateman LA, Willis LH, et al. Effects of exercise training alone vs a combined exercise and nutritional lifestyle intervention on glucose homeostasis in prediabetic individuals: a randomised controlled trial. Diabetologia 2016;59: 2088–98.
56. Tjonna AE, Lee SJ, Rognmo O, et al. Aerobic interval training versus continuous moderate exercise as a treatment for the metabolic syndrome: a pilot study. Circulation 2008;118:346–54.
57. Chiang TL, Chen C, Hsu CH, et al. Is the goal of 12,000 steps per day sufficient for improving body composition and metabolic syndrome? The necessity of combining exercise intensity: a randomized controlled trial. BMC Public Health 2019;19:1215.
58. Son WM, Park JJ. Resistance band exercise training prevents the progression of metabolic syndrome in obese postmenopausal women. J Sports Sci Med 2021; 20:291–9.

Intervention with Therapeutic Agents, Understanding the Path to Remission in Type 2 Diabetes
Part 1

Shuai Hao, MD[a], Guillermo E. Umpierrez, MD[b], Tanicia Daley, MD[a], Priyathama Vellanki, MD[b],*

KEYWORDS

- Type 2 diabetes mellitus • Diabetes remission • β-cell preservation
- Drug-free remission

KEY POINTS

- At the time of type 2 diabetes (T2D) diagnosis, β-cell function is reduced to 50% of normal function. Thereafter, adults have a decline of β-cell function by about 4% to 5% per year. Children and adolescents have a more rapid decline in β-cell function, about 20% to 35% per year.
- Early intensive insulin in adults with T2D may pause or reverse glucose toxicity in β-cells, increasing odds of diabetes remission, whereas significant improvements are not seen in youth with T2D.
- The improvement in β-cell function is lost after cessation of antihyperglycemic medications.

The prevalence and incidence of diabetes is increasing in adults and children. As of 2022, the Centers for Disease Control and Prevention estimates that 37.3 million people in the United States (or 11.3% of the population) have diabetes, and 96 million people aged greater than or equal to 18 years have prediabetes (38% of the population).[1] From 2001 to 2017, there was an increase of 0.32 per 1000 youths with type 2 diabetes (T2D) in the United States, with 18% of adolescents ages 12 to 18 years having prediabetes.[2,3]

[a] Division of Pediatric Endocrinology, Children's Healthcare of Atlanta, Emory University School of Medicine, 1400 Tullie Road Northeast, Atlanta, GA 30329, USA; [b] Division of Endocrinology, Metabolism & Lipids, Emory University School of Medicine, 69 Jesse Hill Jr Drive Southeast, Glenn Building, Room 205, Suite 200, Atlanta, GA 30303, USA
* Corresponding author.
E-mail address: priyathama.vellanki@emory.edu

Endocrinol Metab Clin N Am 52 (2023) 27–38
https://doi.org/10.1016/j.ecl.2022.07.003
0889-8529/23/© 2022 Elsevier Inc. All rights reserved.

T2D has been characterized by progressive loss of irreversible β-cell function, resulting in the need for more medications over time.[4] The United Kingdom Prospective Diabetes Study showed that at the time of T2D diagnosis, β-cell function has already declined by 50%.[4] Thereafter, adults have a decline of their β-cell function by about 4% to 7% per year.[5] Children and adolescents have a more rapid decline in β-cell function, about 20% to 35% per year.[6,7] Studies have shown that a deficit in β-cell mass or dedifferentiation of pancreatic β-cells is likely to lead to failure of insulin secretion.[8,9] Furthermore, major stressors of β-cell function, such as glucotoxicity, islet cell inflammation, and amyloid deposition, may lead to apoptosis.[10] Therefore, preservation of β-cell function aimed at reducing glucose toxicity has been of interest to reverse or delay the clinical course of diabetes.

Growing evidence shows reversible and irreversible defects in pancreatic β-cells in people with T2D, and various studies have been performed to halt the destructive processes.[11] Such treatments as weight loss can augment pancreatic β-cell function, leading to diabetes remission.[12] Several studies have attempted to ameliorate glucotoxicity to preserve β-cell function in adult and pediatric populations. In part one of this review, we discuss studies aiming to achieve diabetes remission with insulin and oral antidiabetic medications (OAD).

The definition of diabetes remission has varied in different studies. In 2021, a consensus report from the American Diabetes Association (ADA) defined remission in subjects with T2D as those who can achieve and maintain a glycosylated hemoglobin (HbA$_{1c}$) concentration less than 6.5% (48 mmol/mol) for at least 3 months after cessation of glucose-lowering therapy.[13] Drug washout is critical because it allows for assessment of glycemic control without the confounding effects of medications.

STUDIES OF DIABETES REMISSION IN ADULTS
Short-Term Intensive Insulin Therapy

Intensive insulin therapy (IIT) has been the most studied intervention to achieve diabetes remission (**Table 1**). Early insulin therapy leading to optimal glycemic control has been shown to improve β-cell dysfunction by reversing glucotoxicity.[10] IIT may have effects independent of glucotoxicity including redifferentiation of β-cells, which can restore insulin secretion and responsiveness to antidiabetic drugs.[14,15] In rats with streptozotocin-induced diabetes, 3 to 10 weeks of IIT had a regenerative effect restoring endogenous insulin production, inhibiting β-cell apoptosis, and promoting β-cell proliferation.[16]

Several studies have aimed to achieve diabetes remission with IIT. The meta-analysis by Kramer and colleagues pooled seven studies comprising 839 patients with newly diagnosed T2D to assess the effects of short-term IIT on diabetes remission, β-cell function, insulin resistance, and long-term drug-free remission.[17] Five of the studies were nonrandomized interventional trials with one arm,[18–22] and two studies compared IIT delivered through multiple doses of insulin (MDI) or continuous subcutaneous insulin infusion (CSII) and OADs.[23,24] In some studies, subjects received 14 days of IIT irrespective of length of glycemic control,[18–20,23,24] whereas in other studies, IIT was maintained for 3 to 7 days then continued for another 14 days of IIT.[21,22] Mean baseline ages were between 45 and 59 years and baseline HbA$_{1c}$ was 9.7% to 11.7% (83–104 mmol/mol). Four of the studies in the meta-analysis assessed glycemic remission, which was defined as the ability to maintain targets of fasting plasma glucose (FPG) greater than 126 to 162 mg/dL (7–9 mmol/L) or postprandial plasma glucose levels less than 180 mg/dL (10 mmol/L) without

Table 1
Intensive insulin therapy

Year of Publication	Sample Size	Inclusion Criteria	Design	Intervention	Duration of Therapy	Study End Point	Duration of Follow-up	Remission, %
Kramer et al,[17] 2013	839	Newly diagnosed	Meta-analysis	CSII and MDI	2–3 wk	Assess HOMA-IR and HOMA-β; Long-term drug-free remission	Up to 24 mo	66.2 after 3 mo; 58.9 after 6 mo; 46.3 after 12 mo; 42.1 after 24 mo
Li et al,[18] 2004	126	Newly diagnosed FPG >200 mg/dL (11.1 mmol/L)	Interventional, 1 arm	CSII	2 wk	Assess HOMA-IR and HOMA-β; Rates of remission (FPG <110 mg/dL or 6.1 mmol/L, PPG <144 mg/dL or 8.0 mmol/L)	24 mo	72.6 after 3 mo; 67.0 after 6 mo; 47.1 after 12 mo; 42.3 after 24 mo
Chen et al,[19] 2007	138	Newly diagnosed FPG >200 mg/dL (11.1 mmol/L)	Interventional, 1 arm	CSII	2 wk	Assess HOMA-IR and HOMA-β	None	Did not assess
Zhao et al,[20] 2007	120	Newly diagnosed	Interventional, 1 arm	CSII	2 wk	Assess HOMA-IR, HOMA-β	None	Did not assess
Chen et al,[24] 2008	22	Newly diagnosed FPG >300 mg/dL (16.6 mmol/L) PPG >400 mg/dL (22.2 mmol/L)	Randomized controlled trial after 2 wk IIT via MDI	Insulin + Insulin or OAD	6 mo	Evaluate β-cell function and insulin sensitivity	12 mo	Did not assess

(continued on next page)

Table 1
(continued)

Year of Publication	Sample Size	Inclusion Criteria	Design	Intervention	Duration of Therapy	Study End Point	Duration of Follow-up	Remission, %
Weng et al,[23] 2008	251	Newly diagnosed FPG 126–300 mg/dL (7–16.7 mmol/L)	Randomized controlled trial	CSII, MDI, or OAD	2–4 wk	Ability to achieve target glycemic control Remission at 12 mo FPG <126 mg/dL or 2-h PPG <180 mg/dL (7 and 10 mmol/L) Measures of β-cell function	12 mo	51.1 on CSII 44.9 on MDI 26.7 on OAD
Chen et al,[21] 2012	118	Newly diagnosed FPG 126–300 mg/dL (7–16.7 mmol/L)	Interventional, 1 arm	CSII	2–3 wk	Remission at 12 mo FPG <126 mg/dL or 2-h PPG <180 mg/dL (7 and 10 mmol/L) Measures of β-cell function	12 mo	55
Liu et al,[22] 2012	64	Newly diagnosed Ages 25–70 FPG 126–300 mg/dL (7–16.7 mmol/L)	Interventional, 1 arm	CSII	2–3 wk	Remission at 3 mo FPG <126 mg/dL or 2-h PPG <180 mg/dL (7 and 10 mmol/L)	3 mo	66
RESET-IT,[32] *2018*	12	T2DM <5 y duration Age 30–80 y Treatment with metformin or lifestyle only HbA$_{1c}$ between 6% and 9.5% (42 and 80 mmol/mol) if no antidiabetic medications or 5.5% and 9.0% (37–75 mmol/mol) if on metformin	Randomized controlled trial after 3 wk IIT	MDI	1–2 wk every 3 mo	Baseline adjusted ISSI-2 and HbA$_{1c}$ HbA$_{1c}$ ≤6.0% (42 mmol/mol)	12 mo	8.3

Abbreviations: CSII, continuous subcutaneous insulin infusion; FPG, fasting plasma glucose; HOMA-β, homeostasis model assessment of β-cell function; HOMA-IR, reduced HOMA insulin resistance; MDI, multiple doses of insulin; PPG, postprandial plasma glucose.

any diabetes therapy for 3 months in one study and greater than 12 months in three other studies.[18,21–23] Measures of β-cell function were collected at baseline and 12 to 48 hours after stopping treatment via oral glucose tolerance test (OGTT) or intravenous glucose tolerance tests.[18,19,21–24] The meta-analysis reported that 66.2% of participants achieved drug-free remission after their 3-month follow-up, 58.9% after 6 months, 46.3% after 12 months, and 42.1% after 24 months. Overall, IIT improved acute insulin release to glucose load, increased area under the curve of insulin secretion, improved whole body insulin sensitivity, increased homeostasis model assessment of β-cell function (HOMA-β), and reduced HOMA insulin resistance (IR).[18,19,22,24–26] In addition, two studies found that IIT improved lipid and free fatty acid levels,[18,19] whereas one did not.[23]

Several studies have reported whether intensive treatment with OADs compared with IIT resulted in long-term drug-free remission.[23,27,28] One study compared whether initiation of IIT by either CSII or MDI, or OADs resulted in short- and long-term remission in treatment-naive newly diagnosed T2D.[23] Subjects were randomized to CSII (n = 137), MDI (n = 124), or OAD (n = 121). Treatment was actively titrated until glycemic control was achieved (7.9 ± 4.6 days) and continued for 2 weeks. All subjects were assessed for glycemic control (FPG <108 mg/dL [6.0 mmol/L]), 2-hour postprandial plasma glucose less than 144 mg/dL (8 mmol/L), and diabetes remission 1 year after therapy. Measures of β-cell secretion were assessed before initiation of therapy and 2 days after stopping therapy with an intravenous glucose tolerance test. One year after stopping therapy, both insulin groups had higher rates of remission compared with the OAD group. Indices of β-cell secretion improved from baseline to after cessation of therapy in all groups but did not differ between the groups. Another study assessed whether initial IIT (n = 45) or combined metformin and glimepiride (n = 44) at time of diabetes diagnosis resulted in drug-free remission at 104 weeks.[27] Subjects in both groups were initially treated until HbA$_{1c}$ was less than 8% (64 mmol/mol) and then they were followed for lifestyle management for 4 weeks. If HbA$_{1c}$ was greater than 7%, OAD therapy was initiated. The IIT group achieved glycemic control faster than the OAD group. At 104 weeks, 53.3% in the IIT group were able to maintain HbA$_{1c}$ less than 7% (53 mmol/mol) without the need for diabetes medications compared with 18.8% in the OAD group.[29]

These studies showed that early IIT result in improved β-cell function and glycemic control for a variable time period. IIT may have effects on insulin secretion beyond glucose control. Predictors for achieving remission include shorter duration of diabetes, lower HbA$_{1c}$, improvement of HOMA-IR, and lower fasting glucose.[21,26,30,31] The likelihood for maintaining remission of diabetes after short-term IIT depends on when IIT is initiated after diagnosis. One study showed that the likelihood of remission at 1 year declines from 77.8% to 70.6% to 58.3% when initiation of IIT is delayed from the first year after diagnosis to the second year or the third year, respectively.[29] Therefore, early aggressive treatment may restore more β-cell function. The degree of initial improvement of β-cell function after starting IIT plays a role.[18,23]

Oral Antidiabetic Agents

Several studies have assessed whether the initial increases in pancreatic β-cell function after a course of short-term IIT are maintained with OADs. The OADs studied were metformin, sulfonylureas, sitagliptin, sodium-glucose cotransporter-2 inhibitors, and thiazolidinediones. These studies assessed pancreatic β-cell function during treatment, with few studies including a washout period to assess maintenance of remission and β-cell function after OAD discontinuation. The mechanisms by which these OADs reduce glucose levels are varied and the durability of glycemic control after drug discontinuation is unknown.

In one study, newly diagnosed patients presenting with severe hyperglycemia (FPG >300 mg/dL [16.65 mmol/L] or a random glucose >400 mg/dL [22.2 mmol/L]) were treated in the hospital for 10 to 14 days with ITT and then randomized to continued insulin therapy (n = 30) or OAD (n = 20), which included metformin and/or gliclazide for 6 months.[24] After 6 months, all subjects who were randomized to insulin therapy were switched to OADs with 1-year follow-up. The primary aim was the proportion with HbA$_{1c}$ less than or equal to 7% (53 mmol/mol) at 6 months and HbA$_{1c}$ less than or equal to 6.5% (48 mmol/mol) at 12 months. After 6 and 12 months, a greater number of participants in the insulin group achieved HbA$_{1c}$ less than 6.5 (48 mmol/mol) and 7% (53 mmol/mol) than the OAD group. Indices of insulin secretion from OGTT, such as the insulin area under the curve, insulinogenic index, and HOMA-β, were higher in the insulin group compared with the OAD group without changes in HOMA-IR or Matsuda index. However, results from this study must be interpreted with caution relative to remission because there was only 12 hours of drug discontinuation before assessment of β-cell function. Also, not all subjects in the OAD group were able to achieve target glycemic control and only those with an HbA$_{1c}$ less than 7% (53 mmol/mol) were included in comparisons of β-cell function and insulin resistance.

In the Remission Studies Evaluating Type 2 Diabetes: Intermittent Insulin Therapy (RESET-IT) pilot study, subjects with mean T2D duration of 2 years and HbA$_{1c}$ between 5.5% and 9.5% (37–80 mmol/mol) were randomized after receiving 3 weeks of induction IIT to either 2 weeks of intermittent insulin therapy (n = 12) every 3 months or daily metformin (n = 12).[32] β-cell assessment was calculated with serial OGTT every 3 months with metformin held the morning of the OGTT. At 2 years, the primary outcome of baseline adjusted insulin secretion sensitivity index-2 (ISSI-2), a marker of β-cell function, was higher in the metformin group compared with the intermittent insulin therapy group without changes in measures of insulin sensitivity (HOMA-IR and Matsuda index). HbA$_{1c}$, FPG, and other measures of β-cell function were all significantly better in the metformin group than the intermittent insulin therapy group. The metformin group had 66.7% remission (defined as HbA$_{1c}$ ≤6.0% or ≤42 mmol/mol) compared with 8.3% of subjects who received intermittent insulin therapy.

The RESET-IT main study evaluated whether adding intermittent insulin therapy to metformin augmented β-cell function.[25] In subjects with mean diabetes duration of 1.8 years, subjects were randomized after initial IIT to continuous metformin with intermittent insulin therapy for 2 weeks every 3 months (n = 55) or metformin only (n = 53). The metformin only arm had a slight increase in baseline adjusted insulin secretion at 2 years compared with the metformin plus intermittent insulin arm. Only 32.6% of participants in each arm were able to maintain HbA$_{1c}$ less than or equal to 6.0% (42 mmol/mol) at 2 years, with no group differences observed. The authors noted that the potential lack of differences between the metformin plus intermittent insulin therapy group and the metformin group may be caused by the metformin plus intermittent therapy group having a 2.5-year or longer duration of diabetes than the metformin group, or caused by metformin being withheld during intermittent insulin therapy.

One study assessed whether preservation of β-cell function with multiple oral agents was comparable with insulin-based therapy.[28] This study had a lead-in period of metformin and insulin for 3 months in subjects with a T2D diagnosis less than 2 months before study enrollment. The participants were then randomized to continue insulin and metformin (n = 29) or to triple therapy with OADs (n = 29): metformin, glyburide, and pioglitazone. Pancreatic β-cell function was assessed using serial mixed-meal tolerance tests at randomization and in intervals up to 42 months after randomization. Antidiabetic therapy was held for 24 hours before the mixed-meal tolerance test. Both groups had equally preserved β-cell function at 3.5 years without differences in mean HbA_{1c}. The insulin and metformin group had mean HbA_{1c} of 6.4% (46 mmol/mol) compared with mean HbA_{1c} of 6.6% (49 mmol/mol) in the triple oral therapy group.

The results of these studies are likely mixed because of differences in study design and the subjects included in the assessment of β-cell function. The initial insulin therapy period varied from 2 to 3 weeks in the RESET-IT studies,[25,32] compared with 2 weeks in the Chen and colleagues study,[24] whereas the Harrison and colleagues[28] study had 3 months of insulin therapy. Assessment of β-cell function was also performed with little washout period suggesting that augmentation or preservation of β-cell function may be affected by glycemic control of the drug itself. Therefore, results of these studies need to be interpreted with caution with respect to diabetes remission as defined by the new ADA consensus statement.[13] However, these studies show that early aggressive treatment may delay the decline of β-cell function that defines the clinical course of diabetes. The initiation of medications after IIT was done to see whether these medications have an effect after the initial glucose toxicity has been eliminated. It is not clear if 10 to 14 days is enough to eliminate glucose toxicity.

The Remission Evaluation of a Metabolic Intervention in Type 2 diabetes (REMIT) and REMIT with dapagliflozin (dapa) trials studied whether drug-free remission can be achieved with intensive early therapy with a combination of OADs and insulin. The REMIT pilot study trial randomized 83 participants with T2D of up to 3 years duration to 8 weeks (n = 28) or 16 weeks (n = 27) of intensive metabolic intervention (which consisted of weight loss, metformin, acarbose, and insulin glargine) or standard of care (n = 28) with subsequent follow-up of 52 weeks from randomization.[33] Complete remission was defined as FPG less than 110 mg/dL (6.1 mmol/L) and a 2-hour glucose less than 140 mg/dL (7.8 mmol/L) on OGTT, and HbA_{1c} less than 6.0% (42 mmol/mol) without diabetes medications at 52-week follow-up. Partial remission was defined as FPG less than 126 mg/dL (7.0 mmol/L) and a 2-hour glucose less than 200 mg/dL (11.1 mmol/L) on OGTT, and HbA_{1c} less than 6.5% (48 mmol/mol) on no chronic diabetes medications. After a 12-week intervention, complete or partial remission was seen in 21.4% of the 8-week group and 40.7% in the 16-week group compared with 14.3% in the control group without a statistical difference. By Week 52, 25% of the 8-week intervention group, 22.2% of the 16-week intervention group, and 10.7% of the control group had maintained complete or partial diabetes remission. This study showed that multiple diabetic agents achieved glycemic control, with longer duration of therapy having more success. Although duration of therapy did not affect long-term remission rates after stopping medications, the 16-week intervention group was on fewer diabetes medications compared with the 8-week group.

The REMIT-dapa trial studied 154 subjects with T2D for up to 8 years in duration, on zero to two noninsulin glucose-lowering medications.[34] The participants were started on an intensive 12-week regimen of insulin glargine, metformin, and dapagliflozin (n = 77) or standard diabetes care (n = 74). All therapies were stopped in subjects achieving HbA_{1c} less than 7.3% (56 mmol/mol) at that period, which was 100% of the intervention group and 69% of the control group. Both groups were followed for 64 weeks. Remission was defined by HbA_{1c} less than 6% (42 mmol/mol) and partial remission by HbA_{1c} less than 6.5% (48 mmol/mol) without need for antidiabetic medications. At 24 weeks, 24.7% had complete or partial remission in the intervention group and 16.9% in the control group, without a statistical difference. However, at 36 weeks, 28.6% in the intervention group and 11.7% in the control group were in remission, which was statistically significant. At 64 weeks only 14.3% in the intervention group and 7.8% in the control group were in partial or complete remission. The low rates of remission could be caused by the number of subjects with longer duration of diabetes, which was approximately 3 years.

STUDIES OF REMISSION IN YOUTH

T2D is increasing in youth, and youth have a higher decline ($\sim$20%) in β-cell function per year compared with approximately 7% decline per year in adults.[6,7,35,36] Longitudinal data over 15 years showed that 50% of youth and adolescents with T2D had microvascular complications at 3 years of follow-up with the number increasing to 80.1% by 15 years.[37] Therefore, methods to preserve β-cell function in youth is highly important.

The Treatment Options for Type 2 Diabetes in Adolescents and Youth (TODAY) randomized controlled trial studied approximately 1000 children ages 10 to 17 years with diabetes duration of less than 2 years and evaluated the effect of metformin, metformin with a lifestyle intervention, or metformin and rosiglitazone on maintaining glycemic control with a follow-up period of 5 years. At baseline, 38% of the participants were treated with insulin alone or a combination of insulin and metformin.[38] Six hundred ninety-nine participants were randomized to continue the trial to receive metformin alone (n = 232), metformin with rosiglitazone (n = 233), or metformin plus lifestyle intervention (n = 234). Treatment failure, the primary outcome, was defined as HbA$_{1c}$ persistently greater than or equal to 8% (64 mmol/mol) over 6 months, or persistent metabolic decompensation defined as the inability to wean from insulin within 3 months of decompensation during the study period or as a repeat decompensation within 3 months of weaning insulin. Approximately 51.7% of participants on metformin alone, 38.6% on metformin and rosiglitazone, and 46.6% on metformin and lifestyle modification eventually required initiation of insulin with a median time of treatment failure of 11.5 months.[39] Although this study did not perform a washout to assess for durability of β-cell function, baseline HbA$_{1c}$ levels and insulinogenic index predicted durable glycemic control for 48 months.[40] In the participants that failed therapy, there was a rapid decline of β-cell function of approximately 20% per year.[7]

The Pediatric Diabetes Consortium was an observational longitudinal study of T2D in children aged less than 21 years. It started children on insulin at the time of T2D diagnosis and subsequently weaned them off for improved glycemic control and showed treatment failure in about half of the group around 1.2 years.[41] Those on metformin had higher rates of remission than intensive lifestyle intervention alone.[41] In Low's study and colleagues,[42] half of obese children who had presented in diabetic ketoacidosis were rapidly weaned off insulin in 2.2 months. The addition of metformin improved rates of near-normoglycemia remission and glycemic control but most subjects required restarting insulin treatment within 15 months of follow-up.

The RISE Consortium performed partially blinded studies in youth aged 10 to 19 years and greater than 85th percentile weight for age and sex with either impaired glucose tolerance or T2D duration less than 12 months. Subjects were randomized to receive glargine for 3 months followed by metformin (n = 44) or to metformin alone for 12 months (n = 47), after which there were 3 months of drug withdrawal. β-cell function was measured using hyperglycemic clamps at baseline, 12 months, and after 3 months of drug withdrawal. At 12 months, there were no differences in β-cell function between the groups with a decline in β-cell function even while on treatment. After withdrawal of the drug, β-cell function was significantly worse than baseline. This decline in β-cell function is in contrast to adults, where β-cell function improved during treatment.[43] Despite having higher insulin secretion in response to glucose and arginine at baseline than adults,[44] youth had a more rapid decline in insulin secretion over time.[43] These data further support that T2D may have a more insidious course in the pediatric population.

DISCUSSION AND FUTURE DIRECTIONS

The current paradigm of T2D management consists of lifestyle and diet changes, then metformin monotherapy, and progressively adding more complex antidiabetic regimens, which might culminate in permanent insulin therapy. The ability to induce diabetes remission and maintain pancreatic β-cell function off antidiabetic agents may simplify the care of T2D, resulting in improved quality of life and potentially lower complications of diabetes. In adults, IIT initiated early during the duration of diabetes augments β-cell function, potentially through improvements in glucose toxicity and may maintain euglycemia while off antidiabetic medications. However, diabetes remission is variable and may only last for 3 to 12 months. OADs, such as metformin, thiazolidinediones, and SGLT2-I, may preserve the initial increases in β-cell function seen with short-term IIT through various mechanisms. Unfortunately, the effect on β-cell preservation is lost when the OADs are stopped. The duration of diabetes and diabetes control before initiation of intensive therapy seems to predict which subjects achieve and maintain remission. This is seen in studies where diabetes remission from a very-low-calorie diet is higher in subjects with diabetes duration less than 2 years.[12]

Several gaps exist in the literature regarding diabetes remission with medications. Differences exist in study designs, making it difficult to generalize conclusions from these studies and compare other modalities of diabetes remission, such as bariatric surgery and intensive weight loss. The studies had various criteria for definition of diabetes remission. Most of the studies had short follow-up with a few exceptions making it difficult to draw conclusions about the factors that predict longer duration of diabetes remission. Few long-term studies exist and are limited by small sample sizes. Furthermore, not every study assessed remission by stopping medications to allow for drug withdrawal.

More studies need to be conducted in youth with T2D because they experience a more rapid decline in β-cell function compared with adults, and short-term insulin therapy and OADs do not pause or preserve β-cell function. As mentioned in the ADA 2021 consensus, future studies need to be designed with uniform criteria so results can be generalized and compared to inform the best course of treatment.[13] Whether duration of diabetes remission affects long-term diabetic complications is also unknown. Long-term follow-up of subjects showed that bariatric surgery can increase life expectancy and decrease microvascular and macrovascular complications of diabetes.[45] Studies of long-term complications are needed for medication-induced remission.

CLINICS CARE POINTS

- Intensive insulin therapy at early onset of type 2 diabetes in adults can achieve diabetes remission for up to 3 to 12 months.

- Most people who achieve diabetes remission with intensive insulin therapy need oral antidiabetic agents to maintain glycemic control and preserve β-cell function. However, the effects on β-cell preservation are lost when medications are stopped.

- Youth with type 2 diabetes have a more rapid decline in β-cell function than adults. Therefore, youth with type 2 diabetes need more aggressive titration of medications to maintain glycemic control.

DISCLOSURE

S. Hao and P. Vellanki have no disclosures. G.E. Umpierrez has received unrestricted support for research studies to Emory University from AstraZeneca and Dexcom. T. Daley has support from Dexcom for research studies.

REFERENCES

1. Centers for Disease Control and Prevention. National Diabetes Statistics Report Website. Available at: https://www.cdc.gov/diabetes/data/statistics-report/index. html. Accessed April 2, 2022.
2. Lawrence JM, Divers J, Isom S, et al. Trends in prevalence of type 1 and type 2 diabetes in children and adolescents in the US, 2001-2017. JAMA 2021;326(8): 717–27.
3. Andes LJ, Cheng YJ, Rolka DB, et al. Prevalence of prediabetes among adolescents and young adults in the United States, 2005-2016. JAMA Pediatr 2020; 174(2):e194498.
4. UKPDS Group. U.K. prospective diabetes study 16. Overview of 6 years' therapy of type II diabetes: a progressive disease. Diabetes 1995;44(11):1249–58.
5. Wysham C, Shubrook J. Beta-cell failure in type 2 diabetes: mechanisms, markers, and clinical implications. Postgrad Med 2020;132(8):676–86.
6. Bacha F, Gungor N, Lee S, et al. Progressive deterioration of beta-cell function in obese youth with type 2 diabetes. Pediatr Diabetes 2013;14(2):106–11.
7. Today Study (TS) Group. Effects of metformin, metformin plus rosiglitazone, and metformin plus lifestyle on insulin sensitivity and beta-cell function in TODAY. Diabetes Care 2013;36(6):1749–57.
8. Butler AE, Janson J, Soeller WC, et al. Increased beta-cell apoptosis prevents adaptive increase in beta-cell mass in mouse model of type 2 diabetes: evidence for role of islet amyloid formation rather than direct action of amyloid. Diabetes 2003;52(9):2304–14.
9. Talchai C, Xuan S, Lin HV, et al. Pancreatic beta cell dedifferentiation as a mechanism of diabetic beta cell failure. Cell 2012;150(6):1223–34.
10. Wajchenberg BL. Beta-cell failure in diabetes and preservation by clinical treatment. Endocr Rev 2007;28(2):187–218.
11. Retnakaran R, Zinman B. Short-term intensified insulin treatment in type 2 diabetes: long-term effects on beta-cell function. Diabetes Obes Metab 2012; 14(Suppl 3):161–6.
12. Taylor R, Al-Mrabeh A, Sattar N. Understanding the mechanisms of reversal of type 2 diabetes. Lancet Diabetes Endocrinol 2019;7(9):726–36.
13. Riddle MC, Cefalu WT, Evans PH, et al. Consensus report: definition and interpretation of remission in type 2 diabetes. Diabetes Care 2021. https://doi.org/10. 2337/dci21-0034.
14. Wang Z, York NW, Nichols CG, et al. Pancreatic beta cell dedifferentiation in diabetes and redifferentiation following insulin therapy. Cell Metab 2014;19(5): 872–82.
15. Sachs S, Bastidas-Ponce A, Tritschler S, et al. Targeted pharmacological therapy restores beta-cell function for diabetes remission. Nat Metab 2020;2(2):192–209.
16. Li HQ, Wang BP, Deng XL, et al. Insulin improves beta-cell function in glucose-intolerant rat models induced by feeding a high-fat diet. Metabolism 2011; 60(11):1566–74.

17. Kramer CK, Zinman B, Retnakaran R. Short-term intensive insulin therapy in type 2 diabetes mellitus: a systematic review and meta-analysis. Lancet Diabetes Endocrinol 2013;1(1):28–34.
18. Li Y, Xu W, Liao Z, et al. Induction of long-term glycemic control in newly diagnosed type 2 diabetic patients is associated with improvement of beta-cell function. Diabetes Care 2004;27(11):2597–602.
19. Chen H, Ren A, Hu S, et al. The significance of tumor necrosis factor-alpha in newly diagnosed type 2 diabetic patients by transient intensive insulin treatment. Diabetes Res Clin Pract 2007;75(3):327–32.
20. Zhao QB, Wang HF, Sun CF, et al. [Effect of short-term intensive treatment with insulin pump on beta cell function and the mechanism of oxidative stress in newly diagnosed type 2 diabetic patients]. Nan Fang Yi Ke Da Xue Xu Bao 2007;27(12):1878–9.
21. Chen A, Huang Z, Wan X, et al. Attitudes toward diabetes affect maintenance of drug-free remission in patients with newly diagnosed type 2 diabetes after short-term continuous subcutaneous insulin infusion treatment. Diabetes Care 2012;35(3):474–81.
22. Liu L, Wan X, Liu J, et al. Increased 1,5-anhydroglucitol predicts glycemic remission in patients with newly diagnosed type 2 diabetes treated with short-term intensive insulin therapy. Diabetes Technol Ther 2012;14(9):756–61.
23. Weng J, Li Y, Xu W, et al. Effect of intensive insulin therapy on β-cell function and glycaemic control in patients with newly diagnosed type 2 diabetes: a multicentre randomised parallel-group trial. Lancet 2008;371(9626):1753–60.
24. Chen HS, Wu TE, Jap TS, et al. Beneficial effects of insulin on glycemic control and beta-cell function in newly diagnosed type 2 diabetes with severe hyperglycemia after short-term intensive insulin therapy. Diabetes Care 2008;31(10):1927–32.
25. Retnakaran R, Emery A, Ye C, et al. Short-term intensive insulin as induction and maintenance therapy for the preservation of beta-cell function in early type 2 diabetes (RESET-IT Main): a 2-year randomized controlled trial. Diabetes Obes Metab 2021;23(8):1926–35.
26. Kramer CK, Choi H, Zinman B, et al. Determinants of reversibility of beta-cell dysfunction in response to short-term intensive insulin therapy in patients with early type 2 diabetes. Am J Physiol Endocrinol Metab 2013;305(11):E1398–407.
27. Chon S, Rhee SY, Ahn KJ, et al. Long-term effects on glycaemic control and beta-cell preservation of early intensive treatment in patients with newly diagnosed type 2 diabetes: a multicentre randomized trial. Diabetes Obes Metab 2018;20(5):1121–30.
28. Harrison LB, Adams-Huet B, Raskin P, et al. Beta-cell function preservation after 3.5 years of intensive diabetes therapy. Diabetes Care 2012;35(7):1406–12.
29. Kramer CK, Zinman B, Choi H, et al. Predictors of sustained drug-free diabetes remission over 48 weeks following short-term intensive insulin therapy in early type 2 diabetes. BMJ Open Diabetes Res Care 2016;4(1):e000270.
30. Stein CM, Kramer CK, Zinman B, et al. Clinical predictors and time course of the improvement in beta-cell function with short-term intensive insulin therapy in patients with type 2 diabetes. Diabet Med 2015;32(5):645–52.
31. Liu L, Ke W, Wan X, et al. Insulin requirement profiles of short-term intensive insulin therapy in patients with newly diagnosed type 2 diabetes and its association with long-term glycemic remission. Diabetes Res Clin Pract 2015;108(2):250–7.
32. Retnakaran R, Choi H, Ye C, et al. Two-year trial of intermittent insulin therapy vs metformin for the preservation of beta-cell function after initial short-term intensive

insulin induction in early type 2 diabetes. Diabetes Obes Metab 2018;20(6): 1399–407.

33. McInnes N, Smith A, Otto R, et al. Piloting a remission strategy in type 2 diabetes: results of a randomized controlled trial. J Clin Endocrinol Metab 2017;102(5): 1596–605.

34. McInnes N, Hall S, Sultan F, et al. Remission of type 2 diabetes following a short-term intervention with insulin glargine, metformin, and dapagliflozin. J Clin Endocrinol Metab 2020;(8):105. https://doi.org/10.1210/clinem/dgaa248.

35. Kahn SE, Lachin JM, Zinman B, et al. Effects of rosiglitazone, glyburide, and metformin on beta-cell function and insulin sensitivity in ADOPT. Diabetes 2011;60(5): 1552–60.

36. Matthews DR, Cull CA, Stratton IM, et al. UKPDS 26: sulphonylurea failure in non-insulin-dependent diabetic patients over six years. UK Prospective Diabetes Study (UKPDS) Group. Diabet Med 1998;15(4):297–303.

37. Study Group Today, Bjornstad P, Drews KL, et al. Long-term complications in youth-onset type 2 diabetes. N Engl J Med 2021;385(5):416–26.

38. Kelsey MM, Geffner ME, Guandalini C, et al. Presentation and effectiveness of early treatment of type 2 diabetes in youth: lessons from the TODAY study. Pediatr Diabetes 2016;17(3):212–21.

39. Study Group Today, Zeitler P, Hirst K, et al. A clinical trial to maintain glycemic control in youth with type 2 diabetes. N Engl J Med 2012;366(24):2247–56.

40. Zeitler P, Hirst K, Copeland KC, et al. HbA1c after a short period of monotherapy with metformin identifies durable glycemic control among adolescents with type 2 diabetes. Diabetes Care 2015;38(12):2285–92.

41. Wolf RM, Cheng P, Gal RL, et al. Youth with type 2 diabetes have a high rate of treatment failure after discontinuation of insulin: a Pediatric Diabetes Consortium study. Pediatr Diabetes 2022. https://doi.org/10.1111/pedi.13325.

42. Low JC, Felner EI, Muir AB, et al. Do obese children with diabetic ketoacidosis have type 1 or type 2 diabetes? Prim Care Diabetes 2012;6(1):61–5.

43. RISE Consortium, Consortium Investigators RISE. Effects of treatment of impaired glucose tolerance or recently diagnosed type 2 diabetes with metformin alone or in combination with insulin glargine on beta-cell function: comparison of responses in youth and adults. Diabetes 2019;68(8):1670–80.

44. RISE Consortium. Metabolic contrasts between youth and adults with impaired glucose tolerance or recently diagnosed type 2 diabetes: I. Observations using the hyperglycemic clamp. Diabetes Care 2018;41(8):1696–706.

45. Sheng B, Truong K, Spitler H, et al. The long-term effects of bariatric surgery on type 2 diabetes remission, microvascular and macrovascular complications, and mortality: a systematic review and meta-analysis. Obes Surg 2017;27(10): 2724–32.

Intervention with Therapeutic Agents, Understanding the Path to Remission to Type 2 Diabetes
Part 2

Shuai Hao, MD[a], Guillermo E. Umpierrez, MD[b],
Priyathama Vellanki, MD[b],*

KEYWORDS

- Type 2 diabetes mellitus • Diabetes remission • β-Cell preservation
- Drug-free remission

KEY POINTS

- At the time of type 2 diabetes (T2D) diagnosis, pancreatic β-cell function is reduced to 50% of normal function. Thereafter, adult and pediatric patients have a decline of β-cell function.
- Use of newer diabetes medications including glucagon-like peptide-1 receptor agonists (GLP-1RA) and dual incretin agonists, such as glucose-dependent insulinotropic polypeptide (GIP) with GLP-1RA, show promising data for preserving β-cell function. However, the effects are lost after cessation of the medication.
- GLP-1RA and GIP/GLP-1RA can cause significant and sustained weight loss but it is unknown whether the weight loss will lead to sustained diabetes remission.

Type 2 diabetes (T2D) has become a health crisis impacting millions of Americans, with more than 37 million diagnosed with diabetes and 96 million with prediabetes.[1] It is a leading cause of death, blindness, amputation, and cardiovascular disease. T2D is characterized by progressive and irreversible loss of β-cell function.[2] The current treatment of T2D consists of diet and lifestyle changes with progressive addition of more complex antidiabetic regimens (including metformin, sulfonylureas, sodium-glucose cotransporter-2 inhibitors, thiazolidinediones, and so forth) and eventually

[a] Division of Pediatric Endocrinology, Children's Healthcare of Atlanta, Emory University School of Medicine, 1400 Tullie Road Northeast, Atlanta, GA 30329, USA; [b] Division of Endocrinology, Metabolism & Lipids, Emory University School of Medicine, 69 Jesse Hill Jr Drive Southeast, Glenn Building, Atlanta, GA 30303, USA
* Corresponding author.
E-mail address: priyathama.vellanki@emory.edu

Endocrinol Metab Clin N Am 52 (2023) 39–47
https://doi.org/10.1016/j.ecl.2022.07.004
0889-8529/23/© 2022 Elsevier Inc. All rights reserved.

insulin therapy. Therefore, there is interest in the development of therapies to induce long-term diabetes remission in T2D mellitus to improve quality of life and potentially lower complications of diabetes. Diabetes remission is defined by the American Diabetes Association as the ability to achieve and maintain a glycosylated hemoglobin (HbA$_{1c}$) concentration less than 6.5% (48 mmol/mol) for at least 3 months after cessation of glucose-lowering therapy.[3] In part two of this review, we discuss studies aiming to achieve remission with incretin-based therapy.

Glucagon-like peptide-1 (GLP-1) and glucose-dependent insulinotropic polypeptide, also known as gastric inhibitory polypeptide (GIP), are incretin hormones that are secreted in the small intestine in response to nutrient ingestion through regulation of the endocrine pancreas.[4] Incretins stimulate insulin secretion in response to food intake in a glucose-dependent fashion.[5] Dipeptidyl-peptidase-IV then quickly degrades GIP and GLP-1.[6] GLP-1 also inhibits glucagon secretion; consequently, without its effects, there is hyperglucagonemia.[6] Patients with T2D have decreased secretion of GLP-1 along with loss of responsiveness to the insulinotropic actions of GIP and GLP-1.[7,8] When supraphysiologic doses of GLP-1 are given, insulin secretion can be increased in a dose-dependent manner and can increase β-cell responsiveness to normal levels,[9] a potential mechanism by which bariatric surgery can induce diabetes remission.[4]

GLP-1 receptor agonists (GLP-1RA) are resistant to dipeptidyl-peptidase-IV degradation. They improve β-cell function and glycemic control through increasing glucose-dependent release of insulin and by inhibiting glucagon excretion.[10] GLP-1RA also slow gastric emptying, lead to early satiety, reduce food intake, and subsequently cause weight loss.[11] GLP-1RA have been found to have tropic effects in in vitro and animal studies, stimulating β-cell proliferation, enhancing differentiation of new β-cells, and preventing apoptosis.[12] They also have pleotropic effects and positively impact cardiovascular performance, reduce inflammation, and provide neuroprotection.[13] In addition to the antihyperglycemic effects, large randomized clinical trials have shown that liraglutide and semaglutide, at doses higher than used for diabetes treatment, have been approved for weight loss in adults and adolescents.[14–16] Even though the weight loss studies included patients with T2D, they did not assess remission of diabetes especially after discontinuation of drug. A few studies have assessed whether use of a GLP-1RA resulted in durable remission and preservation of β-cell function (**Table 1**).

The LIraglutide and Beta-cell RepAir (LIBRA) double-blind randomized placebo-controlled trial aimed to determine whether liraglutide is able to preserve β-cell function in subjects with T2D duration of less than 7 years. Fifty-one subjects were randomized to liraglutide (n = 26) or placebo (n = 25) after 4 weeks of intensive insulin therapy and continued for 48 weeks.[17] After 48 weeks, medication was stopped. Pancreatic β-cell function was assessed by serial oral glucose tolerance tests every 12 weeks and after 2 weeks of cessation of medication. After intensive insulin therapy, mean HbA$_{1c}$ was 6.2% (44 mmol/mol) and 6.4% (46 mmol/mol) in the liraglutide and placebo groups, respectively. The liraglutide arm showed significant improvement of β-cell function, as measured by oral glucose tolerance tests without differences in insulin sensitivity (Matsuda index). The increase in insulin secretion did not differ from placebo after a 2-week washout period. However, the liraglutide arm had a significant decline in body mass index (BMI) at 12 weeks of treatment compared with placebo.

The Restoring Insulin Secretion (RISE) Consortium performed various interventions in adults and children to preserve β-cell function in subjects with prediabetes and early T2D.[18,19] The adult study randomized 267 subjects with impaired glucose tolerance and 70 subjects with T2D duration less than 12 months to receive the following

Table 1
GLP-1

	Year of Publication	Sample Size	Inclusion Criteria	Design	Intervention	Duration of Therapy	Study End Point	Duration of Follow-up	Remission (%)	Persistence of Drug Effects
LIBRA[17]	2014	51	T2D mellitus ≤7 y Treatment of 0–2 diabetes medications HbA1c <9%–10% (75–86 mmol/mol)	Double blinded, randomized controlled trial after 4 wk IIT	Liraglutide vs placebo	48 wk	ISSI-2 and HbA1c HbA1c ≤7.0% (53 mmol/mol)	50 wk	Liraglutide 88.5 vs placebo 84	Lost after 2 wk off
RISE (Adults)[19]	2019	337	Age 20–65 y BMI 25–50 kg/m² FPG 95–124 mg/dL (5.3–6.9 mmol/L) 2-h PPG >140 mg/dL (7.8 mmol/L) HbA1c ≤7.0% (64 mmol/mol)	Randomized control trial	Metformin vs glargine + metformin vs liraglutide + metformin vs placebo	12 mo	Glucose-stimulated C-peptide	15 mo	Not assessed	Lost after 3 mo
Bunck et al[20]	2009	69	Age 30–75 y HbA1c 6.5%–9.5% BMI 25–40 kg/m² Metformin treatment >2 mo No other diabetic medications	Randomized control trial	Exenatide vs glargine	52 wk	Arginine stimulation C-peptide during hyperglycemic clamp	68 wk	Not assessed	C-peptide effects lost after 4 wk HbA1c and body weight effects lost after 12 wk off
Bunck et al[22]	2011	36	Same as above	Continuation of treatment in Bunck et al 2011	Exenatide vs glargine	52 wk, 4 wk off, then 108 wk	Insulin sensitivity and β-cell function	180 wk	Not assessed	Lost after 4 wk
Ellipse[35,36]	2019	134	Age 10–17 y Randomized BMI >85% HbA1c 6.5%–11%	Double blinded, randomized control trial	Liraglutide vs placebo	52 wk	HbA1c change at 26 wk	52 wk	Not assessed	Not assessed

Abbreviations: BMI, body mass index; FPG, fasting plasma glucose; IIT, intensive insulin therapy; PPG, postprandial plasma glucose.

therapies for 12 months followed by 3 months of medication discontinuation: metformin alone (n = 65), 3 months of insulin glargine followed by 9 months of metformin (n = 67), combined liraglutide and metformin (n = 68), or placebo (n = 67). Pancreatic β-cell function was assessed by hyperglycemic clamps with arginine stimulation. Clamp-derived measures of β-cell secretion, such as steady state C-peptide levels and C-peptide levels in response to arginine at 12 months of therapy, were higher in the liraglutide and metformin group compared with other groups. All groups except placebo lost weight and HbA_{1c} levels decreased, with the lowest HbA_{1c} in the liraglutide and metformin group. However, after 3 months of drug discontinuation, measures of β-cell secretion decreased to that of the placebo group, showing that remission was unsustainable. Of note, all groups except the placebo group gained weight after drug withdrawal, which may have contributed to the loss of maintenance of β-cell function.

Another study assessed whether exenatide therapy for 1 year showed improved β-cell secretion in subjects with T2D already treated with metformin.[20] Subjects on stable metformin therapy were randomized to be given exenatide twice daily with meals (n = 36) or glargine insulin once nightly (n = 33). Insulin and exenatide were titrated to maintain a fasting plasma glucose 72 to 99 mg/dL (4.0–5.5 mmol/L).[21] Insulin secretion was assessed by arginine stimulation C-peptide levels during a hyperglycemic clamp at randomization, at 52 weeks while on treatment, and after 4 weeks of washout. First- and second-phase glucose-stimulated C-peptide levels during the hyperglycemic clamps were increased by approximately 1.5-fold and approximately 2.8-fold, respectively, compared with the insulin glargine group. Arginine-stimulated C-peptide levels increased by approximately 3.2-fold from baseline in the exenatide group compared with approximately 1.3-fold from baseline in the insulin glargine group. The exenatide group also lost an average of 3.6 kg, whereas the insulin glargine group gained 1 kg. However, after 4-weeks of washout, the C-peptide increases seen while on exenatide were back to pretreatment values, and by 12 weeks, HbA_{1c} and body weight also rose to pretreatment values. Insulin sensitivity during the clamp remained improved in the exenatide group compared with pretreatment levels.

A subset of subjects (n = 36) was followed for an additional 104-week treatment period on their previously allocated treatment with exenatide (n = 16) or insulin glargine (n = 20) with hyperglycemic clamps with arginine stimulation performed after 4 weeks of a washout period.[22] Glycemic control was comparable between the exenatide and glargine group, with the exenatide group experiencing a mean weight loss of 7.9 kg, whereas the glargine group experienced a mean weight gain of 2.1 kg. After a 4-week washout, glucose-stimulated and arginine-stimulated C-peptide levels did not differ between the groups. However, the disposition index, a measure of insulin secretion accounting for insulin resistance, was sustained at pretreatment levels for the exenatide group, whereas the glargine group experienced a decline from pretreatment levels. The longer-term data suggest that long-term treatment with GLP-1RA may preserve β-cell function. However, the study was limited to a small number of subjects and there were no differences in glucose-potentiated arginine stimulation tests, the gold standard for β-cell assessment.

The SCALE (Satiety and Clinical Adiposity- Liraglutide Evidence in diabetic and nondiabetic individuals) diabetes study randomized patients with T2D, a BMI greater than or equal to 27 kg/m^2, and an HbA_{1c} between 7% and 10% to liraglutide 3.0 mg daily (n = 423), liraglutide 1.8 mg daily (n = 211), or placebo (n = 212).[23] After initial titration, medications were continued for 56 weeks with a 12-week follow-up after drug cessation. At the end of 56 weeks, the liraglutide 3.0-mg group lost more weight compared with liraglutide 1.8 mg or placebo groups at 6.0%, 4.7%, and 2.2%, respectively. An HbA_{1c} less than 6.5% was achieved in 56.5% of patients in the liraglutide

3.0-mg group, in 45.6% of patients in the liraglutide 1.8-mg group, and in 15.0% in the placebo group at 56 weeks of therapy. However, after cessation of therapy, weight regain was noted in both liraglutide groups. This study did not assess diabetes remission because it did not report the number of patients who were able to discontinue all other oral antidiabetic medications.

The STEP (Semaglutide Treatment Effect in People with Obesity) trials studied the effects of once-weekly injectable GLP-1RA semaglutide on weight loss. Overall, patients in the STEP trials lost more weight than patients in the SCALE trials. There was an average 10% to 15% reduction in bodyweight in obese patients from baseline after 68 weeks of treatment,[14,24] and approximately 70% to 85% of the treatment cohorts were able to have a 5% reduction in body weight.[14,24,25] The STEP 2 trial was a double-blind, randomized, placebo-controlled trial that aimed to assess weight loss and glycemic control in adults who were overweight or obese and had T2D using intensive lifestyle modification and semaglutide.[24] It included 1210 participants with T2D duration of greater than 180 days, who had a BMI of at least 27 kg/m^2, an HbA$_{1c}$ between 7% and 10% (53–86 mmol/mol), and could be on stable doses of up to three oral antidiabetic agents. Participants received 2.4 mg semaglutide (n = 403), 1.0 mg semaglutide (n = 404) which is the dose approved for diabetes treatment, or placebo (n = 403) for 68 weeks. Mean weight loss was 9.6% for the 2.4-mg semaglutide group, 7.0% for the 1.0-mg semaglutide group, and 3.4% for the placebo group. Percentage of participants with at least 5% weight reduction was 68.8%, 57.1%, and 28.5% in the 2.4-mg, 1-mg, and placebo groups, respectively. HbA$_{1c}$ decreased by 1.6% (2.5 mmol/mol), 1.5% (2.4 mmol/mol), and 0.4% (0.6 mmol/mol) in the 2.4-mg, 1-mg, and placebo groups, respectively. The weight loss effects were greater in the 2.4-mg cohort compared with the 1.0-mg cohort, whereas HbA$_{1c}$ effects were similar. An HbA$_{1c}$ less than 6.5% was achieved in 67.5% of the cohort on semaglutide 2.4 mg weekly and in 60.1% of the cohort on semaglutide 1.0 mg weekly compared with 15.5% on placebo. However, HbA$_{1c}$ control was not assessed after discontinuation of drug; therefore, it is not known whether the weight loss in and of itself could induce durable remission.

Dual incretin agonists, such as GIP and GLP-1RA, have been shown to have synergistic effects, with greater weight loss and insulinotropic effects in animal models.[13] Although diabetes remission was not an end point, the SURPASS and SURMOUNT phase 3 trials have shown that the once-weekly GLP/GIP tirzepatide (NCT 04184622) is highly effective for weight loss and glycemic control. Participants on tirzepatide were able to achieve an HbA$_{1c}$ less than 6.5% to 7% (48–53 mmol/mol) in approximately 80% to 90% of participants compared to 10% to 20% on placebo while 31% to 52% on tirzepatide achieved an HbA$_{1c}$ less than 5.7% (39 mmol/mol) compared to 1% on placebo.[26] Tirzepatide was superior to semaglutide, insulin degludec, and insulin glargine in HbA$_{1c}$ reduction.[27–29] Significant weight loss with lifestyle interventions or bariatric surgery has been associated with diabetes remission.[30–32] Whether durable diabetes remission can be achieved because of weight loss from these medications needs to be further studied.

There are limited studies about GLP-1RA in the pediatric population because the drug class was only recently approved.[33,34] One study evaluated the efficacy of liraglutide in youth 10 to 17 years of age with T2D who were controlled on diet, metformin, or on insulin therapy.[35] Subjects were randomized in a double-blind manner to liraglutide (n = 66) or placebo (n = 68) with the primary end point of change in HbA$_{1c}$ from baseline after 26 weeks of therapy. The subjects randomized to liraglutide were then continued on liraglutide for another 26 weeks, whereas the placebo group received standard of care. At 26 weeks, liraglutide reduced HbA$_{1c}$ by 0.64% from baseline, whereas the placebo group had an HbA_{1c} increase of 0.42%. At 52 weeks, the HbA_{1c} decrease was sustained in the liraglutide group, whereas the placebo group showed a steady rise in HbA_{1c}. Both groups had a similar decrease in BMI at 26 weeks. However, at 52 weeks, BMI increased in the placebo group, whereas BMI continued to decrease in the liraglutide group. Although there were no measurements of β-cell function or a washout period, a post hoc analysis showed that more subjects in the placebo group needed insulin at 52 weeks, whereas the liraglutide group had a similar number of subjects needing insulin before and after treatment.[36] Although the numbers are small, the data suggest that liraglutide may preserve β-cell function in youth with T2D.

DISCUSSION AND FUTURE DIRECTIONS

Incretin analogues offer beneficial effects to multiple organ systems including brain, cardiovascular, renal, and anti-inflammatory functions.[6] GLP-1RA can restore the insulinotropic actions that are lost with T2D. In addition, GLP-1RAs can augment β-cell function during therapy. The effects on β-cell augmentation are lost once the drug is discontinued. Besides glycemic control, this class of medications has been shown to have significant weight loss. This is critical, especially early in the T2D diagnosis because weight loss of greater than or equal to 10% can double the likelihood of T2D remission at 5 years.[37] Previous studies on intensive lifestyle modifications show that even modest weight loss is difficult to achieve and sustain.[30,38] However, when intensive lifestyle changes are combined with GIP/GLP-1RA therapy, more participants are able to achieve weight loss.[25] Although weight is gained back after stopping GLP-1RA therapy, participants did not return to pretreatment weight even after 48 weeks of therapy.[39] Whether the weight loss caused by these medications will preserve or augment β-cell function independent of GLP-1RA itself needs to be further studied.

CLINICS CARE POINTS

- Glucagon-like peptide-1 receptor agonists (GLP-1RA) can maintain glycemic control and preserve β-cell function after intensive insulin treatment. However, the effects on β-cell function are lost once GLP-1RA are discontinued.
- Newer GLP-1RA and GIP/GLP-1RA therapy has effects on weight loss, which may prolong remission but data are unknown.

DISCLOSURE

S. Hao and P. Vellanki have no disclosures. G.E. Umpierrez has received unrestricted support for research studies (to Emory University) from AstraZeneca and Dexcom.

REFERENCES

1. Centers for Disease Control and Prevention. National Diabetes Statistics Report Website. Available at: https://www.cdc.gov/diabetes/data/statistics-report/index.html. Accessed April 2, 2022.
2. Turner RC, Cull CA, Frighi V, et al. Glycemic control with diet, sulfonylurea, metformin, or insulin in patients with type 2 diabetes mellitus: progressive

requirement for multiple therapies (UKPDS 49). UK Prospective Diabetes Study (UKPDS) Group. JAMA 1999;281(21):2005–12.

3. Riddle MC, Cefalu WT, Evans PH, et al. Consensus report: definition and interpretation of remission in type 2 diabetes. Diabetes Care 2021. https://doi.org/10.2337/dci21-0034.

4. Gallwitz B. Glucagon-like peptide-1 and gastric inhibitory polypeptide: new advances. Curr Opin Endocrinol Diabetes Obes 2016;23(1):23–7.

5. Creutzfeldt W, Ebert R. New developments in the incretin concept. Diabetologia 1985;28(8):565–73.

6. Holst JJ, Vilsboll T, Deacon CF. The incretin system and its role in type 2 diabetes mellitus. Mol Cell Endocrinol 2009;297(1–2):127–36.

7. Nauck M, Stockmann F, Ebert R, et al. Reduced incretin effect in type 2 (non-insulin-dependent) diabetes. Diabetologia 1986;29(1):46–52.

8. Knop FK, Vilsboll T, Hojberg PV, et al. Reduced incretin effect in type 2 diabetes: cause or consequence of the diabetic state? Diabetes 2007;56(8):1951–9.

9. Kjems LL, Holst JJ, Volund A, et al. The influence of GLP-1 on glucose-stimulated insulin secretion: effects on beta-cell sensitivity in type 2 and nondiabetic subjects. Diabetes 2003;52(2):380–6.

10. Knudsen LB, Lau J. The discovery and development of liraglutide and Semaglutide. Front Endocrinol (Lausanne) 2019;10:155.

11. van Can J, Sloth B, Jensen CB, et al. Effects of the once-daily GLP-1 analog liraglutide on gastric emptying, glycemic parameters, appetite and energy metabolism in obese, non-diabetic adults. Int J Obes (Lond) 2014;38(6):784–93.

12. Wajchenberg BL. Beta-cell failure in diabetes and preservation by clinical treatment. Endocr Rev 2007;28(2):187–218.

13. Muller TD, Finan B, Bloom SR, et al. Glucagon-like peptide 1 (GLP-1). Mol Metab 2019;30:72–130.

14. Wilding JPH, Batterham RL, Calanna S, et al. Once-weekly semaglutide in adults with overweight or obesity. N Engl J Med 2021;384(11):989–1002.

15. Pi-Sunyer X, Astrup A, Fujioka K, et al. A randomized, controlled trial of 3.0 mg of liraglutide in weight management. N Engl J Med 2015;373(1):11–22.

16. Kelly AS, Auerbach P, Barrientos-Perez M, et al. A randomized, controlled trial of liraglutide for adolescents with obesity. N Engl J Med 2020;382(22):2117–28.

17. Retnakaran R, Kramer CK, Choi H, et al. Liraglutide and the preservation of pancreatic beta-cell function in early type 2 diabetes: the LIBRA trial. Diabetes Care 2014;37(12):3270–8.

18. RISE Consortium. Restoring Insulin Secretion (RISE): design of studies of beta-cell preservation in prediabetes and early type 2 diabetes across the life span. Diabetes Care 2014;37(3):780–8.

19. RISE Consortium. Lack of durable improvements in beta-cell function following withdrawal of pharmacological interventions in adults with impaired glucose tolerance or recently diagnosed type 2 diabetes. Diabetes Care 2019;42(9):1742–51.

20. Bunck MC, Diamant M, Corner A, et al. One-year treatment with exenatide improves beta-cell function, compared with insulin glargine, in metformin-treated type 2 diabetic patients: a randomized, controlled trial. Diabetes Care 2009;32(5):762–8.

21. Yki-Jarvinen H, Juurinen L, Alvarsson M, et al. Initiate Insulin by Aggressive Titration and Education (INITIATE): a randomized study to compare initiation of insulin combination therapy in type 2 diabetic patients individually and in groups. Diabetes Care 2007;30(6):1364–9.

22. Bunck MC, Corner A, Eliasson B, et al. Effects of exenatide on measures of beta-cell function after 3 years in metformin-treated patients with type 2 diabetes. Diabetes Care 2011;34(9):2041–7.

23. Davies MJ, Bergenstal R, Bode B, et al. Efficacy of liraglutide for weight loss among patients with type 2 diabetes: the SCALE Diabetes Randomized Clinical Trial. JAMA 2015;314(7):687–99.

24. Davies M, Faerch L, Jeppesen OK, et al. Semaglutide 2.4 mg once a week in adults with overweight or obesity, and type 2 diabetes (STEP 2): a randomised, double-blind, double-dummy, placebo-controlled, phase 3 trial. Lancet 2021; 397(10278):971–84.

25. Wadden TA, Bailey TS, Billings LK, et al. Effect of subcutaneous semaglutide vs placebo as an adjunct to intensive behavioral therapy on body weight in adults with overweight or obesity: the STEP 3 Randomized Clinical Trial. JAMA 2021; 325(14):1403–13.

26. Rosenstock J, Wysham C, Frías JP, et al. Efficacy and safety of a novel dual GIP and GLP-1 receptor agonist tirzepatide in patients with type 2 diabetes (SUR-PASS-1): a double-blind, randomised, phase 3 trial. Lancet 2021;398(10295): 143–55.

27. Frias JP, Davies MJ, Rosenstock J, et al. Tirzepatide versus semaglutide once weekly in patients with type 2 diabetes. N Engl J Med 2021;385(6):503–15.

28. Ludvik B, Giorgino F, Jodar E, et al. Once-weekly tirzepatide versus once-daily insulin degludec as add-on to metformin with or without SGLT2 inhibitors in patients with type 2 diabetes (SURPASS-3): a randomised, open-label, parallel-group, phase 3 trial. Lancet 2021;398(10300):583–98.

29. Dahl D, Onishi Y, Norwood P, et al. Effect of subcutaneous tirzepatide vs placebo added to titrated insulin glargine on glycemic control in patients with type 2 diabetes: the SURPASS-5 Randomized Clinical Trial. JAMA 2022;327(6):534–45.

30. Lean MEJ, Leslie WS, Barnes AC, et al. Durability of a primary care-led weight-management intervention for remission of type 2 diabetes: 2-year results of the DiRECT open-label, cluster-randomised trial. Lancet Diabetes Endocrinol 2019; 7(5):344–55.

31. Kirwan JP, Courcoulas AP, Cummings DE, et al. Diabetes remission in the Alliance of Randomized Trials of Medicine Versus Metabolic Surgery in Type 2 Diabetes (ARMMS-T2D). Diabetes Care 2022. https://doi.org/10.2337/dc21-2441.

32. Taheri S, Zaghloul H, Chagoury O, et al. Effect of intensive lifestyle intervention on bodyweight and glycaemia in early type 2 diabetes (DIADEM-I): an open-label, parallel-group, randomised controlled trial. Lancet Diabetes Endocrinol 2020; 8(6):477–89.

33. Bacha F. FDA approval of GLP-1 receptor agonist (liraglutide) for use in children. Lancet Child Adolesc Health 2019;3(9):595–7.

34. Currie BM, Howell TA, Matza LS, et al. A review of interventional trials in youth-onset type 2 diabetes: challenges and opportunities. Diabetes Ther 2021; 12(11):2827–56.

35. Tamborlane WV, Barrientos-Perez M, Fainberg U, et al. Liraglutide in children and adolescents with type 2 diabetes. N Engl J Med 2019;381(7):637–46.

36. Bensignor MO, Bomberg EM, Bramante CT, et al. Effect of liraglutide treatment on body mass index and weight parameters in children and adolescents with type 2 diabetes: post hoc analysis of the ellipse trial. Pediatr Obes 2021;16(8):e12778.

37. Dambha-Miller H, Day AJ, Strelitz J, et al. Behaviour change, weight loss and remission of type 2 diabetes: a community-based prospective cohort study. Diabet Med 2020;37(4):681–8.

38. Look AHEAD Research Group. Eight-year weight losses with an intensive lifestyle intervention: the look AHEAD study. Obesity (Silver Spring) 2014;22(1):5–13.
39. Rubino D, Abrahamsson N, Davies M, et al. Effect of continued weekly subcutaneous semaglutide vs placebo on weight loss maintenance in adults with overweight or obesity: the STEP 4 randomized clinical trial. JAMA 2021;325(14): 1414–25.

Physiology Reconfigured: How Does Bariatric Surgery Lead to Diabetes Remission?

Vance L. Albaugh, MD, PhD[a,b], Christopher Axelrod, MS[b],
Kathryn P. Belmont, BS[b], John P. Kirwan, PhD[b,*]

KEYWORDS

- Diabetes • Obesity • Metabolic surgery • Cardiovascular risk • Bariatric surgery

KEY POINTS

- Bariatric surgery improves the quality of life of patients with type 2 diabetes by decreasing lifelong medication burden and promoting sustained disease remission.
- Bariatric surgery improves glucose homeostasis in patients with type 2 diabetes, in part, by decreasing body weight, a causative factor in disease onset.
- Surgical manipulation of the gastrointestinal tract also contributes to the improvement in glucose homeostasis by hitherto unknown mechanisms of action.
- Further research is required to delineate the synergy and/or additivity of bariatric surgery to weight loss, of any kind, in the remission of type 2 diabetes and restoration of glucose homeostasis.

INTRODUCTION

Type 2 diabetes affects more than 450 million people worldwide[1] and is a leading cause of death due to increased risk of cardiovascular, liver, and kidney disease, as well as numerous types of cancer.[2] The fiscal burden is also exorbitant, with the global cost of treatment and management estimated at 1.7 trillion dollars annually.[3] Metabolic surgery is an accepted and effective clinical treatment of obesity and concurrently improves glycemic control with ~25 to 40% of patients sustaining complete remission for up to 10 years compared to ~6% following intensive medical therapy.[4] Furthermore, there are >13 randomized controlled trials demonstrating that metabolic surgery is superior to conventional or intensive lifestyle and medical management of type 2 diabetes.[5–21]

[a] Metamor Institute, Pennington Biomedical Research Center, 6400 Perkins Road, Baton Rouge, LA 70808, USA; [b] Integrative Physiology and Molecular Medicine Laboratory, Pennington Biomedical Research Center, Louisiana State University, 6400 Perkins Road, Baton Rouge, LA 70808, USA
* Corresponding author.
E-mail address: John.Kirwan@pbrc.edu

Endocrinol Metab Clin N Am 52 (2023) 49–64
https://doi.org/10.1016/j.ecl.2022.06.003
0889-8529/23/© 2022 Elsevier Inc. All rights reserved.

Weight loss is critically important to diabetes treatment, as 90% of adults with type 2 diabetes are overweight or have obesity. Even though prospective trials (eg, Look-AHEAD) have demonstrated that small but significant decreases in body weight improve cardiovascular profiles in patients with diabetes,[22] these small changes do not translate to meaningful clinical benefits (ie, morbidity, mortality).[23] Only bariatric surgery has been shown in prospective and retrospective clinical studies to be associated with diabetes remission and macrovascular benefit, though definitive randomized clinical trials examining long-term cardiovascular outcomes remain as an essential need.[24]

The focus of this review is to discuss the mechanisms of diabetes remission following bariatric surgery. The endemic nature of obesity and type 2 diabetes is too pervasive to allow for surgical management in patients. As such, a better understanding of the mechanisms underlying type 2 diabetes remission following bariatric surgery may lead to novel therapeutics or preventive strategies for many, including children and adolescents, to keep them from needing surgical management for severe obesity and diabetes.

NATURE OF THE PROBLEM–DIABETES REMISSION FOLLOWING BARIATRIC SURGERY

Surgery as an intentional treatment of weight loss dates to the 1950s, with numerous modifications over the past 70 years to reduce risk and maximize efficacy. In 1995, Pories and colleagues[25] described, for the first time, that bariatric surgery may confer long-term control of type 2 diabetes in patients with obesity. The notion that metabolic surgery exerted a direct influence on type 2 diabetes independent of weight loss was conceptualized from diffuse clinical experience whereby insulin secretion is restored and glycemia normalized within days of operation.[25] Moreover, numerous patients dependent on exogenous insulin could even be liberated from insulin as early as 24–48 hours after surgery.[26]

The observation that surgery has early and direct effects on type 2 diabetes was heavily scrutinized, primarily because of the prolonged recovery from open surgery and liquid diets that were frequently utilized postoperatively, as well as the occasional complete restriction of food intake that, in some cases, may last several days to weeks. With the advent of laparoscopic bariatric surgery and quicker surgical recovery, however, Schauer and others began identifying high remission rates for diabetes–especially in those with a recent diagnosis and less severe disease[26,27]—that could not be attributable to a mere reduction in food intake or other factors.

Over the past 30 years, a significant body of evidence has demonstrated improvements in glucose homeostasis associated with metabolic surgery that appear independent of body weight.[28] However, these weight-independent contributions to type 2 diabetes remission remain controversial. For example, intensive lifestyle approaches that integrate calorie restriction with behavioral and dietary counseling can also produce comparable diabetes remission to metabolic surgery in patients with early-onset type 2 diabetes.[29–31]

Diabetes remission following bariatric surgery is likely driven by both weight-dependent and weight-independent mechanisms. Identification of these mechanisms, however, remains difficult as both occur concurrently over time. Thus, this makes study investigation and interpretation of results challenging. In general, effects independent of weight loss appear to occur or be present within days to weeks of surgery, prior to "significant" weight loss. Typically, most patients may lose at most 10–15 pounds in the first month. On the contrary, the weight-dependent effects are much more dominant as increasing amounts of weight are lost, with many individuals losing 50–100+ pounds within the first 12 months.

Weight Loss-dependent Mechanisms of Metabolic Surgery on the Remission of Type 2 Diabetes

Obesity and inflammatory state

Obesity is the primary risk factor for pre- and type 2 diabetes and is present in 90% or greater of patients.[32] Body weight is the product of net energy balance, or the systemic relationship between food intake, energy expenditure, and metabolic efficiency. Positive energy balance and/or weight gain in the absence of adaptive stimuli (ie, exercise, anabolic hormones) is associated with increased risk, time to onset, and progression of type 2 diabetes.[33] Conversely, negative energy balance or weight loss is associated progressive normalization of glycemic control.[34] For example, every 1 kg of weight loss is associated with a 0.1% reduction in HbA_{1c}, independent of weight loss modality.[35] In this view, obesity, or progressive and recurrent body fat accumulation, is a causative factor in the onset of progression of disease, indicating that subsequent body weight reduction may normalize glycemic function. However, it is more likely that obesity triggers adaptive processes to cope with excess fat accumulation which negatively impacts glucose homeostasis and can be reversed by weight loss.

Adiposity

Adipose tissue plays a central role in the regulation of energy balance by allowing rapid and expansive uptake of excess nutrients via cellular hypertrophy and/or hyperplasia. Adipocytes also directly contribute to glycemic control through insulin-mediated glucose disposal, inhibition of lipolysis, and release of inflammatory factors that reciprocally inhibit insulin signaling/glucose uptake. As such, decreasing body weight can relieve glycemic burden directly via enhancing adipose tissue insulin sensitivity and decreasing inflammation. Metabolic surgery procedures decrease body weight by ~30%[36]; the majority of the weight loss being composed of fat mass.[37] To this end, glucose homeostasis is comparable following equivalent body weight and fat loss by Roux-en-Y gastric bypass (RYGB) or calorie restriction in patients with obesity and type 2 diabetes.[38] Concordantly, type 2 diabetes remission is achieved in ~45%[29] and 61%[30] of patients following intensive calorie restriction and lifestyle intervention, respectively, comparable to that of metabolic surgery.[20] Long-term, the modest regression in glycated hemoglobin HbA_{1c} mirrors weight regain after Sleeve Gastrectomy (SG) and RYGB.[39] RYGB yields greater remission of type 2 diabetes than SG, while simultaneously producing greater body weight and fat mass loss.[37]

Insulin sensitivity

Insulin sensitivity contributes to the maintenance of circulating glucose concentrations by dictating the absolute rate and magnitude of glucose uptake. Obesity decreases peripheral insulin sensitivity by ~65%, independent of the presence of metabolic syndrome risk factors.[40] Seven days of lifestyle intervention with dietary management decreases body weight by ~10% and increases peripheral insulin sensitivity by ~40% in patients with obesity and prediabetes.[41] Insulin sensitivity is unaltered by metabolic surgery in the early postoperative period,[42] but progressively increases with the magnitude and duration of weight loss.[43–45] Furthermore, changes in hepatic and skeletal muscle insulin sensitivity are comparable between RYGB and intensive calorie restriction after equivalent weight loss.[38] As such, the acute restoration of glycemia associated with bariatric surgery is unlikely explained by improvements in peripheral insulin sensitivity. However, the durability of remission and reduction in medication use following surgery is certainly impacted by the dramatic improvements in insulin sensitivity associated with weight loss.

β-cell function

Inadequate maintenance of plasma glucose by insulin-producing pancreatic β-cells is the penultimate step in the onset of type 2 diabetes. Initially, the onset of hyperinsulinemia compensates for increasing peripheral insulin resistance, allowing for the maintenance of glucose homeostasis. Overtime, the rate of insulin secretion inadequately clears glucose from the circulation, resulting in the progressive onset of hyperglycemia. Obesity independently increases the rate of insulin secretion to maintain glycemia pressured by increasing insulin resistance.[46] Weight loss via intensive calorie restriction gradually improves β-cell capacity while diminishing hyperinsulinemia and restoring normoglycemia.[47] However, RYGB purportedly increases insulin secretory capacity as early as 4 weeks after surgery which is not observed in nonsurgical controls with equivalent weight loss.[48] In a contrasting report, the 24h rate of insulin secretion and clearance in response to a mixed meal was comparable between RYGB and intensive calorie restriction following equivalent weight loss.[38] Thus, obesity contributes to impaired β-cell function, which is relieved by progressive and sustained weight loss. Further research is required to determine if metabolic surgery independently enhances β-cell function.

Summary–weight-dependent effects. Obesity is a cause of type 2 diabetes and as such, weight-lowering therapies improve glucose homeostasis. Metabolic surgery produces superior remission of type 2 diabetes, but this may be entirely attributable to more rapid and durable weight loss. More intensive lifestyle approaches that integrate calorie restriction with behavioral and dietary counseling appear to produce comparable diabetes remission to metabolic surgery in patients with type 2 diabetes, challenging the notion of a weight-independent mechanism. To clearly delineate a surgical mechanism of glycemic control in humans, a head-to-head comparison of RYGB and/or SG vs. calorie restriction under fixed duration and magnitude of weight loss is required. Such studies are of value in that if the degree of weight loss is the dominant mechanism shared by RYGB, SG and iCR, then combination therapy would have limited clinical value outside of maximizing weight loss (**Fig. 1**)

Weight Loss-independent Mechanisms of Metabolic Surgery on the Remission of type 2 Diabetes

Caloric restriction

It is difficult to mechanistically distinguish weight loss independent improvements in type 2 diabetes from those mediated by negative energy balance, of any kind. In calorie restriction, negative energy balance is achieved by restricting food intake, typically by short-term, low-calorie diets.[49,50] As surgical patients are typically maintained on a liquid diet for at least 1–2 weeks following surgery, it makes matching caloric intake to nonsurgical patients possible. Studies matching calorie intake in surgical and nonsurgical subjects have led to immensely insightful studies demonstrating the early effects of caloric restriction. A prospective, 10-day inpatient study showed glucose homeostasis improved more with diet alone compared to diet + RYGB, suggesting that the early benefits are driven primarily by reduced caloric intake.[51] Jackness and colleagues[50] confirmed these findings, showing specifically that β-cell function and insulin sensitivity are improved by the low-calorie diet consumed by patients with RYGB. In another study using a very low-calorie diet (VLCD, 600 kcal/day), Lim and colleagues[52] showed both β-cell function and hepatic insulin sensitivity are improved by caloric restriction alone and that many individuals have the capacity for redifferentiation and improvement in β-cell mass.[31] The reasons underlying these benefits have been confirmed in preclinical models demonstrating that short-term

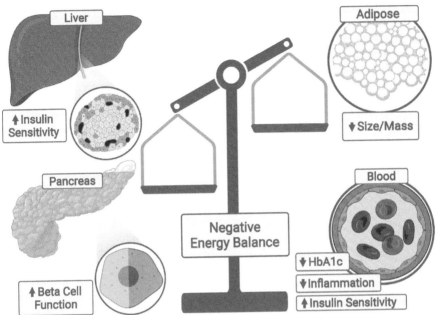

Fig. 1. *Weight-dependent factors that influence remission of type 2 diabetes after bariatric surgery.* Acute or sustained negative energy balance driving a weight-reduced state will improve glucose homeostasis by improving peripheral insulin sensitivity, increasing beta-cell function, and reducing systemic low-grade inflammation.

low-calorie diet improves glucose metabolism prior to weight loss. These changes are associated with reductions in hepatic glycogenolysis, and acetyl-CoA driven pyruvate carboxylase flux and decreased PKCε-mediated insulin resistance.[53]

One of the most marked changes following surgery that is not mimicked by caloric restriction is the increase in postprandial GLP-1 in patients with bariatric surgery. The role of the incretins, namely GLP-1, has been recognized as a potential driver of the early changes in glucose homeostasis in postoperative patients. Interestingly, Isbell[54] examined the contribution of RYGB and caloric restriction in a pre/postmanner and showed that caloric restriction alone was associated with improved insulin sensitivity (as measured by HOMA-IR) at 4 days postoperatively. However, oral glucose tolerance testing was similar in calorie-restricted and RYGB subjects despite significantly augmented GLP-1 responses in the RYGB group. Thus, suggesting that GLP-1 augmentation may not be necessary for the early glycemic improvements in the first week following surgery. Of course, undergoing any surgical operation is associated with a robust inflammatory response that perturbs glycemic control and may mask surgery-specific effects that could not be mimicked in a diet-only intervention group.

Rate and site of intestinal nutrient delivery
The rate and site of intestinal nutrient delivery are altered at the time of surgery, making them leading candidates to alter glucose homeostasis postoperatively. Both rate (VSG and RYGB) and the site of nutrient delivery (RYGB) are altered by either removal of most of the stomach (VSG) or bypass of the stomach and the proximal small intestine (RYGB). In general, the physiologic effects of rapid nutrient delivery have not been widely studied. However, a few studies have demonstrated that intraduodenal nutrient

delivery is associated with altered food intake, gastrointestinal motility, and gastrointestinal hormone secretion.[55,56] In fact, studies using nasoenteric feeding tubes to deliver nutrients into the mid-jejunum can even mimic RYGB-like improvements in glucose tolerance and incretin responses in individuals that have not undergone surgery.[57,58] This ability to essentially recreate the changes in glucose tolerance just by altering the nutrient delivery is highly informative and suggests much of these effects are intrinsic to the anatomical changes in surgery.

Aside from increasing nutrient delivery, RYGB also bypasses the duodenum and proximal portion of the jejunum, creating a relative absence of nutrients within that portion of the intestine. This absence of nutrients has been posited to be responsible for regulating glucose homeostasis in some[59–61] but not all animal models[62] of duodenal-jejunal bypass, an experimental operation focused on isolating the effects of intestinal bypass. Despite some conflicting reports from animals, duodenal-jejunal bypass in humans alleviates insulin resistance and improves glucose homeostasis to underscore the importance of the intestinal tract[63] in the regulation of glycemia and possibly diabetes mission.

The most ideal scenario to study this complex physiology is to be able to measure the effects of normal and surgically altered nutrient delivery in the same individual. To this end, creative studies have taken advantage of the fact that some patients undergoing RYGB have a feeding tube placed into the bypassed stomach, allowing for a randomized "test" of one nutrient route compared to another following surgery. In 2 studies comparing gastric vs. jejunal delivery, the contribution of foregut bypass and rapid nutrient delivery to the jejunum is obvious. Nutrient delivery to the jejunum is associated with a GLP-1 surge that is abrogated by delivery via the bypassed stomach at 1 week following RYGB.[64,65] This effect with jejunal administration is preserved at 6 weeks,[64] though the response changes and is likely affected by other weight-dependent effects. Despite these studies, the findings do not rule out other factors affecting the enteroinsular axis in the postoperative patient.

Further evidence supporting foregut nutrient bypass and diabetes remission has been demonstrated with reversible endoluminal duodenojejunal bypass liner,[66,67] essentially mimicking the foregut bypass portion of RYGB. Placement of the liner is associated with normalized glucose homeostasis in diet-induced obesity rodent models partially by increased energy expenditure that was independent of weight loss.[67] The clinical device typically extends for approximately 65 cm, which likely approaches an area near (though still proximal to) the small bowel transection site where the jejunum is anastomosed to the stomach pouch in a gastric bypass. Another version of the endoluminal sleeve technology is a longer version that includes gastric exclusion to better mimic RYGB surgery. Although the longer device has been trialed in humans,[68] the device has not been studied in preclinical models like the duodeno-jejunal sleeve barrier. Like animal models, human studies demonstrate weight loss and improvement in HbA$_{1c}$.[69,70] Similar approaches to the endoluminal liner include a pharmacologic "coating of the mucosa" with a sucrose-based, octasulfate aluminum complex.[71] Similar to the endoluminal liner device, the chemical complex inhibits nutrient exposure and lowers glucose and ameliorates weight gain in high-fat-fed animal models.[72] Clinical effectiveness of a chemical coating of the intestine is of great interest, though human studies have not yet been published.

Gut-brain Signaling

Gut-brain neural communication via the vagus or other neural pathways is another potential mediator of glucose homeostasis following bariatric surgery. Recent preclinical studies demonstrate neural circuits within the mucosa that detect minuscule amounts of nutrients that directly affect behavior and feeding patterns.[73–75] Although these pathways have yet to be described in humans, the altered intestinal nutrient milieu in the postbariatric surgery patient may also affect these signaling pathways. In preclinical bariatric surgery models, there is a clear alteration of preference for sugar and fat,[76–79] which also occurs clinically.[80–82]

Mechanistically, this type of gut-brain signaling is difficult to identify, but an increasingly studied therapeutic modality suggestive of the importance of these circuits is duodenal mucosal resurfacing. Thermal "resurfacing" of the intestinal lumen is a therapeutic alternative to surgery that has demonstrated improvements in glucose homeostasis and type 2 diabetes status independent of body weight.[83] The underlying mechanism of mucosal resurfacing is unclear, though the procedure likely damages vagal and other centrally projecting nerve endings within the duodenal mucosa. Whether or not this resurfacing mediates its effects through the inhibition of nutrient uptake like a duodenal liner (noted above) or whether it exerts its effects by destroying the signaling pathway that communicates the presence of luminal nutrients remains to be determined. Regardless, in recent years the duodenum has been identified through numerous preclinical and clinical studies as a potential metabolic mediator (reviewed in[84]). Human studies have shown modest, but a significant decrease in body weight that do not necessarily correspond to an improvement in diabetes status (HbA$_{1c}$ or fasting plasma glucose).[83,85] This is highly suggestive of weight-independent effects, but clearly requires further study.

Bile acids

Distinct from anatomic or structural changes inhibiting nutrient contact or exposure within the intestine, circulating hormonal factors are posited to potentially mediate at least some of the early, weight-independent effects of bariatric surgery. In recent years, bile acids and their receptors have been rediscovered as powerful modulators of metabolism that target specific nuclear (eg, farnesoid X receptor, FXR) and membrane-associated receptors (eg, Takeda G-protein Receptor-5, TGR5). In fact, exogenous administration of specific bile acids (eg, ursodeoxycholic acid) is associated with improved hepatic insulin sensitivity[86] and may be associated with liver-protective effects.[87] Bile acids are implicated as an important part of the early metabolic improvements of metabolic surgery, as they modulate energy expenditure in rodents.[88,89] Fasting bile acid concentrations are blunted by obesity and rise following RYGB,[90] with RYGB restoring the prandial bile acid response that is lost with obesity.[90] Perhaps most interestingly, circulating bile acid concentrations are known to surge in postoperative patients[91] and some of these individual bile acids originate from microbial origins that have been shown to have beneficial metabolic effects when given exogenously.[92] The gut microbiota has an active role in shaping the intestinal bile acid milieu, increasing bile acid diversity,[93,94] but the mechanisms driving bile acid synthesis and signaling following surgery remain unknown. Further evidence of bile acids as mechanistic drivers of bariatric surgery-mediated diabetes remission have been elucidated via exploratory metabolic operations in preclinical models. For example, ileal interposition and bile diversion have led to insight regarding the potential of the intestine to regulate insulin sensitivity in a weight-independent manner. Genetic models (eg, Zucker Diabetic Fatty, ZDF, and Zucker rats) have demonstrated weight-independent effects, specifically that ileal interposition improves insulin sensitivity[95] in Zucker rats and even augments β-cell function in ZDF rats.[96] In the presence of these strong genetic models of obesity, increased delivery to the hindgut segments (ileal interposition) or augmented nutrient liberation in the hindgut (bile diversion) are associated with dramatic elevations in circulating bile acids.

Gut Microbiome

In recent years, significant changes in the gut microbiome have been associated with metabolic diseases such as diabetes and obesity. Several studies have implicated *Akkermansia*, a mucin-degrading bacterium that resides in the mucus layer juxtaposed to the intestinal mucosa, in the glycemic benefits related to bariatric surgery. In general, *Akkermansia* species are associated with "metabolic health" and estimates are that these species compose 3–5% of the microbial community in healthy subjects. Notably, the abundance of this "good" bacterium is inversely associated with body weight and is also decreased in patients with diabetes.[97] *Akkermansia* administration in rodents attenuates dietary-induced adiposity, increases intestinal barrier permeability, and improves insulin sensitivity.[98] Probiotic gavage with *Bacteroides thetaiotaomicron* has also been identified as having significant association with clinical states of leanness, also alleviate diet-induced obesity and lead to increased *Akkermansia* abundace.[99] Interestingly, even a prospective clinical study with caloric restriction demonstrated a significantly improved response to caloric restriction for individuals with higher baseline Akkermansia content within the intestinal microbiome,[100] suggesting that Akkermansia is a marker of metabolic health or even potential for reaching a healthier state.

Clinically, Akkermansia and other species increase postbariatric surgery–at least by 3 months,[101] though longer studies are lacking and what long-term effects surgery may have on the intestinal microbiome remains unknown. Bariatric surgery is associated with increased diversity and richness of certain bacteria, though over time improvements in peripheral metabolism, as well as changes in dietary intake, may also affect the gut microbiome. Early changes are difficult to appreciate given that nearly all patients are administered antibiotic prophylaxis at the time of surgery, which may perturb the microbiome for days to weeks. Further evidence for potential benefits of the gut microbiome are observed with other exploratory operations (eg, bile diversion[102]), an exploratory operation that elevates circulating bile acids to mimic the weight loss and improved glucose homeostasis of human bariatric surgery, increases *Akkermansia* species that are associated with weight-independent improvements in glucose tolerance and GLP-1 secretion via the intestine.[103] The crosstalk between bile acids and the gut microbiome is difficult to examine independently of one another but is suggestive of a link between bile acids and gut microbiota that appears to alter incretin levels within the intestinal circulation that may be independent of weight loss.[103]

Bacterially mediated effects of bariatric surgery on metabolism and diabetes remission remain difficult to parse out from those secondary to weight loss. However, there are clear changes in the flux of bile acids and microbiota changes, with increased circulating concentrations of secondary bile acids that only result from microbiome-mediated chemical transformation of human primary bile acids.[91] In this study changes in circulating bile acids were associated with improved hepatic insulin sensitivity during a euglycemic-hyperinsulinemic clamp, consistent with other studies providing these secondary bile acid metabolites via oral administration.[86] Given the plethora of changes in gut microbiota, it remains unclear if underlying microbial changes might be driving metabolic improvements. Both RYGB and Vertical Banded Gastroplasty in humans are associated with long-term alterations in the gut microbiome that are independent of body weight status and modulate long-term changes in adipose tissue mass.[104]

Summary–weight-independent effects

There is significant evidence in support of weight-independent effects of bariatric surgery on remission of type 2 diabetes, though it is inherently difficult to dissect these complex pathways in humans and rodents during a time with concurrent marked weight loss and changes in food intake. As derived from preclinical models, the intestinal tract may harbor a number of possible targets which could be exploited therapeutically for both diabetes as well as obesity management. Further research is needed, especially in humans to identify what is clinically meaningful from preclinical models **(Fig. 2)**

FUTURE DIRECTIONS

As noted, there are likely several weight-dependent and independent mechanisms mediating the remission of diabetes or amelioration of diabetes following bariatric surgery. While the effects secondary to weight loss are very clear and easily tested, the way independent effects represent a huge potential source of targets for pharmacologic therapies that potentially could complement the use of surgery in many individuals for a variety of reasons. Future studies need to continue to explore the weight independent effects of these gastrointestinal operations, and the unexpected improvements that are seen clinically in diabetes status as well as other chronic diseases that remit following surgery.

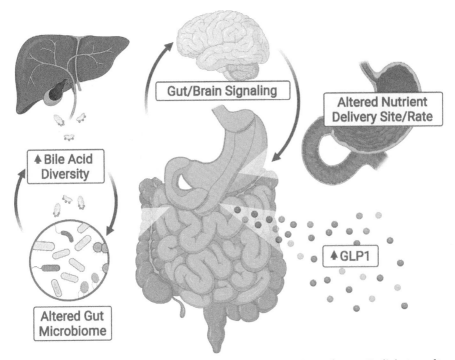

Fig. 2. *Weight-independent factors that influence remission of type 2 diabetes after bariatric surgery.* Structural modification of the gastrointestinal tract during bariatric surgery may directly influence glucose homeostasis by the activation of gastrointestinal hormones that influence insulin secretion, altering the rate and site of nutrient delivery, augmentation gut-brain crosstalk involved in food preference and behavior, and modification of bile acids and bacteria that influence peripheral insulin sensitivity and glycemic control.

CLINICS CARE POINTS

- Weight loss is an important variable to consider in patients undergoing bariatric surgery with an intention to treat type 2 diabetes.
- Pharmacotherapies for obesity with mechanisms of action discrete from that of bariatric surgery should be considered to maximize treatment benefits in patients with type 2 diabetes.
- Similarly, pharmacotherapies for type 2 diabetes with mechanisms of action discrete from that of bariatric surgery should be prioritized to overcome suboptimal patient outcomes related to glucose homeostasis and glycemic control.

DISCLOSURES

The authors have no financial or any other conflicts of interest to disclose concerning this article.

ACKNOWLEDGMENT

This work was supported, in part, by U54GM104940 (JPK).

REFERENCES

1. Saeedi P, Petersohn I, Salpea P, et al. Global and regional diabetes prevalence estimates for 2019 and projections for 2030 and 2045: Results from the International Diabetes Federation Diabetes Atlas, 9th edition. Diabetes Res Clin Pract 2019;157:107843.
2. Heron M. Deaths: leading causes for 2015. Natl Vital Stat Rep 2017;66(5):1–76. Available at: https://pubmed.ncbi.nlm.nih.gov/29235984/.
3. Seuring T, Archangelidi O, Suhrcke M. The economic costs of type 2 diabetes: a global systematic review. Pharmacoeconomics 2015;33(8):811–31.
4. Mingrone G, Panunzi S, Gaetano AD, et al. Metabolic surgery versus conventional medical therapy in patients with type 2 diabetes: 10-year follow-up of an open-label, single-centre, randomised controlled trial. Lancet 2021; 397(10271):293–304.
5. Parikh M, Chung M, Sheth S, et al. Randomized pilot trial of bariatric surgery versus intensive medical weight management on diabetes remission in type 2 diabetic patients Who Do NOT Meet NIH criteria for surgery and the role of soluble rage as a novel biomarker of success. Ann Surg 2014;260(4):617–24.
6. Liang Z, Wu Q, Chen B, et al. Effect of laparoscopic Roux-en-Y gastric bypass surgery on type 2 diabetes mellitus with hypertension: a randomized controlled trial. Diabetes Res Clin Pract 2013;101(1):50–6.
7. Cummings DE, Arterburn DE, Westbrook EO, et al. Gastric bypass surgery vs intensive lifestyle and medical intervention for type 2 diabetes: the CROSSROADS randomised controlled trial. Diabetologia 2016;59(5):945–53.
8. Ding SA, Simonson DC, Wewalka M, et al. Adjustable gastric band surgery or medical management in patients with type 2 diabetes: a randomized clinical trial. J Clin Endocrinol Metab 2015;100(7):2546–56.
9. Dixon JB, O'Brien PE, Playfair J, et al. Adjustable gastric banding and conventional therapy for type 2 diabetes: a randomized controlled trial. JAMA 2008; 299(3):316–23.

10. Ikramuddin S, Korner J, Lee WJ, et al. Roux-en-Y gastric bypass vs intensive medical management for the control of type 2 diabetes, hypertension, and hyperlipidemia: the diabetes surgery study randomized clinical trial. JAMA 2013;309(21):2240–9.

11. Ikramuddin S, Korner J, Lee WJ, et al. Lifestyle intervention and medical management with vs without roux-en-Y gastric bypass and control of hemoglobin A1c, LDL cholesterol, and systolic blood pressure at 5 years in the diabetes surgery study. JAMA 2018;319(3):266–78.

12. Courcoulas AP, Belle SH, Neiberg RH, et al. Three-year outcomes of bariatric surgery vs lifestyle intervention for type 2 diabetes mellitus treatment: a randomized clinical trial. JAMA Surg 2015. https://doi.org/10.1001/jamasurg.2015.1534.

13. Courcoulas AP, Goodpaster BH, Eagleton JK, et al. Surgical vs medical treatments for type 2 diabetes mellitus: a randomized clinical trial. JAMA Surg 2014;149(7):707–15.

14. Halperin F, Ding SA, Simonson DC, et al. Roux-en-Y gastric bypass surgery or lifestyle with intensive medical management in patients with type 2 diabetes: feasibility and 1-year results of a randomized clinical trial. JAMA Surg 2014; 149(7):716–26.

15. Mingrone G, Panunzi S, Gaetano AD, et al. Bariatric-metabolic surgery versus conventional medical treatment in obese patients with type 2 diabetes: 5 year follow-up of an open-label, single-centre, randomised controlled trial. Lancet 2015;386(9997):964–73.

16. Ikramuddin S, Billington CJ, Lee WJ, et al. Roux-en-Y gastric bypass for diabetes (the Diabetes Surgery Study): 2-year outcomes of a 5-year, randomised, controlled trial. Lancet Diabetes Endocrinol 2015;3(6):413–22.

17. Wentworth JM, Playfair J, Laurie C, et al. Multidisciplinary diabetes care with and without bariatric surgery in overweight people: a randomised controlled trial. Lancet Diabetes Endocrinol 2014;2(7):545–52.

18. Mingrone G, Panunzi S, Gaetano AD, et al. Bariatric Surgery versus Conventional Medical Therapy for Type 2 Diabetes. N Engl J Med 2012;366(17): 1577–85.

19. Schauer PR, Bhatt DL, Kirwan JP, et al. Bariatric surgery versus intensive medical therapy for diabetes–3-year outcomes. N Engl J Med 2014;370(21): 2002–13.

20. Schauer PR, Kashyap SR, Wolski K, et al. Bariatric surgery versus intensive medical therapy in obese patients with diabetes. N Engl J Med 2012;366(17): 1567–76.

21. Kirwan JP, Courcoulas AP, Cummings DE, et al. Diabetes remission in the alliance of randomized trials of medicine versus metabolic surgery in type 2 diabetes (ARMMS-T2D). Diabetes Care 2022. https://doi.org/10.2337/dc21-2441.

22. Wing RR, Lang W, Wadden TA, et al. Benefits of modest weight loss in improving cardiovascular risk factors in overweight and obese individuals with type 2 diabetes. Diabetes care 2011;34(7):1481–6.

23. Group TLAR. Cardiovascular effects of intensive lifestyle intervention in type 2 diabetes. N Engl J Med 2013;369(2):145–54.

24. Schauer PR, Nissen SE. After 70 years, metabolic surgery has earned a cardiovascular outcome trial. Circulation 2021;143(15):1481–3.

25. Pories WJ, Swanson MS, MacDonald KG, et al. Who would have thought it? An operation proves to be the most effective therapy for adult-onset diabetes mellitus. Ann Surg 1995;222(3):339–50.

26. Schauer PR, Burguera B, Ikramuddin S, et al. Effect of laparoscopic Roux-En Y gastric bypass on type 2 diabetes mellitus. Trans Meet Am Surg Assoc 2003; 121(NA):160–78.

27. Schauer PR, Ikramuddin S, Gourash W, et al. Outcomes after laparoscopic Roux-en-Y gastric bypass for morbid obesity. Ann Surg 2000;232(4):515–26.

28. Laferrère B, Pattou F. Weight-independent mechanisms of glucose control after Roux-en-Y gastric bypass. Front Endocrinol 2018;9:530.

29. Lean ME, Leslie WS, Barnes AC, et al. Primary care-led weight management for remission of type 2 diabetes (DiRECT): an open-label, cluster-randomised trial. Lancet 2018;391(10120):541–51.

30. Taheri S, Zaghloul H, Chagoury O, et al. Effect of intensive lifestyle intervention on bodyweight and glycaemia in early type 2 diabetes (DIADEM-I): an open-label, parallel-group, randomised controlled trial. Lancet Diabetes Endocrinol 2020;8(6):477–89.

31. Taylor R, Al-Mrabeh A, Zhyzhneuskaya S, et al. Remission of human type 2 diabetes requires decrease in liver and pancreas fat content but is dependent upon capacity for β cell recovery. Cell Metab 2018;28(4):547–56.e3.

32. Prevention C for DC and. National Diabetes statistics report website. national diabetes statistics report. 2020. Available at: https://www.cdc.gov/diabetes/data/statistics-report/index.html. Accessed March 30, 2022.

33. Schulze MB, Manson JE, Ludwig DS, et al. Sugar-sweetened beverages, weight gain, and incidence of type 2 diabetes in young and middle-aged women. JAMA 2004;292(8):927–34.

34. Wing RR, Blair EH, Bononi P, et al. Caloric Restriction Per Se Is a significant factor in improvements in glycemic control and insulin sensitivity during weight loss in obese NIDDM patients. Diabetes Care 1994;17(1):30–6.

35. Gummesson A, Nyman E, Knutsson M, et al. Effect of weight reduction on glycated haemoglobin in weight loss trials in patients with type 2 diabetes. Diabetes Obes Metab 2017;19(9):1295–305.

36. Gloy VL, Briel M, Bhatt DL, et al. Bariatric surgery versus non-surgical treatment for obesity: a systematic review and meta-analysis of randomised controlled trials. BMJ 2013;347(oct22 1):f5934.

37. Hofsø D, Fatima F, Borgeraas H, et al. Gastric bypass versus sleeve gastrectomy in patients with type 2 diabetes (Oseberg): a single-centre, triple-blind, randomised controlled trial. Lancet Diabetes Endocrinol 2019;7(12):912–24. https://doi.org/10.1016/s2213-8587(19)30344-4.

38. Yoshino M, Kayser BD, Yoshino J, et al. Effects of diet versus gastric bypass on metabolic function in diabetes. N Engl J Med 2020;383(8):721–32.

39. Schauer PR, Bhatt DL, Kirwan JP, et al. Bariatric surgery versus intensive medical therapy for diabetes — 5-year outcomes. N Engl J Med 2017;376(7):641–51.

40. Hoddy KK, Axelrod CL, Mey JT, et al. Insulin resistance persists despite a metabolically healthy obesity phenotype. Obesity 2022;30(1):39–44.

41. Solomon TP, Haus JM, Kelly KR, et al. Randomized trial on the effects of a 7-d low-glycemic diet and exercise intervention on insulin resistance in older obese humans. Am J Clin Nutr 2009;90(5):1222–9.

42. Kashyap SR, Daud S, Kelly KR, et al. Acute effects of gastric bypass versus gastric restrictive surgery on |[beta]|-cell function and insulinotropic hormones in severely obese patients with type 2 diabetes. Int J Obes Relat Metab Disord 2010;34(3):462–71.

43. Kashyap SR, Bhatt DL, Wolski K, et al. Metabolic effects of bariatric surgery in patients with moderate obesity and type 2 diabetes. Diabetes Care 2013;36(8): 2175–82.
44. Muscelli E, Mingrone G, Camastra S, et al. Differential effect of weight loss on insulin resistance in surgically treated obese patients. Am J Med 2005; 118(1):51–7.
45. Houmard JA, Tanner CJ, Yu C, et al. Effect of weight loss on insulin sensitivity and intramuscular long-chain fatty Acyl-CoAs in morbidly obese subjects. Diabetes 2002;51(10):2959–63.
46. Rothberg AE, Herman WH, Wu C, et al. Weight loss improves β-Cell function in people with severe obesity and impaired fasting glucose: a window of opportunity. J Clin Endocrinol Metab 2019;105(4):e1621–30.
47. Zhyzhneuskaya SV, Al-Mrabeh A, Peters C, et al. Time course of normalization of functional β-cell capacity in the diabetes remission clinical trial after weight loss in type 2 diabetes. Diabetes Care 2020;43(4):813–20.
48. Laferrère B, Teixeira J, McGinty J, et al. Effect of weight loss by gastric bypass surgery versus hypocaloric diet on glucose and incretin levels in patients with type 2 diabetes. J Clin Endocrinol Metab 2008;93(7):2479–85.
49. Jazet IM, Pijl H, Frölich M, et al. Two days of a very low calorie diet reduces endogenous glucose production in obese type 2 diabetic patients despite the withdrawal of blood glucose–lowering therapies including insulin. Metabolism 2005;54(6):705–12.
50. Jackness C, Karmally W, Febres G, et al. Very low–calorie diet mimics the early beneficial effect of roux-en-Y gastric bypass on insulin sensitivity and β-cell function in type 2 diabetic patients. Diabetes 2013;62(9):3027–32.
51. Lingvay I, Guth E, Islam A, et al. Rapid improvement in diabetes after gastric bypass surgery. Diabetes care 2013;36(9):2741–7.
52. Lim EL, Hollingsworth KG, Aribisala BS, et al. Reversal of type 2 diabetes: normalisation of beta cell function in association with decreased pancreas and liver triacylglycerol. Diabetologia 2011;54(10):2506–14.
53. Perry RJ, Peng L, Cline GW, et al. Mechanisms by which a very-low-calorie diet reverses hyperglycemia in a rat model of type 2 diabetes. Cell Metab 2018; 27(1):210–7.e3.
54. Isbell JM, Tamboli RA, Hansen EN, et al. The importance of caloric restriction in the early improvements in insulin sensitivity after Roux-en-Y gastric bypass surgery. Diabetes care 2010;33(7):1438–42.
55. Chapman IM, Goble EA, Wittert GA, et al. Effects of small-intestinal fat and carbohydrate infusions on appetite and food intake in obese and nonobese men. Am J Clin Nutr 1999;69(1):6–12.
56. Pilichiewicz AN, Chaikomin R, Brennan IM, et al. Load-dependent effects of duodenal glucose on glycemia, gastrointestinal hormones, antropyloroduodenal motility, and energy intake in healthy men. Am J Physiol Endocrinol Metab 2007; 293(3):E743–53.
57. Tamboli RA, Sidani RM, Garcia AE, et al. Jejunal administration of glucose enhances acyl ghrelin suppression in obese humans. Am J Physiol Endocrinol Metab 2016;311(1):E252–9.
58. Breitman I, Isbell JM, Saliba J, et al. Effects of proximal gut bypass on glucose tolerance and insulin sensitivity in humans. Diabetes care 2013;36(4):e57.
59. Rubino F, Forgione A, Cummings DE, et al. The mechanism of diabetes control after gastrointestinal bypass surgery reveals a role of the proximal small intestine in the pathophysiology of type 2 diabetes. Ann Surg 2006;244(5):741–9.

60. Kindel TL, Yoder SM, Seeley RJ, et al. Duodenal-jejunal exclusion improves glucose tolerance in the diabetic, Goto-Kakizaki rat by a GLP-1 receptor-mediated mechanism. J Gastrointest Surg 2009;13(10):1762–72.

61. Angelini G, Castagneto-Gissey L, Casella-Mariolo J, et al. Duodenal-jejunal bypass improves nonalcoholic fatty liver disease independently of weight loss in rodents with diet-induced obesity. Am J Physiol Gastrointest Liver Physiol 2020;319(4):G502–11.

62. Kindel TL, Martins PJF, Yoder SM, et al. Bypassing the duodenum does not improve insulin resistance associated with diet-induced obesity in rodents. Obesity (Silver Spring, Md) 2011;19(2):380–7.

63. Cohen RV, Schiavon CA, Pinheiro JS, et al. Duodenal-jejunal bypass for the treatment of type 2 diabetes in patients with body mass index of 22-34 kg/m2: a report of 2 cases. Surg Obes Relat Dis 2007;3(2):195–7.

64. Hansen EN, Tamboli RA, Isbell JM, et al. Role of the foregut in the early improvement in glucose tolerance and insulin sensitivity following Roux-en-Y gastric bypass surgery. Am J Physiol Gastrointest Liver Physiol 2011;300(5):G795–802.

65. Kirwan JP, Axelrod CL, Kullman EL, et al. Foregut exclusion enhances incretin and insulin secretion after Roux-en-Y gastric bypass in adults with type 2 diabetes. J Clin Endocrinol Metab 2021. https://doi.org/10.1210/clinem/dgab255.

66. Aguirre V, Stylopoulos N, Grinbaum R, et al. An endoluminal sleeve induces substantial weight loss and normalizes glucose homeostasis in rats with diet-induced obesity. - PubMed - NCBI. Obesity 2012;16(12):2585–92.

67. Munoz R, Carmody JS, Stylopoulos N, et al. Isolated duodenal exclusion increases energy expenditure and improves glucose homeostasis in diet-induced obese rats. Am J Physiol Regul Integr Comp Physiol 2012;303(10): R985–93.

68. Sandler BJ, Rumbaut R, Swain CP, et al. One-year human experience with a novel endoluminal, endoscopic gastric bypass sleeve for morbid obesity. Surg Endosc 2015;29(11):3298–303.

69. Patel SRH, Hakim D, Mason J, et al. The duodenal-jejunal bypass sleeve (Endo-Barrier Gastrointestinal Liner) for weight loss and treatment of type 2 diabetes. Surg Obes Relat Dis 2013;9(3):482–4.

70. Rodriguez-Grunert L, Neto MPG, Alamo M, et al. First human experience with endoscopically delivered and retrieved duodenal-jejunal bypass sleeve. Surg Obes Relat Dis 2008;4(1):55–9.

71. Lee Y, Deelman TE, Chen K, et al. Therapeutic luminal coating of the intestine. Nat Mater 2018;17(9):834–42.

72. Lo T, Lee Y, Tseng CY, et al. Daily transient coating of the intestine leads to weight loss and improved glucose tolerance. Metabolis 2022;126:154917.

73. Goldstein N, McKnight AD, Carty JRE, et al. Hypothalamic detection of macronutrients via multiple gut-brain pathways. Cell Metab 2021;33(3):676–87.e5.

74. Buchanan KL, Rupprecht LE, Kaelberer MM, et al. The preference for sugar over sweetener depends on a gut sensor cell. Nat Neurosci 2022;25(2):191–200.

75. Kaelberer MM, Rupprecht LE, Liu WW, et al. Neuropod cells: emerging biology of the gut-brain sensory transduction. Annu Rev Neurosci 2020;43(1):1–17.

76. Shin AC, Zheng H, Pistell PJ, et al. Roux-en-Y gastric bypass surgery changes food reward in rats. Int J Obes 2011;35(5):642–51.

77. Zheng H, Shin AC, Lenard NR, et al. Meal patterns, satiety, and food choice in a rat model of Roux-en-Y gastric bypass surgery. AJP: Regul Integr Comp Physiol 2009;297(5):R1273–82.

78. Chambers AP, Wilson-Perez HE, McGrath S, et al. Effect of vertical sleeve gastrectomy on food selection and satiation in rats. Am J Physiol Endocrinol Metab 2012;303(8):E1076–84.
79. Blonde GD, Price RK, Roux CW le, et al. Meal patterns and food choices of female rats fed a cafeteria-style diet are altered by gastric bypass surgery. Nutrients 2021;13(11):3856.
80. Smith KR, Papantoni A, Veldhuizen MG, et al. Taste-related reward is associated with weight loss following bariatric surgery. J Clin Invest 2020;130(8):4370–81.
81. Zhang Y, Nagarajan N, Portwood C, et al. Does taste preference predict weight regain after bariatric surgery? Surg Endosc 2019;16:1–7.
82. Kapoor N, Najim W al, Menezes C, et al. A comparison of total food intake at a personalised buffet in people with obesity, before and 24 months after Roux-en-Y-gastric bypass surgery. Nutrients 2021;13(11):3873.
83. van Baar ACG, Holleman F, Crenier L, et al. Endoscopic duodenal mucosal resurfacing for the treatment of type 2 diabetes mellitus: one year results from the first international, open-label, prospective, multicentre study. Gut 2020;69(2): 295–303.
84. van Baar ACG, Nieuwdorp M, Holleman F, et al. The duodenum harbors a broad untapped therapeutic potential. Gastroenterology 2018;154(4):773–7.
85. Rajagopalan H, Cherrington AD, Thompson CC, et al. Endoscopic duodenal mucosal resurfacing for the treatment of type 2 diabetes: 6-month interim analysis from the first-in-human proof-of-concept study. Diabetes Care 2016;39(12): 2254–61.
86. Kars M, Yang L, Gregor MF, et al. Tauroursodeoxycholic Acid may improve liver and muscle but not adipose tissue insulin sensitivity in obese men and women. Diabetes 2010;59(8):1899–905.
87. Robles-Díaz M, Nezic L, Vujic-Aleksic V, et al. Role of ursodeoxycholic acid in treating and preventing idiosyncratic drug-induced liver injury. A systematic review. Front Pharmacol 2021;12:744488.
88. Watanabe M, Houten SM, Mataki C, et al. Bile acids induce energy expenditure by promoting intracellular thyroid hormone activation. Nature 2006;439(7075): 484–9.
89. Watanabe M, Horai Y, Houten SM, et al. Lowering bile acid pool size with a synthetic farnesoid X receptor (FXR) agonist induces obesity and diabetes through reduced energy expenditure. J Biol Chem 2011;286(30):26913–20.
90. Ahmad NN, Pfalzer A, Kaplan LM. Roux-en-Y gastric bypass normalizes the blunted postprandial bile acid excursion associated with obesity. Int J Obes 2013;37(12):1553–9.
91. Albaugh VL, Flynn CR, Cai S, et al. Early increases in bile acids post Roux-en-Y gastric bypass are driven by insulin-sensitizing, secondary bile acids. J Clin Endocrinol Metab 2015;100(9):E1225–33.
92. Kim DJ, Yoon S, Ji SC, et al. Ursodeoxycholic acid improves liver function via phenylalanine/tyrosine pathway and microbiome remodelling in patients with liver dysfunction. Sci Rep 2018;8(1):11874.
93. Winston JA, Theriot CM. Diversification of host bile acids by members of the gut microbiota. Gut Microbes 2019;11(2):158–71.
94. Poland JC, Flynn CR. Bile Acids, their receptors, and the gut microbiota. Physiology 2021;36(4):235–45.
95. Culnan DM, Albaugh V, Sun M, et al. Ileal interposition improves glucose tolerance and insulin sensitivity in the obese Zucker rat. Am J Physiol Gastrointest Liver Physiol 2010;299(3):G751–60.

96. Mosinski JD, Aminian A, Axelrod CL, et al. Roux-en-Y gastric bypass restores islet function and morphology independent of body weight in ZDF rats. Am J Physiol Endocrinol Metab 2021;320(2):E392–8.

97. Hasani A, Ebrahimzadeh S, Hemmati F, et al. The role of Akkermansia muciniphila in obesity, diabetes and atherosclerosis. J Med Microbiol 2021;70(10). https://doi.org/10.1099/jmm.0.001435.

98. Everard A, Belzer C, Geurts L, et al. Cross-talk between Akkermansia muciniphila and intestinal epithelium controls diet-induced obesity. Proc Natl Acad Sci U S A 2013;110(22):9066–71.

99. Liu R, Hong J, Xu X, et al. Gut microbiome and serum metabolome alterations in obesity and after weight-loss intervention. Nat Med 2017;510:417–514.

100. Dao MC, Everard A, Aron-Wisnewsky J, et al. *Akkermansia muciniphila* and improved metabolic health during a dietary intervention in obesity: relationship with gut microbiome richness and ecology. Gut 2016;65(3):426–36.

101. Yu D, Shu XO, Howard EF, et al. Fecal metagenomics and metabolomics reveal gut microbial changes after bariatric surgery. Surg Obes Relat Dis 2020;16(11):1772–82.

102. Flynn CR, Albaugh VL, Cai S, et al. Bile diversion to the distal small intestine has comparable metabolic benefits to bariatric surgery. Nat Commun 2015;6(1):7715.

103. Albaugh VL, Banan B, Antoun J, et al. Role of bile acids and GLP-1 in mediating the metabolic improvements of bariatric surgery. Gastroenterology 2019;156(4):1041–51.e4.

104. Tremaroli V, Karlsson F, Werling M, et al. Roux-en-Y gastric bypass and vertical banded gastroplasty induce long-term changes on the human gut microbiome contributing to fat mass regulation. Cell Metab 2015;22(2):228–38.

Remission with an Intervention
Is Metabolic Surgery the Ultimate Solution?

Zubaidah Nor Hanipah, MD[a,b], Francesco Rubino, MD[c],
Philip R. Schauer, MD[a],*

KEYWORDS

- Type 2 diabetes • Metabolic surgery • Bariatric surgery • Cardiovascular risk factor
- Weight loss • Diabetes remission • Diabetes mellitus

KEY POINTS

- Long-term type 2 diabetes (T2D) remission (≥5 years) after lifestyle intervention or pharmacotherapy in patients with mild disease is rare and occurs in less than 5%.
- Long-term T2D remission (≥5 years) occurs in 23% to 98% of patients after metabolic surgery depending on the procedure type, duration, and severity of diabetes.
- Long-term (≥5 years) remission of hypertension (22%–67%), dyslipidemia (21%–80%), and sleep apnea (25%–100%) also occurs after metabolic surgery depending on the procedure type and disease severity.
- Metabolic surgery significantly reduces diabetes complications: microvascular (66%), macrovascular (47%), and all-cause mortality (49%).
- Perioperative morbidity and mortality of metabolic surgery on average is about 2% and 0.1%, respectively.

Curing diabetes has been, perhaps, the most important aspirational priority of diabetes research for ages. The American Diabetes Association (ADA) states that its mission is to "prevent and cure diabetes and to improve the lives of all people affected by diabetes."[1] The timeliness of the topic, "Diabetes Remission," in this issue of Endocrinology and Metabolism Clinics cannot be overstated as 2022 marks the 100th anniversary of the first effective treatment of diabetes—insulin injection. Since the discovery of insulin (1921) and its first use in humans (1922) by Frederick Banting,

[a] Metamor Institute, Pennington Biomedical Research Center, Louisiana State University, 6400 Perkins Road, Baton Rouge, LA 70808, USA; [b] Department of Surgery, Faculty of Medicine and Health Sciences, University Putra Malaysia, Selangor, Malaysia; [c] School of Cardiovascular and Metabolic Medicine & Sciences, King's College London; Bariatric and Metabolic Surgery King's College Hospital, Denmark Hill, London SE5 9RS, UK
* Corresponding author.
E-mail address: philip.schauer@pbrc.edu

Endocrinol Metab Clin N Am 52 (2023) 65–88
https://doi.org/10.1016/j.ecl.2022.09.002
0889-8529/23/© 2022 Elsevier Inc. All rights reserved.

John Macleod, Charles Best and James Collip, investigators have been searching for a cure of diabetes.[2] Banting initially thought he found the cure, but later realized that "insulin is not a cure for diabetes; it is a treatment." [2] Since then, diabetes (and its subtypes 1 and 2) has been defined as an "incurable" chronic disease with treatment goals aimed to ameliorate symptoms and slowdown both disease progression and complications.[3]

DEFINITION, INTERPRETATION, AND CRITERIA FOR DIABETES REMISSION

Despite the century-long interest in curing diabetes, it is interesting that a formal consensus on a standardized definition of a diabetes cure (type 2 diabetes [T2D]) did not emerge until 2009.[4] Before that time, a plethora of definitions of diabetes *resolution* or *cure* appeared in the literature and made comparisons problematic. The expert group organized by the ADA recommended the term "remission" over cure or resolution to reflect the possibility of recurrence. They opined that remission inherently meant restoration to nondiabetic (glycated hemoglobin [HbA1c] <6.5%) glucose levels (partial remission) or normal glucose levels (complete remission) for at least 1 year without the use of glucose-lowering medications.[5] To reflect long-term remission, they recommended the term "prolonged remission," which was defined somewhat arbitrarily as remission for $\geq$ 5 years. Three validated interventions have been identified as yielding remission: (1) lifestyle modification (diet and exercise), (2) short-term intense glucose-lowering medications followed by withdrawal of medications, and (3) gastrointestinal surgery (bariatric/metabolic surgery, peptic ulcer surgery). In an effort to simplify and update the definition of remission for broader use, an international expert group was again recently convened by the ADA and recommended that an HbA1c less than 6.5% (48 mmol/mol) measured at least 3 months after cessation of glucose-lowering pharmacotherapy as the usual diagnostic criterion for diabetes remission.[5] **Table 1** describes criterion for remission based on intervention. Unless otherwise stated, for the purposes of this review, this most recent definition of remission applies.

HISTORY/TIMELINE ON DIABETES REMISSION

Case reports and small observational studies over the last century document at least short-term remission/resolution of diabetes by lifestyle modification, short-term medication use then withdrawal, or gastrointestinal surgery (gastric surgery, bariatric surgery, and metabolic surgery) (**Fig. 1**).[6–21] The observation that gastric surgery for peptic ulcer disease or cancer can yield diabetes remission was first documented in 1925 shortly after the discovery of insulin.[6] Since the 1995 landmark study by Pories and with T2D randomized to a structured colleagues[7] showing 83% diabetes remission (7.6 year mean follow-up) after Roux-en-Y gastric bypass (RYGB) in 146 patients with T2D, a large body of high-quality evidence has accumulated demonstrating the efficacy of bariatric surgery, more appropriately termed metabolic surgery, as a treatment leading to a long-term ($\geq$5 year) remission of diabetes. This review article presents the evidence for metabolic surgery as an evidenced-based treatment of T2D that can often lead to long-term remission especially in patients with early or mild diabetes.

DIABETES INTERVENTIONS
Remission Versus Continuous Treatment

It is well established that reducing HbA1c to achieve long-term glucose control for T2D management reduces both microvascular and macrovascular complications—the

Table 1
Definition of diabetes remission based on interventions

Intervention Note: Documentation of Remission Should Include a Measuement of HbA1c Just Prior to Intervention	Interval Before Testing of HbA$_{1c}$	Subsequent Measurements of HbA$_{1c}$ to Document Continuation of a Remission
Pharmacotherapy	At least 3 months after the cessation of this intervention	Not more often than every 3 months nor less frequent than yearly
Surgery	At leaset 3 months after the procedure and 3 months after cessation of any pharmacotherapy	
Lifestyle	At least 6 months after beginning this intervention and 3 months after cessation of any pharmacotherpy	

From Riddle MC, Cefalu WT, Evans PH, et al. Consensus Report: Definition and Interpretation of Remission in Type 2 Diabetes [published online ahead of print, 2021 Aug 30]. Diabetes Care. 2021;44(10):2438-2444.

major goal of diabetes therapy.[22] The distinction between continuous pharmaco-therapy treatment and long-term remission to achieve glycemic control may have important long-term implications for reducing diabetes complications. Diabetes remission means maintaining glucose control below the threshold for diagnosis

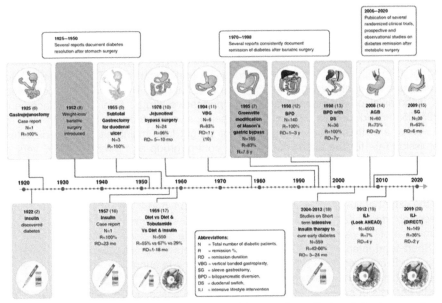

Fig. 1. A century of diabetes remission via surgical (top row), medical and diet interventions (bottom row). AGB = adjustable gastric band.

(HbA1c 6.5%) without ongoing glucose-lowering pharmacotherapy. Thus, beta cell function is restored to normal or near normal function with remission. Conversely, treatment requires ongoing pharmacotherapy to achieve HbA1c targets that are often still in the diabetic range. Organizations such as the ADA recommend treating with glucose-lowering agents to reach HbA1c less than 7.0% or even less than 8.0% for more severe and chronic disease, as more intensive glycemic control with medications may result in higher mortality in some patients presumably due to hypoglycemia.[5,23,24] Although remission achieves sustained near-normal beta cell function and near-normal glucose control, continuous pharmacotherapy does not achieve either. Thus, few would disagree that remission is superior to glucose control achieved by pharmacotherapy and would likely result in greater reduction of diabetes complications, although this is unproven.

Lifestyle and Pharmacologic Interventions May Rarely Lead to Long-Term Remission

Achieving short-term diabetes remission through lifestyle modification using a very low-calorie diet is achievable in patients with early diabetes (<3 years).[18,20,21,25,26] The Look AHEAD (Action for Health in Diabetes) randomized controlled trial (RCT) assessed the effects of intentional weight loss in 5145 patients with mostly mild diabetes (mean HbA1c 7.3%) and obesity. At 4 years, weight loss, and diabetes remission (any remission during the 4 years) were 4.7% and 7.3%, respectively, in the intensive lifestyle intervention (ILI) group and 0.8% and 2%, respectively, in the control group (P < 0.001 for intergroup comparisons).[20] At the end of the trial (approximately 10-year follow-up), weight loss and remission were 6% and 3.5%, respectively, in the ILI group and 3.5% and 2.3%, respectively, in the control group. During the follow-up period, 196 patients elected to have bariatric surgery (RYGB); sleeve gastrectomy [SG]; or laparoscopic adjustable gastric band [LAGB], with weight loss and remission of 19% and 23%, respectively.[25] The Diabetes Intervention Accentuating Diet and Enhancing Metabolism-I trial is an ILI versus usual care study (n = 158) among adult patients with diabetes (duration <3 years) and overweight/obesity. After 1 year of intervention exposure, diabetes remission occurred in 61% of participants compared with 12% of controls; remission beyond 1 year has not been reported.[26] Diabetes Remission Clinical Trial (DiRECT) is an open-label, cluster-RCT conducted at primary care practices in the United Kingdom involving 298 participants with T2D randomized to a structured weight-management program or usual care. The intervention consisted of withdrawal of antidiabetic and antihypertensive drugs, total diet replacement (825–853 kcal/d formula diet for 12–20 weeks), stepped food reintroduction for 2 to 8 weeks, and then structured support for weight loss maintenance. The diabetes remission rate for the intervention versus control group at 1 year was 46% versus 4% (P < 0.0001) and at 2 years was 36% versus 3% (P < 0.0001), respectively.[21] The adjusted mean difference between the control and intervention groups in body-weight change at 2 years was −5·4 kg (P < 0·0001). Sustained remission was linked to the extent of sustained weight loss. Remission beyond 2 years for DiRECT has not been reported. Lifestyle interventions achieving a significant (>30%) and sustained remission of ≥5 years has not been reported in the peer-reviewed literature.

Short-term intensive insulin treatment in patients with newly diagnosed T2D can improve B-cell function, called "B-cell rest," leading to short-term remission on withdrawal of insulin and maintenance of a low-calorie diet.[27–33] A systematic review and meta-analysis of seven studies (N = 839 patients) assessed the effect of short-term (2 weeks) intensive insulin therapy (IIT) in patients with T2D.[19] Follow-up periods ranged from 3 to 24 months after cessation of IIT. Four studies (n = 599) assessed the glycemic remission rate. Participants with drug-free remission were 66% (292 of 441 patients), 59% (222 of 377 patients), 46% (229 of 495 patients), and 42% (53 of 126 patients) at 3, 6, 12, and 24 months of follow-up, respectively.[19] Although short-term remission following intensive pharmacotherapy is possible, long-term remission has not been demonstrated.

Continuous Lifestyle and Pharmacologic Interventions Often Fall Short of Achieving Long-Term Glucose Control

Although long-term sustained remission is rarely achieved after lifestyle with or without pharmacologic treatment, continuous pharmacologic treatment has historically not achieved high success rates for reaching good glucose control globally.[34] A recent meta-analysis (369,251 patients from 20 countries) on the achievement of guideline targets for blood pressure, lipid, and glycemic control in patients with T2D showed suboptimal achievement of these targets over the years.[35] The pooled targets achieved for glycemic control (43%), blood pressure (29%), low-density lipoprotein cholesterol (LDL-C 49%), high-density lipoprotein cholesterol (HDL-C 58%), and tri-glyceride values (62%) were disappointing. According to the US National Health and Nutrition Examination Survey (NHANES), only 51% of patients under T2D treatment with polypharmacy from 2015 to 2018 achieved the ADA recommended glycemic target (HbA1c <7%), which declined from 57% achieved during the 2007 to 2010 period. Moreover, only 22% met all three targets of medical therapy (HbA1c $\leq$ 7.0, LDL-C $\leq$ 100, and blood pressure <130/80 mm Hg).[36] Perhaps greater use of newer agents such as sodium–glucose cotransporter 2 (SGLT2) inhibitors and glucagon-like peptide-1 agonists will improve success in achieving widespread glucose control, but such success remains to be proven.

Metabolic Surgery as Effective Long-Term Treatment of Type 2 Diabetes

Metabolic surgery is another T2D treatment that has been widely available for at least the past 2 decades but underutilized. Less than 1% of patients with obesity and T2D who meet standard criteria undergo metabolic surgery.[37] Metabolic surgery has been shown to result in greater improvements in weight loss, glycemic control, diabetes remission, and cardiovascular (CV) risk factors compared with lifestyle intervention plus pharmacotherapy.[38] Hence, most major international diabetes organizations have endorsed metabolic surgery as a treatment of T2D in patients with obesity.[39]

TYPES OF METABOLIC PROCEDURES

A total of 199,000 metabolic procedures were performed in the United States in 2020, representing a 22% decrease compared with 2019 (256,000 cases) due to the impact of COVID-19.[40] The most common metabolic procedure performed is SG (59%), followed by RYGB (21%), biliopancreatic diversion with duodenal switch (BPD-DS 1.8%), and LAGB (1.2%) (**Fig. 2**). Currently, greater than 95% of metabolic procedures are performed laparoscopically[41]; with typically a 1 to 2-day hospital stay and a 2 to 4-week recovery period after surgery. Postoperative major complications and mortality over the past 25 years have decreased from 11% to 2% and 1% to 0.1%, respectively, approximating a safety profile comparable to cholecystectomy, hysterectomy, and appendectomy.[42,43] Long-term complications requiring medical or surgical intervention such as intestinal obstruction, ulcers, strictures, severe anemia, and nutritional deficiencies occur in 5% to 10% with revisional surgery required in 5% to 10% depending on the specific procedure.[38] BPD-DS is associated with a higher rate of nutritional deficiencies, especially protein calorie malnutrition and metabolic bone

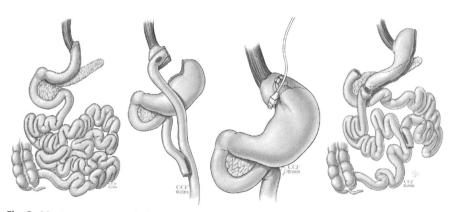

Fig. 2. Most common metabolic procedures in the United States. (From Left to Right) Sleeve Gastrectomy (SG), Roux-en-Y Gastric Bypass (RYGB), Laparoscopic Adjustable Gastric Band (LAGB), Biliopancreatic Diversion with Duodenal Switch (BPD-DS). Reprinted with permission, Cleveland Clinic Foundation 2022. All Rights Reserved.)

disease, and is used less frequently for this reason even though it often yields superior weight loss and metabolic improvement compared with the other surgical options.

EFFICACY OF METABOLIC SURGERY

Both observational studies and RCTs have shown that metabolic surgery results in sustainable weight loss, as well as improvements in glycemic control, CV risk factors, comorbidities, and quality of life and is superior to medical management of T2D. Diabetes remission occurs in 23% to 98% of patients after metabolic surgery at long-term follow-up (≥5 years) depending on the procedure and severity of diabetes (**Tables 2 and 3**).[15,44–81] In addition to remission of diabetes, metabolic surgery is the only known treatment of T2D to result in long-term remission not only of diabetes but also other metabolic comorbidities such as hypertension, dyslipidemia, and sleep apnea that commonly present in patients with T2D (**Table 4**). Patients who do not achieve long-term disease remission after surgery or have recurrence or relapse still have superior disease control compared with medical management or baseline status.[44–53] Thus, recurrence should not be considered a failure. Retrospective observational studies consistently demonstrate an association between metabolic surgery and reduced microvascular and macrovascular events including mortality in patients with T2D compared with nonsurgical treatment.[82,83] These outcomes strongly suggest that metabolic surgery contributes to the major drivers of diabetes improvement including weight loss (adipose tissue reduction), neuroendocrine changes, and ultimately preservation of β cell function to a much greater degree than lifestyle intervention and pharmacologic treatment alone. Although there is much debate regarding mechanisms of diabetes remission and improvement after metabolic surgery, there is little debate that weight loss, directly or indirectly, plays a major mechanistic role. A review of mechanisms of diabetes remission is beyond the scope of this report but has been recently assessed by other investigators.[84–86]

Long-Term Weight Loss

Although few studies of weight loss after lifestyle intervention or anti-obesity medication report long-term weight loss beyond 5 years, many studies report long-term

Table 2
Long-term (≥5 y) diabetes remission after metabolic surgery

Study	Follow-up (Years)	Study Design	Metabolic Surgery	No of Patients	Patients with T2D (%)	Diabetes Remission Criteria	Diabetes Remission (%)	P Value
SOS (Sjöström et al,[44] 2014)	15	Prospective nonrandomized	(Gastric banding/vertical banded gastroplasty/RYGB) vs medical	4047	15	FBG < 110 mg/dL	30 vs 7	<0.001
LABS (Purnell et al,[45] 2020)	7	Prospective study	RYGB vs LAGB	2256	37	HbA1c < 6.5%	57 vs 23	NA
Mingrone et al,[46] 2021	10	Randomized control study	RYGB vs BPD vs medical	60	100	HbA1c ≤ 6.5%	25 vs 50 vs 0	0.002
STAMPEDE (Schauer et al,[47] 2016)	5	Randomized control study	RYGB vs SG vs medical	150	100	HbA1c ≤ 6.0%	22 vs 15 vs 0	< 0.05
Courcoulas et al,[48] 2020	5	Randomized control study	RYGB vs LAGB vs medical	61	100	HbA1c < 6.5%	30 vs 19 vs 0	0.02
DSS (Ikramuddin et al,[49] 2018)	5	Randomized control study	RYGB vs medical	120	100	HbA1c < 6.0%	7 vs 0	0.02
SLEEVEPASS (Salminen et al,[50] 2017)	5	Randomized control study	RYGB vs SG	240	42	HbA1c < 6.0%	25 vs 12	NA
SM-BOSS (Peterli et al,[51] 2018)	5	Randomized control study	RYGB vs SG	205	26	NA	68 vs 62	NA
Brethauer et al,[52] 2013	5	Prospective study	RYGB vs SG vs LAGB	217	100	HbA1c < 6.5%	61 vs 31 vs 9	RYGB vs SG: 0.006 RYGB vs LAGB: <0.001 SG vs LAGB: 0.04

(continued on next page)

Table 2
(continued)

Study	Follow-up (Years)	Study Design	Metabolic Surgery	No of Patients	Patients with T2D (%)	Diabetes Remission Criteria	Diabetes Remission (%)	P Value
Jakobsen et al,[53] 2018)	7	Observational cohort study	(RYGB/SG/other surgery) vs medical	1888	26	Not on diabetic medications	56 vs 22	NA
Madsen et al,[54] 2019	5	Observational cohort study	RYGB	1111	100	HbA1c < 6.5%	70	NA
PCORNet (McTigue et al,[55] 2020)	5	Observational cohort study	RYGB vs SG	9710	100	HbA1c < 6.5%	59 vs 56	<0.001

Abbreviations: BMI, body mass index; BPD, biliopancreatic diversion; FBG, fasting blood glucose; HbA1c, glycated hemoglobin; LAGB, laparoscopic adjustable gastric band; RYGB, Roux-en-Y gastric bypass; SG, sleeve gastrectomy.

Table 3
Randomized control trials of metabolic surgery versus medical treatment for diabetes remission

STUDY	Points with BMI <35 kg/m²	Study Design	No of Points	Follow-up (Months)	Diabetes Remission Criteria	Remission or Change in HbA1c (%)[a]	P Value
Mingrone et al,[46] 2021, Mingrone et al,[56] 2012, Mingrone et al,[57] 2015	0%	RYGB vs BPD vs control	60	120	HbA1c ≤ 6.5%	25 vs 50 vs 0	0.002
Schauer et al,[47] 2017, Schauer et al,[58] 2012, Schauer et al,[59] 2014	36%	RYGB vs SG vs control	150	60	HbA1c ≤ 6.0%	22 vs 15 vs 0	<0.05
Ikramuddin et al,[49] 2018, Ikramuddin et al,[60] 2013, Ikramuddin et al,[61] 2015	59%	RYGB vs control	120	60	HbA1c < 6.0%	7 vs 0	0.02
Courcoulas et al,[48] 2020, Courcoulas et al,[62] 2014, Courcoulas et al,[63] 2015	43%	RYGB vs LAGB vs control	61	60	HbA1c < 6.5%	30 vs 19 vs 0	0.02
Kirwan et al,[64] 2022	35%	(RYGB/LAGB/SG/combined surgery) vs control	256	36	HbA1c ≤ 6.5%	38 vs 3	<0.001
Dixon et al,[15] 2008	22%	LAGB vs control	60	24	HbA1c < 6.2%	73 vs 13	<0.001
Wentworth et al,[65] 2014	100%	LAGB vs control	51	24	FBG < 7.0 mmol/L	52 vs 8	0.001
Shah et al,[66] 2016	85%	RYGB vs control	80	24	HbA1c < 6.5%	60 vs 2.5	<0.001
Cohen et al,[67] 2020	100%	RYGB vs control	100	24	HbA1c < 6.0%	45 vs 24	0.051
Liang et al,[68] 2013	100%	RYGB vs control	101	12	HbA1c < 6.5%	90 vs 0 vs 0[b]	<0.0001
Halperin et al,[69] 2014	34%	RYGB vs control	38	12	HbA1c < 6.5%	58 vs 16	0.03
Ding et al,[70] 2015	34%	LAGB vs control	45	12	HbA1c < 6.5%	33 vs 23[c]	0.46
Cummings et al,[71] 2016	25%	RYGB vs control	43	12	HbA1c < 6.0%	60 vs 5.9	0.002
Parikh et al,[72] 2014	100%	(RYGB/LAGB/SG) vs control	57	6	HbA1c < 6.5%	65 vs 0	0.0001

Abbreviations: BPD, biliopancreatic diversion; BMI, body mass index; FBG, fasting blood glucose; HbA1c, glycated hemoglobin; LAGB, laparoscopic adjustable gastric band; RYGB, Roux-en-Y gastric bypass; SG, sleeve gastrectomy.

Remission criteria:

[a] Remission was primary or secondary end point; HbA1c value without diabetes medications, unless otherwise specific.

[b] Remission was not precisely defined; HbA1c < 6.5% by extrapolation.

[c] Intermittent diabetes medications.

Table 4
Five-year weight loss and disease remission

Outcome	RYGB	BPD ± DS	LSG	LAGB	ILI
Weight loss at 5 y	25.5%[73]	40.3%[75]	18.8%[73]	11.7%[73]	4.7%[20]
Remission of type 2 diabetes	86.1%[74]	98.1%[76]	83.5%[74]	53.6%[78]	7.3%[20]
Remission of dyslipidemia	68.6%[81]	80.0%[80]	55.2%[81]	20.5%[78]	NR
Remission of hypertension	60.1%[81]	66.8%[79]	48.4%[81]	21.7%[78]	NR
Remission of sleep apnea	100.0%[81]	94.9%[79]	75.8%[77]	25.0%[78]	NR

Abbreviations: BPD ± DS, biliopancreatic diversion with or without duodenal switch; LAGB, laparoscopic adjustable gastric band; LSG, laparoscopic sleeve gastrectomy; RYGB; Roux-en-Y gastric bypass.

weight loss after surgery. The Swedish Obese Subjects (SOS) study reported the longest weight loss follow-up (20 years) of any weight loss study. RYGB, gastric banding, or gastroplasty resulted in a 20% to 30% weight loss compared with about 1% for the nonoperative control group.[87] The Look AHEAD study has the longest reported weight loss (10 years) for a lifestyle intervention, 6.0% versus 3.5% for the control group.[88] Adams and colleagues[89] similarly showed significant weight loss 12 years after RYGB compared with two matched nonsurgery groups. The mean change in weight from baseline in the RYGB group was −45 kg (at 2 years), −36 kg (at 6 years), and −35 kg (at 12 years) compared with a mean change in weight in the two nonsurgical groups at 12 years of −3 kg and 0 kg, respectively. Courcoulas and colleagues[90] showed an average weight loss of 28.4% (RYGB) and 14.9% (LAGB) at a 7-year follow-up in 1300 eligible patients. Four RCTs with 5 to 10 year follow-up periods comparing metabolic surgery versus intensive medical management in patients with diabetes showed significant weight loss after metabolic surgery.[46–49] Combined, the studies showed durable weight loss for BPD (29%), RYGB (21.8%–28%), SG (19%), and LAGB (12.7%), whereas a lifestyle intervention yielded 4.2% to 9.6%.

Diabetes Control

The long-term efficacy of metabolic surgery for T2D treatment is well established by an abundance of observational studies and small RCTs (see **Tables 2–4**). Buchwald and colleagues[91,92] conducted a meta-analysis on the impact of bariatric surgery in patients with T2D (621 studies with <5-year follow-up and 135,246 patients) and showed, overall, 78% in complete remission and 87% had either improvement or remission of T2D. In the SOS study, the diabetes remission rate was higher for the surgical compared with nonsurgical group at 2 years (72% vs 16%) and at 15 years (30% vs 7%), respectively (*P* < 0.001).[44] In the Utah RYGB versus matched nonsurgery (control) study, 12-year remission after RYGB was 51% versus 10% and 5% for the two control groups. Remission rates for hypertension and LDL-C were also superior in the surgery versus control groups. The use of antidiabetic medications was reduced after RYGB (−0.3 ± 1.4) but increased in the two control groups by 0.8 ± 1.4 and 1.1 ± 1.3.[89]

Over the past decade, 14 RCTs comparing metabolic surgery to medical treatment of T2D have emerged (see **Table 3**).[46–49,56–72] One RCT by Kirwan and colleagues[64] reports 3-year pooled outcomes from the Alliance of Randomized Trials of Medicine versus Metabolic Surgery in T2D (ARMMS-T2D) studies.[47,48,64,69–71] All 14 RCTs included patients with T2D and obesity (1222 patients) with follow-up from 6 months to 10 years. The severity of T2D among the trials varied significantly from mild (mean

HbA1c 7.7%, <2-year onset, no insulin)[15] to advanced (mean HbA1c 9.3%, 8.3 years duration, 48% on insulin).[38] All the trials included patients with T2D and a body mass index (BMI) ranging from 25 to 53 kg/m^2; 13 of 14 studies included patients with a BMI less than 35 kg/m^2. Surgical procedures included RYGB, LAGB, SG, and BPD. Three studies[49,60,61,66,68] included a significant number of Asian patients. The primary end point for the three RCTs was diabetes remission defined as reaching an HbA1c target (<6.0%–6.5%) without requiring diabetes medications.

Collectively, these RCTs showed that surgery was superior to medical treatment in reaching the designated glycemic target ($P < 0.05$ for all), except the Ding and colleagues[70] study, which showed that diabetes remission for LAGB and medical treatment was 33% and 23%, respectively ($P = 0.46$). This result might be due to patients in the Ding study having advanced T2D (HbA1c 8.2% $\pm$ 1.2%, with 40% on insulin), and they likely had significantly impaired beta cell function. The HbA1c in the LAGB group decreased by 2% to 3.5%, whereas the medical treatment group decreased only 1% to 1.5%. Most of these studies also showed superiority of surgery over medical treatment in achieving secondary end points, such as weight loss, remission of metabolic syndrome, reduction in diabetes and cardiovascular medications, and improvement in triglycerides, HDL-C, and quality of life.[38]

The durability of the effects of surgery is highlighted by three 5-year studies[47–49] and one 10-year study.[46] The surgical groups showed significant and durable weight loss and glycemic control (remission) compared with the medical groups. The RCTs predicted the common factors contributing to remission of diabetes, including the duration of diabetes, weight loss, and the requirement for insulin and disease status (HbA1c).[38]

The Surgical Treatment and Medications Potentially Eradicate Diabetes Efficiently (STAMPEDE) trial[47] reported that at 5 years, patients who underwent either (gastric bypass or SG) had a significantly greater mean percentage reduction from baseline in HbA1c level than patients on medical therapy alone (2.1% vs 0.3%, $P = 0.003$). Both the surgical procedures were superior to intensive medical therapy alone with respect to achieving HbA1c of ≤6% with or without the use of diabetes medications, ≤6.5% without the use of diabetes medications, and ≤7.0% with the use of diabetes medications ($P < 0.05$). Diabetes remission rate (HbA1c ≤ 6.0%) was 22% (gastric bypass), 15% (SG), and none in the medical therapy group. Ikramuddin and colleagues[49] also demonstrated significantly higher diabetes remission in the gastric bypass group compared with lifestyle medical management group at 5 years; 7% versus 0 ($P = 0.02$). The HbA1c less than 7.0% was 55% in the bypass group compared with 14% in the lifestyle-medical management group ($P = 0.002$). Courcoulas and colleagues[48] also reported superior 5-year remission rates for RYGB (30%) and LAGB (19%) compared with medical management (0%) ($P = 0.02$). The ARMMS-T2D study (four pooled RCTs) revealed that 3-year diabetes remission was 38% in the surgical group compared with 3% in the medical group ($P < 0.001$).[64] Mingrone and colleagues[46] had the longest follow-up (10 years), and remission rates were 25% (gastric bypass), 50% (BPD), and none in the medical therapy group ($P < 0.002$). For those patients who achieved remission at 2 years, 20 (58.8%) of 34 had a relapse of hyperglycemia during follow-up (10 [52.6%] of 19 in the BPD group and 10 [66.7%] of 15 in the RYGB group). All patients who had a relapse of hyperglycemia maintained good glycemic control at 10 years (mean HbA1c was 6.7 [standard deviation, 0·2]; all but one patient had HbA1c < 7·0%) despite drastically reduced use of diabetes medications.

These RCTs consistently showed that metabolic surgery decreased diabetes and CV medication requirements while achieving superior glycemic control. In

STAMPEDE,[47] patients in the surgical groups required significantly fewer diabetes and CV medications than patients on medical therapy ($P < 0.05$). At 5 years, approximately 89% of patients in the surgical groups were not on insulin and maintained an average HbA1c of 7.0%, whereas 61% of patients in the medical therapy group were not on insulin, with an average HbA1c of 8.5%. Ikramuddin and colleagues[49] also showed similar reductions in medication usage at the 5-year follow-up. Both insulin and non-insulin diabetes medications were significantly lower in the gastric bypass group compared with lifestyle–medical management group; insulin use was 15% versus 37% ($P = 0.02$) and noninsulin diabetes medication use was 42% versus 88% ($P < 0.001$), respectively. Mingrone and colleagues[46] found that surgically treated patients used significantly less diabetes medications than patients in the medical therapy group at 10 years (mean number of antidiabetes drugs 0.7 in the BPD group, 1.4 in the RYGB group, and 2.9 in the medical therapy group; $P < 0.0001$; see **Table 3**). At 10 years, 53.3% in the medical therapy group required insulin therapy compared with only 2.5% who underwent surgery.[5] ARMMS-T2D similarly showed reductions in diabetes medication use in the surgery group versus medical group.[64]

Most of the RCTs showed improvement in the secondary end points after metabolic surgery compared with medical treatment. There was reduction in the CV medications, improvement in triglyceride, and HDL-C levels after metabolic surgery compared with medical treatment. However, the results showed mixed improvement after metabolic surgery for blood pressure and LDL-C.[38] Ikramuddin and colleagues[49] showed at the 5-year follow-up, 23% in the RYGB group compared with 4% in the medical treatment group achieved the composite triple end points (HbA1c < 7%, systolic blood pressure < 130 mm Hg, and LDL-C < 100 mg/dL, $P = 0.002$). Schauer and colleagues[47] showed similar findings at 5-year follow-up and significant improvement in triglyceride and HDL-C levels after RYGB and SG compared with medical therapy. There was no significant improvement in blood pressure and LDL-C levels among the surgical and medical groups, but there were significantly lower medications required to treat hypertension and hyperlipidemia among the surgical groups compared with the medical group.

Microvascular and Macrovascular Outcomes of Metabolic Surgery

The primary goal of diabetes treatment is to reduce the complications of diabetes. Many large, mostly retrospective cohort studies over the last 25 years have attempted to ascertain the potential for metabolic surgery to reduce macrovascular complications also known as major adverse cardiovascular events (MACE), specifically myocardial infarction (MI), stroke, death, and microvascular complications, specifically retinopathy, neuropathy, and nephropathy. The SOS study (30% with diabetes or prediabetes) reports major reductions in MACE and microvascular complications following surgery.[44] With a median follow-up of 17.6 years, the cumulative incidence of microvascular complications was 41.8/1000 person-years (95% confidence interval [CI], 35.3 to 49.5) for controls and 20.6/1000 person-years (95% CI, 17.0–24.9) for the surgery group (hazard ratio [HR], 0.44; 95% CI, 0.34 to 0.56; $P < 0.001$). Macrovascular complications were observed in 44.2/1000 person-years (95% CI, 37.5–52.1) for controls and 31.7/1000 person-years (95% CI, 27.0–37.2) for the surgical group (HR, 0.68; 95% CI, 0.54–0.85; $P = 0.001$). A subsequent analysis of all-cause mortality in SOS at a median follow-up of 24 years revealed that 457 patients (22.8%) in the surgery group and 539 patients (26.4%) in the control group died (HR, 0.77; 95% CI, 0.68–0.87; $P < 0.001$).[91] The corresponding HR was 0.70 (95% CI, 0.57–0.85) for death from cardiovascular disease and 0.77 (95% CI, 0.61–0.96) for death from cancer. The adjusted median life expectancy in the surgery group was 3.0 years (95% CI, 1.8–4.2) longer than the control group. Another large comparative cohort study at Cleveland Clinic assessed MACE outcomes in patients with T2D who underwent metabolic surgery (n = 2,287) versus a matched cohort who had usual medical care (n = 11,435).[93] Metabolic surgery consisted of RYGB (63%), SG (32%), LAGB (5%), and duodenal switch (1%). At 8-year follow-up, metabolic surgery was associated with reductions in all-cause mortality (41%), heart failure (62%), coronary artery disease (31%), stroke (33%), nephropathy (60%), and atrial fibrillation (22%) when compared with the nonoperative control group.

A very large meta-analysis of CV outcomes after metabolic surgery versus usual care involving 21 population-based cohort studies and 2,857,016 participants was recently reported.[94] The relative risk (RR) of MACE in the metabolic surgery group was 0.53 (95% CI, 0.45–0.62; $P<0.001$) relative to the nonsurgical group. Relative to the nonsurgical group, the risk of MI (RR, 0.40; 95% CI, 0.30–0.52; $P < 0.001$), stroke (RR, 0.60; 95% CI, 0.46–0.79; $P < 0.001$), cardiovascular death (RR, 0.43; 95% CI, 0.35–0.54; $P < 0.001$), and all-cause death (RR, 0.44; 95% CI, 0.32–0.59; $P < 0.001$) was significantly reduced for patients who underwent metabolic surgery. In subgroup analyses, as the proportion of patients with diabetes mellitus increased, lower RRs for MACE, MI, and stroke were observed in the surgery group relative to the nonsurgical group. MACE reduction was more pronounced in patients with diabetes.

Similarly, major reductions in microvascular complications have been reported in large population-based cohort studies. A recent meta-analysis was done with 12 studies involving 32,756 participants with T2D and obesity who underwent metabolic surgery versus nonsurgical treatment.[95] Metabolic surgery reduced the incidence rate of microvascular complications (odds ratios [OR], 0.34; 95% CI, 0.30 to 0.39; $P < 0.001$) compared with nonsurgical treatment. Further, metabolic surgery reduced the incidence of diabetic nephropathy (OR, 0.39; 95% CI, 0.30–0.50; $P < 0.001$), diabetic retinopathy (OR, 0.52; 95% CI, 0.42–0.65; $P < 0.001$), and diabetic neuropathy (OR, 0.27; 95% CI, 0.22–0.34; $P < 0.001$) compared with nonsurgical treatment.

Finally, a large meta-analysis of 16 matched cohort studies and one prospective controlled trial of 174,772 participants assessed mortality reduction after metabolic surgery compared with usual care.[96] Metabolic bariatric surgery was associated with a reduction in the hazard rate of death of 49.2% (95% CI, 46.3–51.9; $P < 0.0001$) and the median life expectancy was 6.1 years (95% CI, 5.2–6.9 years) longer than usual care. In the subgroup analyses, both individuals with baseline diabetes (HR, 0.409; 95% CI, 0.370–0.453; $P < 0.0001$) or without baseline diabetes (HR, 0.704; 95% CI, 0.588–0.843; $P < 0.0001$) who underwent metabolic-bariatric surgery had lower rates of all-cause mortality, but the treatment effect was considerably greater for those with diabetes (between-subgroup I^2 95.7%, $P < 0.0001$). Median life expectancy was 9.3 years (95% CI, 7.1–11.8) longer for patients with diabetes in the surgery group than the nonsurgical group, whereas the life expectancy gain was 5.1 years (2.0–9.3 years) for patients without diabetes. The treatment effects did not seem to differ between RYGB, LAGB, and SG (I^2 3.4%, $P = 0.36$).

Mingrone and colleagues[46] were the first and only to show reductions in microvascular and macrovascular complications after metabolic surgery compared with medical management in an RCT (N = 60) with a 10-year follow-up. Medically treated patients had a significantly higher incidence of diabetes-related complications than surgically treated patients (72.2%; 95% CI, 49.1–87.5 vs. 5.0%, 95% CI, 0.9–23.6). Participants in both the RYGB and the BPD groups had less diabetes-related complications throughout the 10-year study than participants in the medical therapy group (RR, 0.07; 95% CI, 0.01–0.48 for both comparisons). Participants in the medical therapy group had both macrovascular (two MIs, one fatal) and microvascular diabetic complications (retinopathy [n = 2], nephropathy [n = 5], and neuropathy [n = 4]). Only two patients among surgically treated patients developed diabetic complications (one case of macroalbuminuria in each surgical group). Otherwise, none of the other small RCTs comparing metabolic surgery to medical management were powered sufficiently to detect differences in macrovascular or microvascular complications or death especially at relatively short follow-up.

Large observational studies with long-term follow-up suggest that metabolic surgery significantly reduces macrovascular complications by 47%, microvascular complications by 66%, and all-cause mortality by 49%. To put this into perspective, the effect size of these reductions in complications and mortality are enormous compared with highly effective CV drugs such as antihypertensive agents, statins, and SGLT2 inhibitors, which produce mortality reductions around 5% to 15%.[97–99] However, such observational studies are subject to inherent limitations from bias and confounding factors. Thus far, just one small RCT by Mingrone and colleagues[46] demonstrates diabetes complication reductions after surgery versus medical treatment. Nevertheless, these mostly observational studies are the best evidence available to inform medical decision-making, short of a large multicenter RCT. Most of these large observational cohort studies recommend a multicenter RCT, and some suggest only an RCT will end doubt about the role of metabolic surgery in treating diabetes and obesity.[100] In the 70-year history of bariatric/metabolic surgery, no large multicenter cardiovascular trial has been conducted.

CURRENT GUIDELINES FOR TYPE 2 DIABETES MANAGEMENT

International guidelines for T2D management in patients with T2D and obesity have endorsed metabolic surgery as a treatment with significant potential for remission.[5,27] Metabolic surgery has historically been recommended based on the patient's body weight using BMI [101]; patients with obesity and BMI greater than 40 or BMI greater than 35 with comorbidity are candidates for surgery if they are psychologically stable and have no active substance abuse. However, metabolic surgery in patients with T2D should be tailored based on the class of obesity and inadequate glycemic control despite optimal medical treatment. Based on strong evidence from RCTs, metabolic surgery was recommended in the treatment algorithm for T2D in the second Diabetes Surgery Summit.[39] This guideline was published in collaboration with six international

Table 5
Treatment options for overweight and obesity in type 2 diabetes

Treatment	BMI Category, kg/m²		
	25.0-26.9 (or 23.0-24.9[a])	27.0-29.9 (or 25.0-27.4[a])	≥ 30.0 (or ≥ 27.5[a])
Diet, physical activity, and behavioral counselling	b	b	b
Pharmacortherapy		b	b
Metabolic surgery			b

[a] Recommended cut points for Asian-American individuals (expert opinion).
[b] Treatment may be indicated for select motivated patients.

From Rubino F, Nathan DM, Eckel RH, et al. Metabolic Surgery in the Treatment Algorithm for Type 2 Diabetes: A Joint Statement by International Diabetes Organizations. Diabetes Care. 2016;39(6):861-877. Reprinted with permission from The American Diabetes Association. Copyright 2022 by the American Diabetes Association.

Table 6
Studies on diabetes remission scoring model

	Surgical-Based Model				Nonsurgical Model	
Remission Model	ABCD[104]	DiaRem2[106]	Duke Diabetes Remission[107]	IMS[103]	DiRECT[106]	Kramer et al,[109] 2016
Procedure or Method	RYGB/mini gastric bypass	RYGB	RYGB/SG/ LAGB/BPD/DS	RYGB/SG	Intensive lifestyle therapy	Intensive insulin therapy
Number of patients	63	307	602	900	149	25
Predictor variables:						
1) HbA1c	Yes	Yes	Yes	Yes	Yes	Yes
2) Duration of diabetes	Yes	Yes	NA	Yes	NA	Yes
3) Insulin usage	NA	Yes	Yes	Yes	NA	NA
4) Diabetes medications	NA	NA	Yes (type of meds)	Yes (number of meds)	Yes (number of meds)	NA
5) Age	Yes	Yes	Yes	NA	NA	NA
6) BMI	Yes	NA	Yes	NA	NA	NA
7) Type of surgery	NA	NA	Yes	NA	NA	NA

Abbreviations: BMI, body mass index; BPD, biliopancreatic diversion; DS, duodenal switch; HbA1c, glycated hemoglobin; LAGB, laparoscopic adjustable gastric band; NA, not assessed or mentioned; RYGB, Roux-en-Y gastric bypass; SG, sleeve gastrectomy.
Data from Chumakova-Orin M, Vanetta C, Moris DP, Guerron AD. Diabetes remission after bariatric surgery. World J Diabetes. 2021;12(7):1093-1101.

diabetes organizations and was endorsed by 53 leading professional diabetes and surgical societies worldwide including the ADA. Since 2017, the ADA has endorsed metabolic surgery as a treatment for T2D.

The indication for metabolic surgery was extended for patients with diabetes and a BMI between 30 and 34.9 and lowered the BMI threshold by 2.5 in patients of Asian origin. These current guidelines provide greater emphasis on surgical treatment of patients with BMI greater than 40 regardless of glycemic control (**Table 5**).[5,39,102] Metabolic surgery should be performed in high-volume centers by a multidisciplinary team, including the bariatric surgeon, endocrinologist/diabetologist, cardiologist, anesthesiologist, psychologist, and dietician with expertise in diabetes care.

Predictors of Diabetes Remission/Improvement

Prediction models are available to access the probability of diabetes remission after metabolic surgery, lifestyle intervention, or intensive short-term insulin treatment (**Table 6**).[103–109] They can assist with clinical decisions regarding medical versus surgical treatment of T2D and surgical procedure selection. The Individualized Metabolic Surgery (IMS) Score (http://riskcalc.org/Metabolic_Surgery_Score/) predicts the success of diabetes remission after metabolic surgery (SG and RYGB).[103] This scoring system was generated from a database of approximately 900 patients with diabetes who had greater than 5-year follow-up after SG or RYGB. This score predicts diabetes remission based on preoperative diabetes severity, including the duration of T2D ($P < 0.0001$), number of diabetes medications ($P < 0.0001$), insulin use ($P = 0.002$), and HbA1c <7% ($P = 0.002$). The scores assist in choosing the metabolic procedures (SG or RYGB) based on a specific patient's diabetes severity. The probability of remission is greater than 90% in patients with mild T2D with either RYGB or SG. With moderate disease, remission reduces to 60% to 70% for RYGB and 25% to 56% for SG. For long-standing T2D, remission is less than 12% for either RYGB or SG. Other predictive models available for diabetes remission after surgery include the ABCD, DiaRem, and Duke models.[104–107] In the DiRECT study, remission after lifestyle intervention was associated with fewer diabetes medications, lower HbA1c and triglycerides levels, better quality of life, and less depression at baseline.[108] Kramer and colleagues[109] studied intensive insulin treatment and found baseline HbA1c and duration of diabetes were key predictors of remission. Whether for surgical or medical intervention, all of these remission predictors are essentially markers of beta cell function. Regardless of the treatment, what is clear is that early intervention, when beta cell function has not permanently deteriorated, is the key to achieving remission.

SUMMARY

Since the discovery of insulin, the quest for a "cure" for diabetes (T2D) has come very close to reality. Although a treatment that guarantees a "cure" for 10 years or more in 100% of patients clearly has not materialized, the evidence is strong that a significant percentage of patients with T2D and obesity undergoing metabolic surgery can achieve long-term remission and become "nondiabetic." Thus far, long-term remission following lifestyle intervention or pharmacotherapy even in patients with very mild diabetes has not been demonstrated with significant frequency. Based on evidence from mostly observational studies, diabetes remission following surgery equates to excellent glycemic control without relying on pharmacotherapy and is associated with improvements in quality of life, major reductions in microvascular and macrovascular complications, and enhanced long-term survival with reasonably low rates of short- and long-term complications of surgery. Moreover, metabolic surgery uniquely results in remission of other key comorbidities such as hypertension, dyslipidemia, and sleep apnea. These benefits of diabetes remission call into question why remission is not considered a standard therapeutic goal of diabetes treatment. Powerful evidence indicates that early intervention with metabolic surgery, when beta cell function is robust, provides the greatest probability of long-term remission as high as 90% or more. Long-term diabetes remission with surgery is as close to "curing" diabetes that may ever emerge. Accordingly, it is remarkable how underutilized metabolic surgery is given the degree of high-quality evidence supporting its ability to achieve long-term remission. A large multicenter RCT comparing metabolic surgery to medical management that assesses macrovascular and microvascular complications would be helpful in addressing any doubt about long-term clinical benefits of surgery.

CLINICS CARE POINTS

- Metabolic surgery should be prioritized for diabetes patients with type 2 diabetes (T2D) and body mass index (BMI) ≥ 40 regardless of glycemic control.
- Patients with BMI ≥ 30 with uncontrolled T2D despite on optimal pharmacotherapy should be considered for metabolic surgery.
- Consider early intervention with metabolic surgery to increase the possibility of long-term diabetes remission.

DISCLOSURE

Dr P.R. Schauer has the following relationships Consultancy Agreements: GI Dynamics; Keyron; Persona; Mediflix, Metabolic Health International, LTD, Novo Nordisk and Lilly Ownership Interest: SE Healthcare LLC, Mediflix, Metabolic Health International, LTD Research Funding: Ethicon; Medtronic; Pacira; Persona Honoraria: Ethicon; Medtronic; BD Surgical; Gore Scientific Advisor or Membership: SE Healthcare Board of Directors; GI Dynamics; Keyron; Persona; Mediflix. Dr Z.N. Hanipah has consultancy agreement with Novo Nordisk. Dr F. Rubino has the following relationships Research grants: Ethicon and Medtronic Consulting fees: Ethicon, Novo Nordisk, and Medtronic Scientific advisory board: GI Dynamics and Keyron.

REFERENCES

1. American Diabetes Association. American diabetes Association website. 1995. Available at: https://diabetes.org/about-us. Accessed 16 August 2022.
2. Bliss M. The discovery of insulin. 25th Anniversary Edition. The University of Chicago; 2007.
3. Hallberg SJ, Gershuni VM, Hazbun TL, et al. Reversing type 2 diabetes: a narrative review of the evidence. Nutrients 2019;11(4):766.
4. Buse JB, Caprio S, Cefalu WT, et al. How do we define cure of diabetes? Diabetes Care 2009;32(11):2133–5.
5. Riddle MC, Cefalu WT, Evans PH, et al. Consensus report: definition and interpretation of remission in type 2 diabetes. J Clin Endocrinol Metab 2022; 107(1):1–9.

6. Leyton O. Diabetes and operation.: a note on the effect of gastro-jejunostomy upon a case of mild diabetes mellitus with a low renal threshold. Lancet 1925; 206(5336):1162–3.

7. Pories WJ, Swanson MS, MacDonald KG, et al. Who would have thought it? an operation proves to be the most effective therapy for adult-onset diabetes mellitus. Ann Surg 1995;222(3):339–50.

8. Henrikson V. Can small bowel resection be defended as therapy for obesity? Nordisk Medicin 1952;47:744.

9. Henrikson V. Can small bowel resection be defended as therapy for obesity? Obes Surg 1994;1(4):54–5.

10. Friedman MN, Sancetta AJ, Magovern GJ. The amelioration of diabetes mellitus following subtotal gastrectomy. Surg Gynecol Obstet 1955;100(2):201–4.

11. Ahmad U, Danowski TS, Nolan S, et al. Remissions of diabetes mellitus after weight reduction by jejunoileal bypass. Diabetes Care 1978;1(3):158–65.

12. Bourdages H, Goldenberg F, Nguyen P, et al. Improvement in obesity-associated medical conditions following vertical banded gastroplasty and gastrointestinal bypass. Obes Surg 1994;4(3):227–31.

13. Scopinaro N, Adami GF, Marinari GM, et al. Biliopancreatic diversion. World J Surg 1998;22(9):936–46.

14. Hess DS, Hess DW. Biliopancreatic diversion with a duodenal switch. Obes Surg 1998;8(3):267–82.

15. Dixon JB, O'Brien PE, Playfair J, et al. Adjustable gastric banding and conventional therapy for type 2 diabetes: a randomized controlled trial. JAMA 2008; 299:316–23.

16. Rosenthal R, Li X, Samuel S, et al. Effect of sleeve gastrectomy on patients with diabetes mellitus. Surg Obes Relat Dis Off J Am Soc Bariatric Surg 2009;5: 429–34.

17. Harwood R. Severe diabetes with remission: report of a case and review of the literature. N Engl J Med 1957;257(6):257–61.

18. Bloom A. Remission in diabetes. Br Med J 1959;2(5154):731.

19. Kramer CK, Zinman B, Retnakaran R. Short-term intensive insulin therapy in type 2 diabetes mellitus: a systematic review and meta-analysis. Lancet Diabetes Endocrinol 2013;1(1):28–34.

20. Gregg EW, Chen H, Wagenknecht LE, et al. Association of an intensive lifestyle intervention with remission of type 2 diabetes. Jama 2012;308(23):2489–96.

21. Lean ME, Leslie WS, Barnes AC, et al. Durability of a primary care-led weight-management intervention for remission of type 2 diabetes: 2-year results of the DiRECT open-label, cluster-randomised trial. Lancet Diabetes Endocrinol 2019;7(5):344–55.

22. Skyler JS, Bergenstal R, Bonow RO, et al. American diabetes association; american college of cardiology foundation; american heart association. intensive glycemic control and the prevention of cardiovascular events:implications of the accord, advance, and va diabetes trials. a position statement of the american diabetes association and a scientific statement of the american college of cardiology foundation and the american heart association. Diabetes Care 2009; 32:187–92.

23. Gerstein HC, Miller ME, Byington RP, et al. Action to control cardiovascular risk in diabetes study group. effects of intensive glucose lowering in type 2 diabetes. N Engl J Med 2008;358:2545–59.

24. Duckworth WC, Abraira C, Moritz TE, et al. Investigators of the VADT. the duration of diabetes affects the response to intensive glucose control in type 2 subjects: the VA Diabetes Trial. J Diabetes Complications 2011;25:355–61.

25. Wadden TA, Chao AM, Bahnson JL, et al. The Look AHEAD research group. end-of-trial health outcomes in look ahead participants who elected to have bariatric surgery. Obesity (Silver Spring) 2019;27(4):581–90.

26. Taheri S, Zaghloul H, Chagoury O, et al. Effect of intensive lifestyle intervention on Body weight and glycaemia in early type 2 diabetes (DIADEM-I): an open-label, parallelgroup, randomised controlled trial. Lancet Diabetes Endocrinol 2020;8:477–89.

27. Weng J, Li Y, Xu W, et al. Effect of intensive insulin therapy on β-cell function and glycaemic control in patients with newly diagnosed type 2 diabetes: a multicentre randomised parallel-group trial. Lancet 2008;371(9626):1753–60.

28. Wajchenberg BL. β-cell failure in diabetes and preservation by clinical treatment. Endocr Rev 2007;28:187–218.

29. Ilkova H, Glaser B, Tunckale A, et al. Induction of long-term glycaemic control in newly diagnosed type 2 diabetic patients by transient intensive insulin treatment. Diabetes Care 1997;20:1353–6.

30. McFalane SI, Chaiken RL, Hirsch S, et al. Near-normoglycaemic remission in African-Americans with Type 2 diabetes mellitus is associated with recovery of beta cell function. Diabet Med 2001;18:10–6.

31. Ryan EA, Imes S, Wallace C. Short-term intensive insulin therapy in newly diagnosed type 2 diabetes. Diabetes Care 2004;27:1028–32.

32. Li YB, Xu W, Liao ZH, et al. Induction of long-term glycaemic control in newly diagnosed type 2 diabetic patients is associated with improvement of beta-cell function. Diabetes Care 2004;27:2597–602.

33. Li Y, Xu W, Liao Z, et al. The effect of continuous subcutaneous insulin infusion (CSII) on glucose metabolism and induction of long-term glycemic control in newly diagnosed type 2 diabetic patients (Abstract). Diabetes 2004;53(Suppl 2):A112.

34. Kahn SE, Cooper ME, Del Prato S. Pathophysiology and treatment of type 2 diabetes: perspectives on the past, present, and future. Lancet 2014;383(9922): 1068–83.

35. Khunti K, Ceriello A, Cos X, et al. Achievement of guideline targets for blood pressure, lipid, and glycaemic control in type 2 diabetes: a meta-analysis. Diabetes Res Clin Pract 2018;137:137–48.

36. Fang M, Wang D, Coresh J, et al. Trends in diabetes treatment and control in U.S. adults, 1999-2018. N Engl J Med 2021;384(23):2219–28.

37. American Society for Metabolic and Bariatric Surgery. Estimate of bariatric surgery numbers, 2011-2020. Available at: https://asmbs.org/resources/estimate-of-bariatric-surgery-numbers. Accessed Oct 31, 2022.

38. Schauer PR, Mingrone G, Ikramuddin S, et al. Clinical Outcomes of Metabolic Surgery: Efficacy of Glycemic Control, Weight Loss, and Remission of Diabetes. Diabetes Care 2016;39(6):902–11.

39. Rubino F, Nathan DM, Eckel RH, et al. Metabolic surgery in the treatment algorithm for type 2 diabetes: a joint statement by international diabetes organizations. Diabetes care 2016;39(6):861–77.

40. Clapp B, Ponce J, DeMaria E, et al. American society for metabolic and bariatric surgery 2020 estimate of metabolic and bariatric procedures performed in the United States. Surg Obes Relat Dis 2022;18(9):1134–40.

41. Brethauer SA, Chand B, Schauer PR. Risks and benefits of bariatric surgery: current evidence. Cleve Clin J Med 2006;73(11):993.

42. Aminian A, Brethauer SA, Kirwan JP, et al. How safe is metabolic/diabetes surgery? Diabetes Obes Metab 2015;17:198–201.

43. Campos GM, Khoraki J, Browning MG, et al. Changes in utilization of bariatric surgery in the United States from 1993 to 2016. Ann Surg 2020;271(2):201–9.

44. Sjöström L, Peltonen M, Jacobson P, et al. Association of bariatric surgery with long-term remission of type 2 diabetes and with microvascular and macrovascular complications. JAMA 2014;311:2297–304.

45. Purnell JQ, Dewey EN, Laferrère B, et al. Diabetes remission status during seven-year follow-up of the longitudinal assessment of bariatric surgery study. J Clin Endocrinol Metab 2021;106(3):774–88.

46. Mingrone G, Panunzi S, De Gaetano A, et al. Metabolic surgery versus conventional medical therapy in patients with type 2 diabetes: 10-year follow-up of an open-label, single-centre, randomised controlled trial. Lancet 2021;397(10271): 293–304.

47. Schauer PR, Bhatt DL, Kirwan JP, et al. STAMPEDE investigators. metabolic surgery vs. intensive medical therapy for diabetes: 5-year outcomes. N Engl J Med 2017;376:641–51.

48. Courcoulas AP, Gallagher JW, Neiberg RH, et al. Bariatric surgery vs lifestyle intervention for diabetes treatment: 5-year outcomes from a randomized trial. J Clin Endocrinol Metab 2020;105(3):866–76.

49. Ikramuddin S, Korner J, Lee WJ, et al. lifestyle intervention and medical management with vs without roux-en-y gastric bypass and control of hemoglobin A1c, LDL cholesterol, and systolic blood pressure at 5 years in the diabetes surgery study. JAMA 2018;319(3):266–78.

50. Salminen P, Grönroos S, Helmiö M, et al. Effect of laparoscopic sleeve gastrectomy vs roux-en-y gastric bypass on weight loss, comorbidities, and reflux at 10 years in adult patients with obesity: the sleevepass randomized clinical trial. JAMA Surg 2022;157(8):656–66.

51. Peterli R, Wölnerhanssen BK, Peters T, et al. Effect of laparoscopic sleeve gastrectomy vs laparoscopic Roux-en-Y gastric bypass on weight loss in patients with morbid obesity: the SM-BOSS randomized clinical trial. JAMA 2018; 319(3):255–65.

52. Brethauer SA, Aminian A, Romero-Talamás H, et al. Can diabetes be surgically cured?: long-term metabolic effects of bariatric surgery in obese patients with type 2 diabetes mellitus. Ann Surg 2013;258(4):628.

53. Jakobsen GS, Småstuen MC, Sandbu R, et al. Association of bariatric surgery vs medical obesity treatment with long-term medical complications and obesity-related comorbidities. JAMA 2018;319(3):291–301.

54. Madsen LR, Baggesen LM, Richelsen B, et al. Effect of Roux-en-Y gastric bypass surgery on diabetes remission and complications in individuals with type 2 diabetes: a Danish population-based matched cohort study. Diabetologia 2019;62(4):611–20.

55. McTigue KM, Wellman R, Nauman E, et al. Comparing the 5-year diabetes outcomes of sleeve gastrectomy and gastric bypass: the National Patient-Centered Clinical Research Network (PCORNet) Bariatric Study. JAMA Surg 2020;155(5): e200087.

56. Mingrone G, Panunzi S, De Gaetano A, et al. Bariatric surgery versus conventional medical therapy for type 2 diabetes. N Engl J Med 2012;366:1577–85.

57. Mingrone G, Panunzi S, De Gaetano A, et al. Bariatric-metabolic surgery versus conventional medical treatment in obese patients with type 2 diabetes: 5 year follow-up of an open-label, single-centre, randomized controlled trial. Lancet 2015;386:964–73.

58. Schauer PR, Kashyap SR, Wolski K, et al. Bariatric surgery versus intensive medical therapy in obese patients with diabetes. N Engl J Med 2012;366: 1567–76.

59. Schauer PR, Bhatt DL, Kirwan JP, et al. STAMPEDE Investigators. Bariatric surgery versus intensive medical therapy for diabetes—3-year outcomes. N Engl J Med 2014;370:2002–13.

60. Ikramuddin S, Korner J, Lee WJ, et al. Roux-en-Y gastric bypass vs intensive medical management for the control of type 2 diabetes, hypertension, and hyperlipidemia: the Diabetes Surgery Study randomized clinical trial. JAMA 2013;309:2240–9.

61. Ikramuddin S, Billington CJ, Lee WJ, et al. Roux-en-Y gastric bypass for diabetes (the Diabetes Surgery Study): 2-year outcomes of a 5-year, randomized, controlled trial. Lancet Diabetes Endocrinol 2015;3:413–22.

62. Courcoulas AP, Goodpaster BH, Eagleton JK, et al. Surgical vs medical treatments for type 2 diabetes mellitus: a randomized clinical trial. JAMA Surg 2014;149:707–15.

63. Courcoulas AP, Belle SH, Neiberg RH, et al. Three-year outcomes of bariatric surgery vs. lifestyle intervention for type 2 diabetes mellitus treatment: a randomized clinical trial. JAMA Surg 2015;150:931–40.

64. Kirwan JP, Courcoulas AP, Cummings DE, et al. Diabetes Remission in the Alliance of Randomized Trials of Medicine Versus Metabolic Surgery in Type 2 Diabetes (ARMMS-T2D). Diabetes Care 2022;45(7):1574–83.

65. Wentworth JM, Playfair J, Laurie C, et al. Multidisciplinary diabetes care with and without bariatric surgery in overweight people: a randomised controlled trial. Lancet Diabetes Endocrinol 2014;2:545–52.

66. Shah SS, Todkar J, Phadake U, et al. Gastric bypass vs. medical/lifestyle care for type 2 diabetes in South Asians with BMI 25-40 kg/m2: the COSMID randomized trial [261-OR]. Presented at the American Diabetes Association's 76th Scientific Session; June 10–14, 2016; New Orleans, LA.

67. Cohen RV, Pereira TV, Aboud CM, et al. Effect of gastric bypass vs best medical treatment on early-stage chronic kidney disease in patients with type 2 diabetes and obesity: a randomized clinical trial. JAMA Surg 2020;155(8):e200420.

68. Liang Z, Wu Q, Chen B, et al. Effect of laparoscopic Roux-en-Y gastric bypass surgery on type 2 diabetes mellitus with hypertension: a randomized controlled trial. Diabetes Res Clin Pract 2013;101:50–6.

69. Halperin F, Ding SA, Simonson DC, et al. Roux-en-Y gastric bypass surgery or lifestyle with intensive medical management in patients with type 2 diabetes: feasibility and 1-year results of a randomized clinical trial. JAMA Surg 2014; 149:716–26.

70. Ding SA, Simonson DC, Wewalka M, et al. Adjustable gastric band surgery or medical management in patients with type 2 diabetes: a randomized clinical trial. J Clin Endocrinol Metab 2015;100:2546–56.

71. Cummings DE, Arterburn DE, Westbrook EO, et al. Gastric bypass surgery vs. intensive lifestyle and medical intervention for type 2 diabetes: the CROSSROADS randomized controlled trial. Diabetologia 2016;59:945–53.

72. Parikh M, Chung M, Sheth S, et al. Randomized pilot trial of bariatric surgery versus intensive medical weight management on diabetes remission in type 2

diabetic patients who do not meet NIH criteria for surgery and the role of soluble RAGE as a novel biomarker of success. Ann Surg 2014;260:617–22.

73. Arterburn D, Wellman R, Emiliano A, et al. PCORnet Bariatric Study Collaborative. Comparative Effectiveness and Safety of Bariatric Procedures for Weight Loss: A PCORnet Cohort Study. Ann Intern Med 2018;169(11):741–50.

74. McTigue KM, Wellman R, Nauman E, et al. PCORnet Bariatric Study Collaborative. Comparing the 5-Year Diabetes Outcomes of Sleeve Gastrectomy and Gastric Bypass: The National Patient-Centered Clinical Research Network (PCORNet) Bariatric Study. JAMA Surg 2020;155(5):e200087.

75. Risstad H, Søvik TT, Engström M, et al. Five-year outcomes after laparoscopic gastric bypass and laparoscopic duodenal switch in patients with body mass index of 50 to 60: a randomized clinical trial. JAMA Surg 2015;150(4):352–61.

76. Goriparthi RG, Martins A, Yerragorla P, et al. Long-term resolution of type 2 diabetes after biliopancreatic diversion and duodenal switch procedure: a retrospective analysis from a high-volume institution. Surg Obes Relat Dis 2022; S1550-7289(22):00181-2.

77. Juodeikis Ž, Brimas G. Long-term results after sleeve gastrectomy: a systematic review. Surg Obes Relat Dis 2017;13(4):693–9.

78. Boza C, Gamboa C, Perez G, et al. Laparoscopic adjustable gastric banding (LAGB): surgical results and 5-year follow-up. Surg Endosc 2011;25(1):292–7.

79. Bianchi A, Pagan-Pomar A, Jimenez-Segovia M, et al. Biliopancreatic diversion in the surgical treatment of morbid obesity: long-term results and metabolic consequences. Obes Surg 2020;30(11):4234–42.

80. Marceau P, Biron S, Marceau S, et al. Long-term metabolic outcomes 5 to 20 years after biliopancreatic diversion. Obes Surg 2015;25(9):1584–93.

81. Sharples AJ, Mahawar K. systematic review and meta-analysis of randomised controlled trials comparing long-term outcomes of roux-en-y gastric bypass and sleeve gastrectomy. Obes Surg 2020;30(2):664–72.

82. Sheng B, Truong K, Spitler H, et al. The long-term effects of bariatric surgery on type 2 diabetes remission, microvascular and macrovascular complications, and mortality: a systematic review and meta-analysis. Obes Surg 2017;27(10): 2724–32.

83. Billeter AT, Scheurlen KM, Probst P, et al. Meta-analysis of metabolic surgery versus medical treatment for microvascular complications in patients with type 2 diabetes mellitus. BJS 2018;105(3):168–81.

84. Martin WP, Docherty NG, Le Roux CW. Impact of bariatric surgery on cardiovascular and renal complications of diabetes: a focus on clinical outcomes and putative mechanisms. Expert Rev Endocrinol Metab 2018;13(5):251–62.

85. Yoshino M, Kayser BD, Yoshino J, et al. Effects of diet versus gastric bypass on metabolic function in diabetes. N Engl J Med 2020;383(8):721–32.

86. Laferrère B, Pattou F. A gut check explains improved glucose metabolism after surgery. Cell Metab 2019;30(5):852–4.

87. Sjöström L, Peltonen M, Jacobson P, et al. Bariatric surgery and long-term cardiovascular events. JAMA 2012;307:56–65.

88. Wing RR, Bolin P, Brancati FL, et al. For the look ahead research group. cardiovascular effects of intensive lifestyle intervention in type 2 diabetes. N Engl J Med 2013;369:145–54.

89. Adams TD, Davidson LE, Litwin SE, et al. Weight and metabolic outcomes 12 years after gastric bypass. N Engl J Med 2017;377(12):1143–55.

90. Courcoulas AP, King WC, Belle SH, et al. Seven-year weight trajectories and health outcomes in the longitudinal assessment of bariatric surgery (LABS) study. JAMA Surg 2017;153(5):427–34.
91. Buchwald H, Estok R, Fahrbach K, et al. Weight and type 2 diabetes after bariatric surgery: systematic review and meta-analysis. Am J Med 2009;122:248–56.
92. Carlsson LMS, Sjöholm K, Jacobson P, et al. Life expectancy after bariatric surgery in the Swedish obese subjects study. N Engl J Med 2020;383(16):1535–43.
93. Aminian A, Al-Kurd A, Wilson R, et al. Association of bariatric surgery with major adverse liver and cardiovascular outcomes in patients with biopsy-proven nonalcoholic steatohepatitis. JAMA 2021;326(20):2031–42.
94. Borui T, Zhang Y, Wang Y, et al. Effect of bariatric surgery on long-term cardiovascular outcomes: a systematic review and meta-analysis of population-based cohort studies. Surg Obes Relat Dis 2022;18(8):1074–86.
95. Chen X, Zhang J, Zhou Z. The effects of metabolic surgery on microvascular complications in obese patients with type 2 diabetes: a meta-analysis. Surg Obes Relat Dis 2021;17(2):434–43.
96. Syn NL, Cummings DE, Wang LZ, et al. Association of metabolic-bariatric surgery with long-term survival in adults with and without diabetes: a one-stage meta-analysis of matched cohort and prospective controlled studies with 174 772 participants. Lancet 2021;397(10287):1830–41.
97. Brunström M, Carlberg B. Association of blood pressure lowering with mortality and cardiovascular disease across blood pressure levels: a systematic review and meta-analysis. JAMA Intern Med 2018;178(1):28–36.
98. Zinman B, Wanner C, Lachin JM, et al. EMPA-REG outcome investigators. empagliflozin, cardiovascular outcomes, and mortality in type 2 diabetes. N Engl J Med 2015;373(22):2117–28.
99. Taylor F, Huffman MD, Macedo AF, et al. Statins for the primary prevention of cardiovascular disease. Cochrane Database Syst Rev 2013;2013(1):CD004816.
100. Schauer PR, Nissen SE. After 70 years, metabolic surgery has earned a cardiovascular outcome trial. Circulation 2021;143(15):1481–3.
101. Consensus Development Conference Panel. NIH conference. gastrointestinal surgery for severe obesity. Ann Intern Med 1991;115:956–61.
102. American Diabetes Association Professional Practice Committee. American diabetes association professional practice committee:. 8. obesity and weight management for the prevention and treatment of type 2 diabetes: standards of medical care in diabetes—2022. Diabetes Care 2022;45(Supplement_1):S113–24.
103. Aminian A, Brethauer SA, Andalib A, et al. individualized metabolic surgery score: procedure selection based on diabetes severity. Ann Surg 2017;266(4):650–7.
104. Lee WJ, Hur KY, Lakadawala M, et al. Predicting success of metabolic surgery: age, body mass index, C-peptide, and duration score. Surg Obes Relat Dis 2013;9(3):379–84.
105. Still CD, Wood GC, Benotti P, et al. Preoperative prediction of type 2 diabetes remission after Roux-en-Y gastric bypass surgery: a retrospective cohort study. Lancet Diabetes Endocrinol 2014;2:38–45.
106. Still CD, Benotti P, Mirshahi T, et al. DiaRem2: Incorporating duration of diabetes to improve prediction of diabetes remission after metabolic surgery. Surg Obes Relat Dis 2019;15:717–24.

107. Guerron AD, Perez JE, Risoli T Jr, et al. Performance and improvement of the DiaRem score in diabetes remission prediction: a study with diverse procedure types. Surg Obes Relat Dis 2020;16:1531–42.

108. Thom G, Messow CM, Leslie WS, et al. Predictors of type 2 diabetes remission in the Diabetes Remission Clinical Trial (DiRECT). Diabetic Med 2021;38(8): e14395.

109. Kramer CK, Zinman B, Choi H, et al. Predictors of sustained drug-free diabetes remission over 48 weeks following short-term intensive insulin therapy in early type 2 diabetes. BMJ Open Diabetes Res Care 2016;4(1):e000270.

Can the Future be Bright with Advances in Diabetic Eye Care?

Samantha Paul, MD[a], Christian Kim, MD[a],
Mohamed Kamel Soliman, MD[b,c], Warren Sobol, MD[a,c],
Jose J. Echegaray, MD[a,c], Shree Kurup, MD[a,c],*

KEYWORDS

- Diabetic • Retinopathy • Diabetic macular edema • Ophthalmic imaging

KEY POINTS

- The growing population of patients with diabetic retinopathy highlights the importance of timely diagnosis, evidence-based management, and personalized treatment plans for patients.
- Improvements in ophthalmic imaging and pharmacologic agents have all contributed to improved visual outcomes in patients with diabetic retinopathy over the past decade.
- Novel therapies targeting different pathways in the pathogenesis of diabetic retinopathy are in the pipeline.

INTRODUCTION

Diabetic retinopathy is a major complication of diabetes mellitus and is a leading cause of visual impairment among working-age adults.[1] The number of individuals diagnosed with diabetes mellitus is growing at a rapid pace and there is an accompanying increase in the prevalence of diabetic retinopathy. Globally, there are estimated to be over 200 million individuals with diabetes mellitus. Nearly one-third of these patients have some form of diabetic retinopathy, and one-third of these patients have vision-threatening diabetic retinopathy.[2] By 2050, it is estimated that 14.6 million Americans will be affected by diabetic retinopathy.[3] In patients with Type 1 DM, 99% of patients have some stage of diabetic retinopathy by 20 years after diagnosis,

[a] University Hospitals Eye Institute/Department of Ophthalmology and Visual Sciences, Case Western Reserve University, 11100 Euclid Avenue, Cleveland, OH 44106, USA; [b] Department of Ophthalmology, Assiut University Hospitals, Al Walideyah Al Qebleyah, Asyut 2, Assiut Governorate 2074020, Egypt; [c] Case Western Reserve University, Vitreoretinal Diseases & Surgery, Ocular Immunology & Uveitis, Department of Ophthalmology, University Hospitals, 11100 Euclid Avenue, Cleveland, OH 44106, USA
* Corresponding author. Case Western Reserve University, Vitreoretinal Diseases & Surgery, Ocular Immunology & Uveitis, Department of Ophthalmology, University Hospitals, 11100 Euclid Avenue, Cleveland, OH 44106.
E-mail address: Shree.Kurup@UHhospitals.org

Endocrinol Metab Clin N Am 52 (2023) 89–99
https://doi.org/10.1016/j.ecl.2022.06.004
0889-8529/23/© 2022 Elsevier Inc. All rights reserved.

and 50% have proliferative diabetic retinopathy (PDR) by 20 years after diagnosis. In patients with Type II DM, 60% of patients have some stage of diabetic retinopathy by 20 years after diagnosis, and 25% have PDR by 20 years after diagnosis.[4] Untreated, diabetic retinopathy progresses to advanced stages that can be sight-threatening resulting in irreversible blindness. However, over the past two decades, advances in diagnostic imaging, therapeutic treatments, and surgical techniques have led to improved visual outcomes in patients with diabetic retinopathy.

PATHOPHYSIOLOGY AND STAGES OF DIABETIC RETINOPATHY

The retina is particularly vulnerable to the effects of prolonged hyperglycemia as glucose uptake in the retina is not dependent on insulin activity. Retinal tissue appears to have a higher level of sensitivity to long-term elevated glucose levels than most other tissues in the body.[5] The hallmark of pathological changes in DR is microangiopathy in the form of microvascular leakage and occlusion. Accumulation of advanced glycosylation end-products in small blood vessels secondary to long-standing hyperglycemia results in endothelial cell damage and pericyte loss, which in turn cause disruption of the blood–retina barrier and leakage of interstitial fluid into the retina.[6] Increased capillary basement membrane thickness and hematological changes such as platelet aggregation and leukocyte activation lead to microvascular occlusion and retinal ischemia.[7]

Diabetic retinopathy is classified into nonproliferative and proliferative DR based on the presence or absence of neovascularization.[8] In nonproliferative diabetic retinopathy (NPDR), microangiopathy results in microaneurysms, leakage of hard exudates, intraretinal "dot-blot" hemorrhages, venous beading, or intraretinal microvascular abnormalities. NPDR is further subdivided into different stages which vary from mild to severe depending on the severity of retinal findings. With long-standing retinopathy and progressive retinal ischemia, various cytokines and growth factors are released, particularly vascular endothelial growth factor (VEGF) which induces neovessel formation.[9] The development of neovascularization heralds the onset of PDR.[8] These abnormal, newly proliferating vessels lack the structural integrity of normal blood vessels and therefore are prone to leak fluid and bleed, causing intraretinal edema as well as preretinal and vitreous hemorrhage. Furthermore, the cytokines and growth factors released induce cellular proliferation and extracellular matrix expansion resulting in fibrous tissue formation.[10] This milieu leads to the development of fibrovascular tissue which may proliferate on the retinal surface and into the vitreous cavity. Contraction of this tissue leads to severe complications including vitreous hemorrhage, tractional retinal detachments, and macular edema.

DIABETIC MACULAR EDEMA

Diabetic macular edema (DME) is the leading cause of vision loss in patients with diabetic retinopathy.[11] DME represents the accumulation of fluid in the extracellular space within the retina. It may occur at any stage of diabetic retinopathy, but is more often seen in severe stages of DR. The etiology of DME is multifactorial and is mediated by increased vascular permeability, dysfunctional blood-retinal barrier, inflammatory cytokines, and proangiogenic factors.[12] Abnormal accumulation of fluid causing retinal edema may occur anywhere in the central or peripheral retina. The center area of the retina, the macula, is of particular importance as it has the most profound effect on vision. Long-standing DME may cause irreversible damage to photoreceptors and permanent visual loss.[13] Treatment of DME has evolved substantially over the past few decades to include numerous medications with different modes of action and routes of delivery. Currently, intravitreal anti-VEGF is a preferred first-line therapy while intravitreal or periocular steroids are typically reserved for patients not responding to anti-VEGF.[14]

TIMING OF REFERRAL TO OPHTHALMOLOGY

Diabetic retinopathy rarely develops within the first 5 years after diagnosis in patients with Type 1 DM; however, the incidence of DR increases substantially thereafter and therefore ophthalmologic examination is warranted after 5 years from diagnosis.[15] In patients diagnosed with Type 2 DM, ophthalmic referral should be conducted at the time of diagnosis as the duration of diabetes may be unknown and about 30% of these patients will have some manifestations of DR by the time of diagnosis.[16] Pregnant women with an existing diagnosis of DM should undergo examination in the first trimester and the timing of follow-up is determined on initial exam findings.[17] Even though there are well-established guidelines on the timing of referral to ophthalmology for patients with diabetes, there is underutilization of care by these patients. Socioeconomic status, delayed referrals, and poor understanding of the implications of diabetic retinopathy are important factors that lead to delayed ophthalmological evaluation. In a cross-sectional analysis of the National Health and Nutrition Examination Survey, Bressler and colleagues[18] reported that more than half of patients with DME were not informed by their physician that diabetes had affected their eyes or that they had retinopathy. Another study by Bresnick and colleagues[19] showed that only 5% of patients attended the initial ophthalmology referral within the recommended time interval, 15% in twice the recommended time interval, and 51% within one year of referral. At the time of diagnosis, 28.7% of patients with DME already had a visual acuity of less than 20/40.[18] Ensuring patient understanding of the importance of ophthalmology evaluation is critical to avoid unnecessary delays in care that often result in irreversible vision loss.

PATIENT EVALUATION OVERVIEW

Patients with diabetes should have a comprehensive ocular exam at their initial visit. The patient's current glycemic control, hemoglobin A1c, presence of complications such as nephropathy or neuropathy are important variables in evaluating patients with diabetes. History of decreased vision, floating spots, and flashes of light are particularly important in ruling in those who might have DR. Ophthalmological exam involves the assessment of ocular vital signs including visual acuity, pupillary responses, and intraocular pressure. Examination of the anterior segment of the eye is necessary to rule out early cataract formation and anterior segment neovascularization and ocular surface disease which may occur due to impaired wound healing. Dilated fundus exam is of paramount importance to assess the stage of diabetic retinopathy, if any, and determine follow-up intervals and whether treatment is necessary.

Ancillary tests are highly useful in ruling out sight-threatening complications. Optical coherence tomography (OCT) is a noninvasive imaging modality that uses low-coherence light to obtain high-resolution cross-sectional images of the retina. Prior to the widespread use of OCT, DME was a clinical diagnosis;[8] however, OCT is more sensitive than clinical examination and it allows for quantitative measurements of retinal thickening.[20] Currently, OCT is the most commonly used test to evaluate patients with DR and is invaluable in diagnosing and monitoring treatment response of DME. Intravenous fluorescein angiography is used in selected cases to highlight the retinal vascular integrity and confirm suspected neovascularization. OCT-angiography is another imaging modality that highlights the vascular abnormalities without the need for the injection of dye intravenously.[21] In case of media opacity obscuring the view to the posterior pole of the eye (ie, dense cataract or vitreous hemorrhage), B-scan ultrasonography may be utilized to characterize any vitreous opacities or retinal detachments.

TREATMENT
Laser Photocoagulation Treatment

Retinal photocoagulation by laser has been the mainstay of treatment of diabetic retinopathy since the 1970s for about four decades.[22] The Early Treatment Diabetes Retinopathy Study (ETDRS) and Diabetic Retinopathy Study (DRS) are 2 landmark clinical trials that demonstrated the benefits of laser treatment in preventing visual loss in patients with DR.[8,23] The exact mechanism of action of laser photocoagulation in DR remain unclear. In PDR, destruction of the metabolically demanding photoreceptors in the peripheral retina reduces the overall oxygen demand and the hypoxic surface area of the retina and subsequently decreases the release of cytokines and growth factors that induce neovascularization.[24] In DME, focal laser photocoagulation may obliterate the leaking microaneurysm and thus reduce fluid accumulation in the retina. Despite demonstrating great potential in preventing visual loss, there is limited potential for laser to restore visual acuity. In addition, laser photocoagulation is destructive to the retina and is associated with various complications, including decreased vision, visual field, color, and contrast sensitivity.[25] The latter shortcomings of laser photocoagulation emphasized the need for better therapeutic options and as a consequence, the introduction of new pharmacological agents led to minimizing the role of laser in DR. Nevertheless, nearly 50% of patients undergoing treatment of DME may require laser photocoagulation during the course of anti-VEGF treatment.[26,27] Furthermore, in PDR, panretinal laser photocoagulation was comparable to anti-VEGF but with much less treatment burden.[28]

Surgical treatment

Vitreoretinal surgery has evolved over the past few years; smaller gauge vitrectomy with valved ports, improved visualization systems, and more versatile surgical instruments are important advancements that allow safer surgery with less morbidity and faster recovery for patients with DR.

Surgical treatment is typically indicated for complications of PDR including non-clearing or recurrent vitreous hemorrhage, tractional retinal detachment involving or threatening to involve the macula, combined tractional and rhegmatogenous retinal detachment, or progressive fibrovascular proliferation.[46]

Intravitreal Pharmacotherapy

Antivascular endothelial growth factors

Anti-VEGF agents provide superior visual outcomes and fewer complications compared to laser photocoagulation. In 2006, Spaide and colleagues reported the first off-label use of bevacizumab in 2 patients with vitreous hemorrhage due to PDR. Anti-VEGF injection was associated with regression of neovascularization and rapid resolution of vitreous hemorrhage.[29] Subsequently, several reports have demonstrated the safety and effectiveness of anti-VEGF in DR.[30,31]

The RISE and RIDE, VIVID and VISTA were pivotal phase III randomized clinical trials that demonstrated the safety and efficacy of Ranibizumab and Aflibercept, respectively, in the treatment of DME leading to their FDA approval in 2012 and 2014.[31,32] Ranibizumab is a monoclonal antibody that binds with high affinity to all isoforms of VEGF-A, whereas Aflibercept is a recombinant fusion protein that acts against multiple growth factors including VEGF-A, VEGF-B and placental growth factor.[33] Bevacizumab remains an off-label low-cost monoclonal antibody against VEGF that provides comparable efficacy and safety to the latter FDA approved drugs.[30,34] The use of anti-VEGF was extended to include PDR and any level of DR with DME.[35,36] In PDR, anti-VEGF not only induces regression of neovascularization and reduces the incidence of proliferative complications, but can even downgrade the severity of retinopathy.[37,38] The PANORAMA and the Diabetic Retinopathy Clinical Research (DRCR) Protocol W studies evaluated the use of ranibizumab and aflibercept, respectively, in subjects with moderate to severe NPDR without DME. Both studies have reported meaningful improvement in DR Severity Scores of these patients.[39,40] Nevertheless, the role of prophylactic anti-VEGF injections in patients with moderate to severe NPDR without DME is yet to be defined.

Steroids
The development of DME is not solely dependent on VEGF release; several inflammatory cytokines are implicated in the pathogenesis of DME. Triamcinolone acetonide (TA) was evaluated in patients with DR in the early 2000s.[41,42] Subsequently numerous clinical trials were conducted to evaluate its safety and efficacy compared to laser photocoagulation or anti-VEGF in patients with DME. TA combined with prompt laser treatment was shown to produce greater visual gain versus laser alone and comparable gains to anti-VEGF in pseudophakic eyes.[43] Intravitreal dexamethasone implant (IDI) is a sustained-release steroid implant that was initially FDA approved to treat macular edema secondary to retinal vein occlusion.[44] In DME, IDI was associated with superior visual gains compared to sham treatment.[45] Although IDI and TA are efficacious in the treatment of DME, they are associated with increased incidence of cataract and glaucoma, thus their use is typically reserved to cases where anti-VEGF is contraindicated or associated with suboptimal response.[14]

Newer pharmaceutical agents: a breakthrough toward reducing the burden of treatment
Intravitreal anti-VEGF injections have dramatically changed the landscape of treatment options for diabetic retinopathy. Clinical trials evaluating anti-VEGF agents have demonstrated their impressive potential to restore and preserve vision. However, in most of these clinical trials, patients were intensively treated with monthly anti-VEGF.[30–32] The majority of patients who showed substantial visual gains in the original trials lost this initial gain in the extension studies when treatment frequency was reduced.[47,48] Similarly, the outcomes of anti-VEGF in real-world studies were inferior to those obtained in clinical trials.[49] In the real-world clinical setting, frequent injections are often not feasible due to the significant burden placed on patients, caregivers, doctors, and health care resources. Transportation and time off from work are required, and scheduling regular appointments can be difficult as patients with diabetes frequently have complications involving other organ systems that require management by other specialists. A 2012 Medical Expenditure Panel Survey found that people with diabetes reported a mean of 10.5 outpatient visits in a 12-month period.[50] Patients with diabetes often struggle to meet all their appointments with primary care physicians, endocrinologists, nephrologists, ophthalmologists, and other specialists, highlighting the growing need for longer-lasting treatments for patients with diabetic retinopathy. Fortunately, there are several pharmacological agents in development that aim to decrease the treatment burden on patients.

Faricimab is a novel monoclonal antibody with 2 distinct targets, VEGF-A and angiopoietin-2, designed with the intent of extending the length of treatment intervals.

It is hypothesized that its multiple modes of action may enhance its durability.[51] Faricimab is currently FDA-approved for the treatment of neovascular age-related macular degeneration (nAMD).[52] The YOSEMITE and RHINE are 2 Phase III randomized trials that evaluated intravitreal faricimab vs aflibercept in patients with DME. They showed that treatment intervals with faricimab could be extended to every 4 months in up to 60% of patients and to up to every 3 months in about 80% of patients while achieving meaningful gains in visual acuity and anatomic improvements.[53]

Brolucizumab is a humanized monoclonal single-chain variable fragment that inhibits VEGF-A and is also FDA-approved for the treatment of nAMD. The relatively low-molecular-weight of brolucizumab allows a higher amount of drug to be administered per injection compared to other anti-VEGF agents.[54] The KESTREL and KITE are 2 Phase III trials that demonstrated that brolucizumab was noninferior to aflibercept at 1 year in terms of visual acuity gains. Furthermore, more than half of the patients that received brolucizumab were successfully maintained on 3-month dosing after initial loading doses.[55]

A port-delivery system (PDS) for ranibizumab is a novel refillable drug delivery system that maintains continuous release of ranibizumab into the vitreous. The PDS was approved by the FDA in October 2021 for nAMD.[56] The PAGODA study is a Phase III trial evaluating the safety and functional outcomes of PDS refilled every 6 months with ranibizumab compared to monthly treatment in patients with DME. PAVILION is another Phase III trial investigating the PDS in patients with DR without DME.[57] The potential for the PDS to significantly extend the duration of treatment to every 6–9 months is an exciting prospect for patients with DR.

Fluocinolone acetonide (FAc) intravitreal insert is another option for longer-lasting treatment in patients with DME. These inserts consist of polymers impregnated with FAc that are contained within nonbiodegradable tubes 3.5 × 0.37 mm in size. The efficacy of intravitreal FAc inset in patients with persistent DME was investigated in the Phase III FAME study. The study demonstrated robust visual improvement for up to 3 years after a single intravitreal injection of FAc inset.[58]

Novel gene therapies are currently in the pipeline for the treatment of DR. RGX-314 is a gene therapy developed by REGENXBIO that utilizes an adenoviral vector containing a gene encoding for a monoclonal antibody that inhibits VEGF. This gene therapy is delivered to the retinal pigment epithelium through injection into the suprachoroidal space. RGX-314 was investigated in the Phase II ALTITUDE study in patients with DR without DME. Early results showed a significant reduction in anti-VEGF injection treatment burden while maintaining stable vision.[59]

TELEMEDICINE AND ARTIFICIAL INTELLIGENCE IN DIABETIC RETINOPATHY

The use of artificial intelligence, namely machine learning, in the world of diabetic retinopathy is quickly growing. Deep learning models have been developed that can classify stages of diabetic retinopathy on fundus photographs with high accuracy.[60] In addition to fundus photographs, OCT, OCT angiography, and fluorescein angiography are imaging modalities that have been used for training deep learning models to identify stages of diabetic retinopathy, features of diabetic retinopathy, and distinguish diabetic retinopathy from other retinal vascular diseases.[61] The implementation of artificial intelligence with retinal telehealth has vast potential to expand care to patients with diabetes. The COVID-19 pandemic rapidly accelerated the use of telemedicine. Retinal telemedicine allowed for screening for retinopathy in patients with diabetes living in underserved areas. The development of cost-effective and portable retinal imaging devices will be a significant achievement that can further increase access to care for those who need it most. Ensuring that the most vulnerable populations can participate in telemedicine will rely on accessible high-speed, broadband internet, and available electronic devices. Lack of high-speed internet and appropriate devices may result in retinal telemedicine perpetuating existing health disparities if only patients of higher socioeconomic status are able to participate in retinal telehealth visits.

SUMMARY

The management of diabetes is becoming increasingly complex. With more therapeutic approaches to target end-organ damage, much more coordination and communication between specialists and inter-specialty care will be required. These new developments afford an opportunity but also pose a challenge to care for patients already stressed by multiple clinic visits. With all of the aforementioned advances in the diagnosis and treatment of diabetic retinopathy, as well as the new treatments on the horizon, the future does appear brighter for patients with diabetes.

DISCLOSURE

The authors have nothing to disclose.

REFERENCES

1. Zhang X, Gregg EW, Cheng YJ, et al. Diabetes mellitus and visual impairment: national health and nutrition examination survey, 1999-2004. Arch Ophthalmol 2008;126(10):1421–7.
2. Yau JW, Rogers SL, Kawasaki R, et al. Meta-Analysis for Eye Disease (META-EYE) Study Group. Global prevalence and major risk factors of diabetic retinopathy. Diabetes Care 2012;35(3):556–64.
3. National Eye Institute. Diabetic Retinopathy Data and Statistics. Www.Nei.Nih.-Gov. 2020. Available at: https://www.nei.nih.gov/learn-about-eye-health/outreach-campaigns-and-resources/eye-health-data-and-statistics/diabetic-retinopathy-data-and-statistics. Accessed May 7, 2022.
4. Klein R, Klein BE, Moss SE, et al. the wisconsin epidemiologic study of diabetic retinopathy. VII. Diabetic nonproliferative retinal lesions. Ophthalmology 1987; 94(11):1389–400.
5. Rajah TT, Olson AL, Grammas P. Differential glucose uptake in retina- and brain-derived endothelial cells. Microvasc Res 2001;62(3):236–42.
6. Ejaz S, Chekarova I, Ejaz A, et al. Importance of pericytes and mechanisms of pericyte loss during diabetes retinopathy. Diabetes Obes Metab 2008;10(1): 53–63.
7. Cai J, Boulton M. The pathogenesis of diabetic retinopathy: old concepts and new questions. Eye 2002;16:242–60. https://doi.org/10.1038/sj.eye.6700133.
8. Grading diabetic retinopathy from stereoscopic color fundus photographs–an extension of the modified Airlie House classification. ETDRS report number 10. Early Treatment Diabetic Retinopathy Study Research Group. Ophthalmology 1991;98(5 Suppl):786–806.
9. Ban CR, Twigg SM. Fibrosis in diabetes complications: pathogenic mechanisms and circulating and urinary markers. Vasc Health Risk Manag 2008;4(3):575–96.
10. Friedlander M. Fibrosis and diseases of the eye. J Clin Invest 2007;117(3): 576–86.

11. Varma R, Bressler NM, Doan QV, et al. Prevalence of and risk factors for diabetic macular edema in the United States. JAMA Ophthalmol 2014;132(11):1334–40.
12. Romero-Aroca P, Baget-Bernaldiz M, Pareja-Rios A, et al. Diabetic macular edema pathophysiology: vasogenic versus inflammatory. J Diabetes Res 2016; 2016:2156273.
13. El-Baha SM, Abdel Hadi AM, Abouhussein MA. Submacular Injection of Ranibizumab as a New Surgical Treatment for Refractory Diabetic Macular Edema. J Ophthalmol 2019;2019:6274209.
14. Downey L, Acharya N, Devonport H, et al. Treatment choices for diabetic macular oedema: a guideline for when to consider an intravitreal corticosteroid, including adaptations for the COVID-19 eraBMJ Open. Ophthalmology 2021;6:e000696.
15. Wang SY, Andrews CA, Gardner TW, et al. Ophthalmic screening patterns among youths with diabetes enrolled in a large US managed care network. JAMA Ophthalmol 2017;135(5):432–8.
16. Nentwich MM, Ulbig MW. Diabetic retinopathy - ocular complications of diabetes mellitus. World J Diabetes 2015;6(3):489–99.
17. Mallika P, Tan A, Aziz S, et al. Diabetic retinopathy and the effect of pregnancy. Malays Fam Physician 2010;5(1):2–5.
18. Bressler NM, Varma R, Doan QV, et al. Underuse of the health care system by persons with diabetes mellitus and diabetic macular edema in the United States. JAMA Ophthalmol 2014;132(2):168–73.
19. Bresnick G, Cuadros JA, Khan M, et al. Adherence to ophthalmology referral, treatment and follow-up after diabetic retinopathy screening in the primary care settingBMJ Open. Diabetes Res Care 2020;8:e001154.
20. Yang CS, Cheng CY, Lee FL, et al. Quantitative assessment of retinal thickness in diabetic patients with and without clinically significant macular edema using optical coherence tomography. Acta Ophthalmol Scand 2001;79(3):266–70.
21. Kashani AH, Chen CL, Gahm JK, et al. Optical coherence tomography angiography: a comprehensive review of current methods and clinical applications. Prog Retin Eye Res 2017;60:66–100.
22. Beetham WP, Aiello LM, Balodimos MC, et al. Ruby laser photocoagulation of early diabetic neovascular retinopathy: preliminary report of a long-term controlled study. Arch Ophthalmol 1970;83(3):261–72.
23. Aiello LM, Berrocal J, Davis MD, et al. The diabetic retinopathy study. Arch Ophthalmol 1973;90(5):347–8.
24. Kumar V, Ghosh B, Raina U, et al. Subthreshold diode micropulse panretinal photocoagulation for proliferative diabetic retinopathy. Eye 2009;23:2122–3. https://doi.org/10.1038/eye.2008.416.
25. Fong DS, Girach A, Boney A. Visual side effects of successful scatter laser photocoagulation surgery for proliferative diabetic retinopathy: a literature review. Retina 2007;27(7):816–24.
26. Boyer DS, Hopkins JJ, Sorof J, et al. Anti-vascular endothelial growth factor therapy for diabetic macular edema. Ther Adv Endocrinol Metab 2013;4(6):151–69.
27. Wells JA, Glassman AR, Ayala AR, et al. Aflibercept, bevacizumab, or ranibizumab for diabetic macular edema: two-year results from a comparative effectiveness randomized clinical trial. Ophthalmology 2016;123(6):1351–9.
28. Gross JG, Glassman AR, Liu D, et al. Diabetic retinopathy clinical research network. five-year outcomes of panretinal photocoagulation vs intravitreous ranibizumab for proliferative diabetic retinopathy: a randomized clinical trial. JAMA Ophthalmol 2018;136(10):1138–48 [Erratum in: JAMA Ophthalmol. 2019 Apr 1;137(4):467. PMID: 30043039; PMCID: PMC6233839].

29. Spaide RF, Fisher YL. Intravitreal bevacizumab (Avastin) treatment of proliferative diabetic retinopathy complicated by vitreous hemorrhage. Retina 2006;26(3): 275–8.

30. Wells JA, Glassman AR, Ayala AR, et al, Diabetic Retinopathy Clinical Research Network. Aflibercept, bevacizumab, or ranibizumab for diabetic macular edema. N Engl J Med 2015;372(13):1193–203.

31. Nguyen QD, Brown DM, Marcus DM, et al, RISE and RIDE Research Group. Ranibizumab for diabetic macular edema: results from 2 phase III randomized trials: RISE and RIDE. Ophthalmology 2012;119(4):789–801.

32. Korobelnik JF, Do DV, Schmidt-Erfurth U, et al. Intravitreal aflibercept for diabetic macular edema. Ophthalmology 2014;121(11):2247–54.

33. Papadopoulos N, Martin J, Ruan Q, et al. Binding and neutralization of vascular endothelial growth factor (VEGF) and related ligands by VEGF Trap, ranibizumab and bevacizumab. Angiogenesis 2012;15(2):171–85.

34. Vader MJC, Schauwvlieghe ASME, Verbraak FD, et al. Comparing the efficacy of bevacizumab and ranibizumab in patients with diabetic macular edema (BRDME): the brdme study, a randomized trial. Oph Retina 2020;4(8):777–88.

35. Writing Committee for the Diabetic Retinopathy Clinical Research Network, Gross JG, Glassman AR, Jampol LM, et al. Panretinal Photocoagulation vs Intravitreous Ranibizumab for Proliferative Diabetic Retinopathy: A Randomized Clinical Trial. JAMA 2015;314(20):2137–46 [Erratum in: JAMA. 2016 Mar 1;315(9): 944. Erratum in: JAMA. 2019 Mar 12;321(10):1008. PMID: 26565927; PMCID: PMC5567801].

36. Genentech, Inc.. FDA approves Genentech's Lucentis (ranibizumab injection) for diabetic retinopathy, the leading cause of blindness among working age adults in the United States. 2015. Available at: https://www.gene.com/media/press-releases/14661/2017-04-17/fda-approves-genentechs-lucentis-ranibiz.   Accessed May 30, 2018.

37. Wykoff CC, Shah C, Dhoot D, et al. Longitudinal retinal perfusion status in eyes with diabetic macular edema receiving intravitreal aflibercept or laser in VISTA study. Ophthalmology 2019;126(8):1171–80.

38. Ip MS, Domalpally A, Sun JK, et al. Long-term effects of therapy with ranibizumab on diabetic retinopathy severity and baseline risk factors for worsening retinopathy. Ophthalmology 2015;122(2):367–74.

39. Brown DM, Wykoff CC, Boyer D, et al. Evaluation of intravitreal aflibercept for the treatment of severe nonproliferative diabetic retinopathy: results from the PANORAMA randomized clinical trial. JAMA Ophthalmol 2021;139(9):946–55.

40. Maturi RK, Glassman AR, Josic K, et al. Effect of intravitreous anti–vascular endothelial growth factor vs sham treatment for prevention of vision-threatening complications of diabetic retinopathy: the protocol w randomized clinical trial. JAMA Ophthalmol 2021;139(7):701–12.

41. Jonas JB, Hayler JK, Söfker A, et al. Intravitreal injection of crystalline cortisone as adjunctive treatment of proliferative diabetic retinopathy. Am J Ophthalmol 2001;131(4):468–71.

42. Jonas JB, Söfker A. Intraocular injection of crystalline cortisone as adjunctive treatment of diabetic macular edema. Am J Ophthalmol 2001;132(3):425–7.

43. Elman MJ, Aiello LP, Beck RW, et al, Diabetic Retinopathy Clinical Research Network. Randomized trial evaluating ranibizumab plus prompt or deferred laser or triamcinolone plus prompt laser for diabetic macular edema. Ophthalmology 2010;117(6):1064–77.e35.

44. Allergan receives FDA approval for Ozurdex biodegradable, injectable steroid implant with extended drug release for retinal disease. Drugs.com. 2009. Available at:https://www.drugs.com/newdrugs/allergan-receives-fda-approval-ozurdex-biodegradable-injectable-steroid-implant-extended-release-1473.html. Accessed May 7, 2022.

45. Boyer DS, Yoon YH, Belfort R Jr, et al, Ozurdex MEAD Study Group. Three-year, randomized, sham-controlled trial of dexamethasone intravitreal implant in patients with diabetic macular edema. Ophthalmology 2014;121(10):1904–14.

46. Berrocal MH, Acaba LA, Acaba A. Surgery for diabetic eye complications. Curr Diab Rep 2016;16(10):99.

47. Glassman AR, Wells JA 3rd, Josic K, et al. Five-year outcomes after initial aflibercept, bevacizumab, or ranibizumab treatment for diabetic macular edema (protocol t extension study). Ophthalmology 2020;127(9):1201–10.

48. Elman MJ, Ayala A, Bressler NM, et al. Diabetic Retinopathy Clinical Research Network. Intravitreal Ranibizumab for diabetic macular edema with prompt versus deferred laser treatment: 5-year randomized trial results. Ophthalmology 2015;122(2):375–81.

49. Ciulla TA, Pollack JS, Williams DF. Visual acuity outcomes and anti-VEGF therapy intensity in diabetic macular oedema: a real-world analysis of 28 658 patient eyes. Br J Ophthalmol 2021;105(2):216–21.

50. McEwen LN, Herman WH. Health Care Utilization and Costs of Diabetes. In: Cowie CC, Casagrande SS, Menke A, et al, editors. Diabetes in America. 3rd edition. Bethesda (MD: National Institute of Diabetes and Digestive and Kidney Diseases (US); 2018. CHAPTER 40. Available at: https://www.ncbi.nlm.nih.gov/books/NBK567979/. Accessed 7 May 2022.

51. Sahni J, Patel SS, Dugel PU, et al. Simultaneous Inhibition of Angiopoietin-2 and Vascular Endothelial Growth Factor-A with Faricimab in Diabetic Macular Edema. Ophthalmology 2019. https://doi.org/10.1016/j.ophtha.2019.03.023.

52. FDA accepts application for Roche's faricimab for the treatment of neovascular age-related macular degeneration (nAMD) and diabetic macular edema (DME). Roche. Available at: www.roche.com/investors/updates/inv-update-2021-07-29b.htm. Accessed December 29, 2021.

53. Wykoff CC, Abreu F, Adamis AP, et al. YOSEMITE and RHINE Investigators. Efficacy, durability, and safety of intravitreal faricimab with extended dosing up to every 16 weeks in patients with diabetic macular oedema (YOSEMITE and RHINE): two randomised, double-masked, phase 3 trials. Lancet 2022; 399(10326):741–55.

54. Tadayoni R, Sararols L, Weissgerber G, et al. Brolucizumab: a newly developed anti-VEGF molecule for the treatment of neovascular age-related macular degeneration. Ophthalmologica 2021;244(2):93–101.

55. Brown DM, Emanuelli A, Bandello F, et al. KESTREL and KITE: 52-week results from two Phase III pivotal trials of brolucizumab for diabetic macular edema. Am J Ophthalmol 2022;13. https://doi.org/10.1016/j.ajo.2022.01.004.

56. FDA approves Genentech's Susvimo, a first-of-its-kind therapeutic approach for wet age-related macular degeneration (AMD) [press release]. San Francisco,CA: Genentech; 2021. Available at: www.gene.com/media/press-releases/14935/2021-10-22/fda-approves-genentechs-susvimo-a-first-. Accessed January 2, 2022.

57. Bryn Mawr Communications. Genentech initiates phase 3 trial for port delivery system with ranibizumab in diabetic retinopathy. Eyewire+. Available at: https://eyewire.news/articles/late-stage-trial-starts-for-port-delivery-system-with-

ranibizumab-in-diabetic-retinopathy/?c4src=article%3Ainfinite-scroll. Accessed May 7,2022.

58. Campochiaro PA, Brown DM, Pearson A, et al. Sustained delivery fluocinolone acetonide vitreous inserts provide benefit for at least 3 years in patients with diabetic macular edema. Ophthalmology 2012;119(10):2125–32.

59. RegenxBio presents additional positive interim data from trials of RGX-314 in wet AMD and diabetic retinopathy using suprachoroidal delivery at AAO 2021 [news release]. Rockville, MD: RegenxBio; 2021. regenxbio.gcs-web.com/news-releases/news-release-details/regenxbio-presents-additional-positive-interim-data-trials-rgx.

60. Gulshan V, Peng L, Coram M, et al. Development and validation of a deep learning algorithm for detection of diabetic retinopathy in retinal fundus photographs. JAMA 2016;316(22):2402–10.

61. Retinal Physician - An Update on Artificial Intelligence and Deep Learning in Retina. Retinal Physician. Available at: https://www.retinalphysician.com/issues/2021/november-december-2021/an-update-on-artificial-intelligence-and-deep-lear. Accessed May 8, 2022.

Diabetic Kidney Care Redefined with a New Way into Remission

Nour Hammad, MD[a,1], Mohamed Hassanein, MD[b],
Mahboob Rahman, MD[a,c,d,*]

KEYWORDS

- Diabetic nephropathy • Albuminuria • Remission

KEY POINTS

- Glycemic control, blood pressure control, and renin angiotensin system (RAS) inhibition are the traditional interventions to slow diabetic kidney disease progression.
- Sodium–glucose co-transporter 2 inhibitors and finerenone are the most recent additions to diabetic kidney disease management with promising results.
- Diabetes remission remains to be a challenging target to achieve, and therefore, various targets are currently being investigated.

Diabetic kidney disease (DKD) is the leading cause of chronic kidney disease (CKD) and end-stage renal disease (ESRD).[1] In this article, the authors briefly review the epidemiology and pathophysiology of DKD and focus on therapeutic interventions, both established and experimental, to slow decline in the glomerular filtration rate (GFR) and to reduce albuminuria.

Remission of DKD, measured by clinical and morphologic parameters, remains the holy grail of this field. Given the complex pathophysiology of DKD, a comprehensive multipronged strategy will likely be needed to achieve and maintain remission. Although such strategies do not currently exist, there is an armamentarium of interventions available and others being evaluated that make the likelihood of achieving remission feasible. The authors summarize the current state of interventional strategies in

[a] Division of Nephrology and Hypertension, University Hospitals Cleveland Medical Center, 11100 Euclid Avenue, Cleveland, OH 44106, USA; [b] Division of Nephrology, University of Mississippi Medical Center, 2500 North State Street, Jackson, MS 39216, USA; [c] Louis Stokes Cleveland VA Medical Center, 10701 East Boulevard, Cleveland, OH 44106, USA; [d] Case Western Reserve University, 10900 Euclid Avenue, Cleveland, OH 44106, USA
[1] Present address: 1127 Euclid Avenue, Apartment 919, Cleveland, OH 919.
* Corresponding author. Division of Nephrology and Hypertension, University Hospitals Cleveland Medical Center, 11100 Euclid Avenue, Cleveland, OH 44106.
E-mail address: Mahboob.Rahman@UHhospitals.org
Twitter: @nourhammad92 (N.H.); @kidneymo (M.H.); @MRrenaldoc (M.R.)

Endocrinol Metab Clin N Am 52 (2023) 101–118
https://doi.org/10.1016/j.ecl.2022.08.002
0889-8529/23/© 2022 Elsevier Inc. All rights reserved.

this article. The wealth of exciting new, recent research supports our optimism that many of these can be translated to meaningful clinical benefit for patients with DKD.

DKD is the most common attributable condition resulting in renal replacement therapy, including dialysis and renal transplantation in the United States and worldwide.[2] An estimated 10.5% of the US population, or 34.2 million individuals, have DKD.[3] This represents a substantial increase in the prevalence of DKD, which was 3.3% between 2005 and 2008, and likely related to the increase in diabetes prevalence.[2] DKD affects between 20% and 40% of all patients with diabetes.[4] Although DKD is more common among patients with type 1 diabetes, more than half of patients with type 2 diabetes mellitus (T2D) are on hemodialysis given the higher prevalence of T2D.[5] The importance of DKD lies in its high prevalence and its association with higher cardiovascular risk and mortality.[6] It is also associated with incremental socioeconomic and humanistic burden as the disease progresses. Therefore, early recognition and slowing progression are crucial.[7]

DKD is defined as either increased urine albumin excretion or decreased GFR or both.[3] Approximately a quarter of patients with diabetes develop microalbuminuria after 15 years of disease duration, and less than 50% develop diabetic nephropathy.[8] Higher excretion of urinary albumin is associated with a faster rate of kidney function loss in both type 1 and type 2.[9,10] Once in the macroalbuminuria range greater than 300 mg/d, the GFR decline rate is often faster.[11] A GFR decline can also occur in patients with non-proteinuric DKD. This phenomenon is seen those with T2D who usually do not suffer from retinopathy, implying different mechanisms of DKD.[12]

The pathophysiology of diabetic nephropathy is multifactorial and includes structural, physiologic, hemodynamic, and inflammatory processes that result in worsening kidney function. Hyperglycemia is a major driver for diabetic nephropathy[13]; hyperglycemia triggers multiple intracellular and biochemical pathways causing the development of glomerulosclerosis, mesangial expansion, podocyte loss, and tubulointerstitial damage, eventually resulting in decreased GFR and albuminuria.[13]

TRADITIONAL INTERVENTIONS TO SLOW DIABETIC KIDNEY DISEASE PROGRESSION

Adequate glycemic and blood pressure control and use of agents that inhibit the renin–angiotensin axis have been the bedrock of efforts to slow decline in kidney function in DKD.

Glycemic Control

Substantial evidence supports that poor glycemic control is associated with increased risk for worsening microalbuminuria and decline in GFR over time.[13] In addition, improving glycemic control in clinical trials has been associated with improved kidney outcomes. The Diabetes Control and Complications Trial showed that intensive glycemic control achieved approximately a 50% decline in the incidence of albuminuria.[14] A study in the United Kingdom reduced hemoglobin A1c (HbA1c) by 1% and observed a decrease of microvascular complications by 37% and microalbuminuria by 33%.[15] Such data support optimization of glycemic control as an important therapeutic target in DKD. Target HbA1c levels are based on an individual's age and other comorbid conditions. The 2020 Kidney Disease Improving Global Outcomes (KDIGO) guidelines recommend that the HbA1c target may range between less than 6.5 mg/dL and less than 8.0 mg/dL based on the clinical characteristics of individuals.[16]

Blood Pressure Control

Hypertension is also a major contributor to DKD development and decline.[17] Blood pressure control is an established effective way to decrease albuminuria, delaying the progression of DKD, decreasing the occurrence of cardiovascular disease in patients with DKD.[18] The various proposed mechanisms by which hypertension develops in patients with diabetes include inappropriate activation of the renin–angiotensin–aldosterone system (RAAS) and the sympathetic nervous system, increased sodium reabsorption resulting in volume expansion, peripheral vasoconstriction, endothelin-1 upregulation, production of reactive oxygen species, and inflammation.[18] The American Heart Association and American College of Cardiology joint 2017 guidelines recommend blood pressure less than 130/80 mm Hg for all patients with diabetes and CKD.[19] The American Diabetes Association standards also support a target blood pressure less than 130/80 mm Hg for patients with diabetes, cardiovascular risk factors, or kidney disease, if it can be achieved safely.[20]

Cardiovascular Risk Reduction

Hyperlipidemia may contribute to DKD development and progression as it can cause apoptosis of podocytes, macrophage infiltration, and overproduction of extracellular matrix.[21] Diet, physical activity, smoking cessation, and weight management are all also important risk factors for DKD.[16] Therefore, DKD management requires a multidisciplinary team to help control the risk factors to slow DKD progression.

Renin–Angiotensin Axis Inhibition

Targeting the renin–angiotensin pathway has been one of the mainstays of DKD management. In rats with streptozotocin-induced diabetes mellitus, mesangial expansion was reversed and regressed after the use of losartan. Sclerotic lesions affecting the Bowman's capsule occurred at a similar frequency between the control and losartan groups, but the severity of lesions was milder in the losartan arm.[22] Similarly, losartan treatment was associated with the regression and reversal of sclerosis in Sprague Dawley rats, perhaps mediated by reduction in plasminogen activator inhibitor-1.[22]

Angiotensin-converting enzyme (ACE) inhibitors and angiotensin receptor blockers (ARBs) have been studied extensively for blood pressure control and found superior in patients with diabetes as these agents preserve kidney function and improve proteinuria (**Table 1**). Their renal protective effects are attributed to lowering the intraglomerular pressure and decreasing hyperfiltration.[23] In 2001, the RENAAL trial results showed the superiority of losartan for lowering the rate of creatinine doubling and the progression to ESRD over placebo. Losartan reduced proteinuria by 35% compared with placebo over the 3.4-year study.[24] Similarly, irbesartan showed the decreased progression of kidney disease when compared with placebo in the IRMA-2 study of 590 patients who were followed for 2 years.[25] Some data suggest that the protective effect of ARBs is independent of blood pressure,[26] and similar beneficial effects seen with both ACE inhibitors and ARBs.[27,28] However, the combination of an ACE inhibitor and ARB may not have an additive benefit and, in fact, may increase the risk of adverse events.[29] Combination therapy of losartan and lisinopril for diabetic nephropathy was studied in the veterans affairs (VA) nephron-D trial; the study was terminated early after the combination therapy arm experienced higher risk of hyperkalemia and acute kidney injury.[30]

RECENT INTERVENTIONS FOR DIABETIC KIDNEY DISEASE

Multiple glucose-lowering agents have been studied in CKD. As of the 2022 KIDGO guidelines, sodium–glucose cotransporter-2 (SGLT2) inhibitors and metformin are still the first-line recommended agents after lifestyle modifications.[31]

Table 1
Major clinical trials studying the renal protective effects of angiotensin-converting enzyme inhibitors and angiotensin receptor blockers

Trial	Design and Population Characteristics	Follow-up	Kidney Outcomes
RENAAL[24]	1513 patients randomized to losartan vs placebo	3.4 y	Losartan decreased proteinuria by 35% ($P < .001$), risk of serum creatinine doubling by 25% ($P = .006$) and ESRD by 28% ($P = .002$)
IRMA-2[25]	590 patients randomized to irbesartan vs placebo	2 y	Irbesartan decrease renal disease progression (HR 0.3; 95% CI 0.14–0.61; $P < .001$ for 300 mg irbesartan)
MARVAL[26]	332 patients randomized to valsartan vs amlodipine	24 wk	Albuminuria was reduced by 44% with valsartan compared with 5% with amlodipine
CALM[28]	199 patients randomized to candesartan vs lisinopril vs combination therapy	12 wk	Both are equally effective in decreasing albuminuria. The ACR were 30% (95% CI 15% to 42%, $P < .001$) and 46% (35% to 56%, $P < .001$) for candesartan and lisinopril, respectively
DETAIL[27]	250 patients randomized to telmisartan vs enalapril	5 y	Telmisartan is non-inferior to enalapril. (The change in the GFR difference between two groups was -3.0 mL per minute per 1.73 m^2 [95% CI, -7.6–1.6 mL per minute per 1.73 m^2])
ONTARGET[29]	25,577 patients randomized to telmisartan vs enalapril vs combination therapy	56 mo	Both had similar reduction in cardiovascular outcomes. Combination therapy had higher risk of adverse outcomes. The death from cardiovascular causes, myocardial infarction, stroke, or hospitalization for heart failure had occurred in 1412 patients in the ramipril group (16.5%), as compared with 1423 patients in the telmisartan group (16.7%; relative risk, 1.01; 95% confidence interval [CI], 0.94–1.09). While in the combination arm, the primary outcome was seen in 1386 patients (16.3%; relative risk, 0.99; 95% CI, 0.92–1.07)

(continued on next page)

Trial	Design and Population Characteristics	Follow-up	Kidney Outcomes
Table 1 (*continued*)			
VA NEPHRON-D[30]	1448 patients randomized to combination of losartan and lisinopril vs losartan	2.2 y	Combination therapy had higher risk of adverse events: hyperkalemia (6.3 events per 100 person-years vs 2.6 events per 100 person-years with monotherapy; *P* < .001) and acute kidney injury (12.2 vs 6.7 events per 100 person-years, *P* < .001)

Abbreviations: ACR, albumin-to-creatinine ratio; CI, confidence interval.

Sodium–Glucose Cotransporter-2 Inhibitors

These agents were initially approved solely as hypoglycemic agents by the Food and Drug Administration in 2013.[32] Since then, several clinical trials established the nephro-protective effects of SGLT2 inhibitors as secondary outcomes, paving the way for major clinical trials (**Table 2**) that proved the substantial effects of these drugs in halting the progression of DKD.[33–37] The nephro-protective effects of SGLT2 are primarily related to their effect on tubulo-glomerular feedback (TGF), which depends on the distal sodium delivery to the macula densa. Poor distal sodium delivery to the macula densa in early DKD abolishes TGF leading to afferent arteriolar dilatation, glomerular hyperfiltration, and increased glomerular filtration pressure. SGLT2 inhibitors block the proximal absorption of sodium and glucose, increasing distal tubular sodium delivery and, hence, restoring TGF-mediated afferent arteriolar tone, inhibiting hyperfiltration and proteinuria.[38] In 2020, the KDIGO updated their guidelines to recommend initiating SGLT2 inhibitors in patients with T2D, CKD (estimated [eGFR] $\geq$ 30 mL/min/1.73 m^2) at any level of glycemic control.[39]

The kidney-protective effects of SGLT2 inhibitors may extend beyond TGF. SGLT2 inhibitor-induced osmotic diuresis and natriuresis lead to improved glycemic control, blood pressure control, and weight loss.[40] In addition, SGLT2 inhibitors offer cardio-protection by reducing preload, afterload, arterial stiffness, and risk of arrhythmias and increasing cardiac efficiency.[40] SGLT2 inhibitors stimulate erythropoietin production,[41] leading to protection from oxidative stress.[40] Indeed, SGLT2 inhibitors are thought to enhance mitochondrial-mediated kidney protection through the reduction of reactive oxygen species[42] and, hence, potentially reduce inflammation and fibrosis.[43] SGLT2 inhibitors increase uric acid excretion and, thus, help control hyperuricemia, an important risk factor for CKD progression.[44,45] More recently, we have learned that SGLT2 inhibitors improve hypomagnesemia: a risk factor for CKD progression through increasing paracellular magnesium reabsorption in the kidney.[46,47] Moreover, SGLT2 inhibitors may reduce the risk of calcium-containing kidney stones through changes in urine supersaturation mediated by acidification of the urine, promoting citraturia.[48]

Finerenone

Mineralocorticoid receptor activation is one of the key factors that promote DKD progression by increasing intraglomerular pressure in addition to pro-inflammatory and pro-fibrotic effects.[49] Thus, mineralocorticoid receptor blockade reduces proteinuria

Table 2
Major clinical trials studying the nephron-protective effects of sodium–glucose cotransporter-2 inhibitors

Trial	Year	Agent	Design and Population Characteristics	Kidney Outcomes
EMPA-REG OUTCOME[34,65]	2015/2016	Empagliflozin	7020 patients with eGFR $\geq$ 30 mL/min/1.73 m² randomized to empagliflozin or placebo	44% reduction in doubling of serum Cr and 55% reduction in KRT in the empagliflozin group compared with placebo
CANVAS CANVAS-R[36]	2017	Canagliflozin	10,142 patients with eGFR $\geq$ 30 mL/min/1.73 m² randomized to canagliflozin or placebo	40% sustained reduction in eGFR, KRT and death from kidney-related causes, and 27% reduction in progression of albuminuria with canagliflozin
DECLARE-TIMI 58[37]	2019	Dapagliflozin	17,160 patients with CrCl $\geq$ 60 mL/min randomized to dapagliflozin or placebo	47% reduction in ESKD, kidney-related mortality, and $\geq$ 40% decrease in eGFR <60 mL/min/1.73 m² with dapagliflozin
CREDENCE[66]	2019	Canagliflozin	4401 patients with eGFR $\geq$ 30 mL/min/1.73 m² randomized to canagliflozin or placebo	30% reduction in ESKD, doubling of serum Cr or kidney/CV-related mortality with canagliflozin
VERTIS-CV[67]	2020	Ertugliflozin	8246 patients with eGFR $\geq$ 30 mL/min/1.73 m² randomized to ertugliflozin or placebo	19% reduction in ESKD, doubling of serum Cr or kidney-related mortality with ertugliflozin
EMPEROR Reduced[35]	2020	Empagliflozin	3730 patients with EF $\leq$ 40% and eGFR $\geq$ 20 mL/min/1.73 m² randomized to empagliflozin or placebo	50% reduction in sustained $\geq$ 40% decrease in eGFR, ESKD, or kidney transplant with empagliflozin
DAPA-CKD[68]	2020	Dapagliflozin	4304 patients with eGFR $\geq$ 25 mL/min/1.73 m² randomized to dapagliflozin or placebo	39% reduction in sustained $\geq$ 50% decrease in eGFR, ESKD, or kidney/CV-related mortality with dapagliflozin
EMPA-Kidney[69]	2022	Empagliflozin	6000 patients with eGFR $\geq$ 20 mL/min/1.73 m² randomized to empagliflozin or placebo	Study halted in March 2022 due to evidence of efficacy. Results pending Endpoints: ESKD, sustained $\geq$ 40% GFR reduction, or eGFR < 10 mL/min/1.73 m,² kidney-related mortality

Abbreviations: CKD, chronic kidney disease; CV, cardiovascular; EF, ejection fraction; ESKD, end-stage kidney disease; seGFR, estimated glomerular filtration rate; KRT, kidney replacemenyt therapy.

and DKD progression.[50] Finerenone is a relatively novel, nonsteroid, selective mineralocorticoid receptor antagonist that has recently proved to reduce cardiovascular morbidity and progression of DKD in patients with T2D.[50] The early animal studies of finerenone showed anti-proteinuric, anti-inflammatory, antioxidant, and antifibrotic effects in mice, halting the progression of DKD.[51–53] Accumulating evidence confirmed the efficacy of finerenone in delaying progression of DKD. Bakris and colleagues evaluated the efficacy and safety of finerenone in patients with T2D and albuminuria on RAAS blockade; 823 patients were randomized to finerenone versus placebo with a 90-day follow-up. Compared with placebo, finerenone exerted a dose-dependent reduction in albuminuria especially in doses $\geq$ 7.5 mg/d. There were no differences in adverse events between the groups.[54] Katayama and colleagues reported similar findings in a Japanese trial of 96 patients randomized to finerenone versus placebo with no incidence of hyperkalemia.[55] These findings were later confirmed in the finerenone in Reducing Kidney Failure and Disease Progression in Diabetic Kidney Disease landmark trial in DKD. Bakris and colleagues randomized 5734 patients on RAAS blockade with an eGFR of 25 to less than 60 mL/min/1.73 m^2, urine albumin-to-creatinine ratio (ACR) of 30 to 300 mg/g or those with diabetic retinopathy or urine ACR greater than 300 mg/g with an eGFR 25 to 75 mL/min/1.73 m^2. The results were very promising over 2.6 years of follow-up, with an 18% reduction in primary outcomes, a sustained decrease $\geq$40% in eGFR, kidney-related mortality, and kidney failure in the finerenone group. Moreover, finerenone reduced the incidence of secondary outcomes (cardiovascular mortality, myocardial infarction, stroke, or hospitalization from heart failure) by 14% compared with placebo. Despite the similar frequency of adverse events among the two groups, the incidence of hyperkalemia-induced discontinuation of the drug was higher in the finerenone group (2.3%) compared with placebo (0.9%).[56] The Finerenone in Reducing Cardiovascular Mortality and Morbidity in Diabetic Kidney Disease trial further evaluated finerenone in reducing cardiovascular morbidity and mortality in patients with CKD stage 1 to 2 with urine ACR 300 to 5000 mg/g or CKD stage 2 to 4 with urine ACR 30 to 300 mg/g. Compared with placebo, finerenone reduced cardiovascular morbidity and mortality, with a slightly higher incidence of hyperkalemia-induced drug discontinuation (1.2% vs 0.4%). The beneficial results of finerenone were irrespective of baseline use of SGLT2 inhibitors or dipeptidyl peptidase-4 (DPP-4) agonists, suggesting a possible role of combination therapy, which needs further validation in clinical trials.[57]

Dipeptidyl Peptidase-4 Inhibitors

Following the ingestion of a glucose load, several hormones are produced by the intestine, promoting an insulinotropic effect. Glucagon-like peptide 1 (GLP-1) and glucose-dependent insulinotrophic polypeptide (GIP) are two hormones that together comprise the "incretin system." The physiologic action of GLP-1 is short due to inactivation by DPP-4 enzymes.[58] In the kidney, DPP-4 has been postulated to play a role in the pathogenesis of DKD by influencing collagen metabolism and promoting fibrosis.[59] DPP-4 has also been discovered in the proximal tubular cells and podocytes and suggested to play a role in ischemic-reperfusion injury and glomerular injury of the kidney.[60]

DPP-4 inhibitors are oral antihyperglycemic drugs that extend the half-life of incretins (GLP-1 and GIP) by inhibiting DPP-4 enzymes, increasing insulin and improving glycemic control. Clinical data supporting the use of DPP-4 inhibitors in DKD are limited with many clinical trials in the pipeline. A secondary analysis of the Saxagliptin Assessment of Vascular Outcomes Recorded in Patients with Diabetes Mellitus–

Thrombolysis in Myocardial Infarction 53 trial reported improvement in proteinuria with no difference in safety kidney-related outcomes, including doubling of creatinine or creatinine greater than 6 mg/dL, the initiation of dialysis, or kidney transplantation.[61] The Trial Evaluating Cardiovascular Outcomes with Sitagliptin and Cardiovascular and Renal Microvascular Outcome Study with Linagliptin trial reported similar outcomes, with improvement in albuminuria without a change in eGFR or kidney-related outcomes.[62,63] Furthermore, a meta-analysis of 217 patients, including 4 randomized controlled trials, showed a 32% reduction of proteinuria in patients with DKD on RAAS blockade.[64] Long-term clinical trials are needed to assess the efficacy of DPP-4 inhibitors in delaying the progression of DKD. **Table 2** summarizes the major clinical trials studying the nephron-protective effects of SGLT2 inhibitors.[65–69]

EXPERIMENTAL/INNOVATIVE STRATEGIES IN PROGRESS FOR WAYS TO SLOW DIABETIC KIDNEY DISEASE PROGRESSION AND INDUCE REMISSION

There are several innovative approaches under the study for slowing the decline in kidney function and inducing remission. Although not in clinical use, these represent exciting opportunities for the future. The authors briefly summarize these interventions below (**Table 3**).

Pancreatic Transplant

Pancreas transplant allows a unique opportunity to evaluate the long-term effects of normoglycemia on diabetic nephropathy. In a post-pancreas transplant study, kidney biopsies at 0, 5, and 10 years showed that the total mesangial volume per glomerulus and the total mesangial matrix volume per glomerulus were relatively constant in the first 5 years, but remarkably decreased at 10 years. Serum creatinine improved 1 year posttransplant and was stable thereafter. Albuminuria did not significantly change; however, patients with more advanced albuminuria at baseline showed improvement throughout the study period.[70]

Transforming Growth Factor-Beta Inhibition

Transforming growth factor beta (TGF-β) has been extensively studied as a mediator of CKD. As a key element for renal fibrosis, inhibition of TGF-β has been considered as a potential target for slowing the progression of CKD. However, TGF-β has an anti-inflammatory effect and blocking it can worsen inflammation.[71] In an animal model, administration of pirfenidone, an agent that decreases TGF-β production, showed a decline in mesangial matrix expansion resulting in improvement in 50% of glomerular lesions from grade 4 to 2 after 4 weeks of therapy with improved GFR; however there was no change in albuminuria.[72] A double-blinded, placebo-controlled trial by Sharma and colleagues evaluated the use of pirfenidone in 77 patients with DKD with GFR ranging between 20 and 75 mL/min per 1.73 m^2. The study tested two doses of pirfenidone (1200 and 2400 mg), and patients were on ACE inhibitor/ARB therapy. Participants taking pirfenidone 1200 mg daily showed a GFR increase of +3.3 ± 8.5 mL/min per 1.73 m^2 compared with both placebo and the higher dose of pirfenidone at 2400 mg. The improvement in GFR was appreciated after 3 to 6 months into therapy, although no refinement in albuminuria was found on follow-up and no renal biopsies were performed for histologic evaluation.[73] Pirfenidone is currently undergoing a Phase 3 trial to evaluate change in GFR and albuminuria as primary endpoints in patients with DKD (NCT02689778).[74]

Table 3
Experimental/innovative strategies in progress ways to slow diabetic kidney disease progression and remission

Trial	Phase	Agent	Mechanism of Action	Subjects	Kidney Outcomes
SONAR- 2019[76]	3	Atrasentan (ET$_A$) 0.75 mg/d	Endothelin receptor (ETR) antagonism	3668	Decrease of relative risk of kidney disease progression across all GFR and albuminuria subgroups, with the highest absolute risk reduction in lower GFRs and higher degree of albuminuria.
B7A-MC-MBBR(c) 2015[78]	3	Ruboxistaurin	PKC inhibitor	707	May lower rates of DKD progression and development
NCT01683409[82]	2	Baricitinib	JAK1/JAK2 inhibitor	126	Decreased albuminuria
PF-00489791[83]	2	PF-00489791	PDE-5 inhibitor	256	Reduced albuminuria
PREDIAN[85]	4	Pentoxifylline	Methylxanthine phosphodiesterase inhibitor	169	Reduce albuminuria and GFR decline
Cilostazol[89]	4	Cilostazol	Antiplatelet/anti-inflammatory	156	Improves albuminuria

Endothelin Antagonists

Endothelin contributes to CKD progression—higher levels of endothelin are associated with proteinuria and acidosis. Activation of endothelin receptor 1 leads to mesangial expansion, podocyte effacement, renal vasculature vasoconstriction, and tissue inflammation.[75] Atrasentan, an endothelin receptor antagonist, was developed to prevent endothelin effects of worsening renal function and albuminuria. The Study of Diabetic Nephropathy with Atrasentan trial was conducted in DKD patients with stage 2 to 4 kidney disease and varying degrees of albuminuria. Atrasentan was associated with lower relative risk of kidney disease progression across all GFR and albuminuria subgroups, with the highest absolute risk reduction in lower GFRs and a higher degree of albuminuria. It is relevant to mention that atrasentan has been associated with water retention and heart failure exacerbation with similar risk across the subgroups of patients with varying GFRs and albuminuria. Further studies are needed to balance the risk and benefit of atrasentan use in DKD.[76]

Inhibition of Protein Kinase C-β

Protein kinase C-β (PKC-β) is a second messenger that is activated by hyperglycemia and can lead to glomerular hypertrophy and fibrosis. It also leads to the increased production and activation of TGF-β.[77] Ruboxistaurin mesylate is a selective antagonist of PKC-β. Ruboxistaurin mesylate has been shown to evaluate its effects on urine ACR and eGFR. After 1 year, the urinary ACR decreased substantially in the ruboxistaurin-treated arm ($-24 \pm 9\%$, $P = .020$) and to lesser extent in the placebo-treated arm ($-9 \pm 11\%$, $P = .430$). In terms of eGFR decline after 1 year, a lesser decline was seen in the ruboxistaurin group (-2.5 ± 1.9 mL/min per 1.73 m2) ($P = .185$) when compared with the placebo group (-4.8 ± 1.8 mL/min per 1.73 m2) ($P = .009$).[78]

Advanced Glycation End Product Inhibition

The Maillard reaction to glucose, lipids, and nucleic acid produces advanced glycation end products (AGE) as a byproduct that interacts with AGE receptors resulting in pro-inflammatory cytokines (interleukin [IL]-6, IL-8, and tumor necrosis factor (TNF)-alpha) and pro-fibrotic cytokines (TGF-β) leading to renal inflammation, fibrosis, and renal cell apoptosis.[79] Sevelamer, a phosphorus binder, was found to decrease absorption of AGE acting as an anti-inflammatory drug in DKD.[80]

Janus kinase-Signal Transducer and Activator of Transcription Pathway Inhibition

Another pathway targeted for its potential benefit in DKD is the Janus kinase (JAK)-signal transducer and activator of transcription (STAT) pathway. In laboratory studies, the activation of the JAK-STAT pathway led to worsening glomerular function, proteinuria, mesangial expansion, decreased podocyte density, and glomerular sclerosis in diabetic mice. Those were markedly improved after the use of JAK1 and JAK2 inhibitors for 2 weeks.[81] Baricitinib was developed as a JAK1 and JAK2 inhibitor and was previously studied in autoimmune diseases for its anti-inflammatory properties. In DKD, Baricitinib showed a decrease in urine ACR by 41% when compared with placebo at week 24. Whether it affects the progression of DKD is still unknown and needs further study.[82]

Pentoxifylline

Pentoxifylline is a methylxanthine phosphodiesterase inhibitor that has been used for peripheral arterial disease and was identified to have anti-inflammatory and immuno-regulatory properties. Previous studies demonstrated that pentoxifylline acts by increasing intracellular cyclic adenosine monophosphate (cAMP) and cyclic guanosine monophosphate (cGMP), leading to enhanced glucose metabolism by increasing nitric oxide.[83] Pentoxifylline also inhibits the expression of TNF-alpha giving it its antiinflammatory characteristics and leads to downregulation of monocyte chemoattractant protein-1 gene expression, suppression of mitogenic and profibrogenic genes expression, and suppression of interstitial fibroblast and glomerular mesangial cells proliferation.[84] The Pentoxifylline for Renoprotection in Diabetic kidney disease trial showed that pentoxifylline decreases proteinuria and slows the eGFR decline in diabetic patients with stage 3–4 CKD.[85]

Cilostazol

Cilostazol is a phosphodiesterase 3 inhibitor used as an antiplatelet and antithrombotic drug for treating chronic peripheral arterial occlusive disease and preventing cerebral infarction, with properties similar to pentoxifylline. In streptozotocin-induced diabetic rats, the use of cilostazol resulted in increases of intracellular second messengers, such as cAMP and cGMP, which are associated with multiple cellular processes including mitogenesis, inflammation, and extracellular matrix synthesis. Cilostazol has been shown to decrease superoxide generation in situ.[86] Reactive oxygen species in patients with diabetes result from increased cellular respiration in the setting of hyperglycemia and associated with disruption of vascular endothelium and damage of extracellular matrix proteins.[87] Reactive oxygen species stimulate inflammatory pathways including TGF-β1 and tumor necrosis factor alpha, leading to mesangial extracellular matrix expression. After cilostazol therapy, mesangial expansion regressed in streptozotocin-induced diabetic rats.[86] Cilostazol has been shown to slow down basal membrane thickening, restore mitochondrial morphology, and prevent cellular apoptosis.[88] Based on these potentially beneficial effects, a clinical trial was conducted by Tang and colleagues to evaluate whether cilostazol has similar effects of slowing diabetic nephropathy in human subjects. The study population included 156 patients with T2D and proteinuria who were randomized to cilostazol versus placebo and followed for 52 weeks. When compared with placebo, cilostazol reduced urinary microalbumin to creatinine ratio at the end of the study ($P = .02$).[89] Additional studies are needed to evaluate the role of cilostazol in DKD.

Phospdodiesterase-5 Inhibitor

PF-00489791 is a phospdodiesterase (PDE)-5 inhibitor that showed improved albuminuria in preclinical studies. In a Phase 2 trial, PF-00489791 showed reduction in albuminuria in 256 participants with DKD and albuminuria on ACE inhibitor/ARB therapy. Further studies have yet to confirm results.[83] A similar medication, roflumilast, a PDE-4 inhibitor, is currently being investigated on DKD (NCT04755946).[90]

Apoptosis Signal-Regulating Kinase 1 Inhibition

Apoptosis signal-regulating kinase 1 (ASK1) is a member of the mitogen-activated protein (MAP) kinase family. ASK1 is activated in the presence of oxidative stress,[91] leading to the serial activation of MAP kinases (p38 and c-Jun N-terminal kinase) resulting in inflammation, apoptosis, and fibrosis. High levels of oxidative stress in diabetic patients lead to the continuous activation of ASK1. Selonsertib is a selective ASK1 inhibitor that was developed to reduce inflammation. In the Phase 2 trial, selonsertib did not result in improving GFR as the difference was not significant between selonsertib doses and placebo. Despite the study not reaching its primary end point, exploratory post hoc analyses suggest that selonsertib may slow DKD progression.[92] More studies are needed to confirm the beneficial effects of selonsertib on DKD.

Rho Kinase (ROCK) Inhibitor

RhoA/Rho kinase (ROCK) pathway results in NF-kB activation leading to inflammation seen in DKD. In animal studies, the ROCK inhibitor fasudil was found to modulate eNOS activity and nitric oxide production in renal endothelial cells and eventually improved endothelial dysfunction that is one of the key elements in DKD.[93] In another animal model, the inhibitory effect of fasudil on ROCK and neutralization of oxidative stress resulted in prevention of albuminuria and glomerular sclerosis.[94] Fasudil is yet to be explored in human studies.

Leukotriene Inhibitors

Given the importance of inflammation in the pathogenesis of DKD, leukotriene inhibitors such as montelukast were thought to decrease disease progression. Montelukast improved retinopathy in diabetic rats. A new clinical trial currently underway will include patients with stage 3 CKD with types I and II diabetes with albuminuria (NCT05362474).[95,96] BI 703704 is a soluble guanylate cyclase activator that was studied in diabetic rats that showed decreased proteinuria and reduction in the incidence of glomerulosclerosis and interstitial lesions, seen on pathologic specimens post-15 weeks of therapy.[91] Human clinical trials are planned (NCT04750577).[97]

DKD is a complex disease with multiple targets that promise efficacy in slowing progression of the disease and, in some cases, resolution of albuminuria. The exciting portfolio of products discussed above is an important step in achieving the goal of remission of DKD. Future research will need to design and evaluate combinations and implementation strategies for the new therapies that are developed. Finally, social determinants of health remain an important barrier in the development and progression of DKD. Comprehensive population health-based programs that incorporate solutions for socioeconomic barriers along with novel therapies will be required for the large, global at-risk population to benefit from these advances.

CLINICS CARE POINTS

- When managing patient with diabetic kidney disease, a multistep approach is used to achieve remission starting with blood pressure and diabetic control.
- Angiotensin axis inhibitors are still the first agents to be used in diabetic kidney disease management. If tolerated by glomerular filtration rate and potassium levels, finerenone and sodium glucose inhibitors are incrementally added to improve proteinuria and slow decline in kidney function.
- Other potential advances are still in process, and one should be aware of data available to aid in using in the future in diabetic kidney disease patients.

DISCLOSURE

Dr M. Rahman has research grants from Bayer and Duke Clinical Research Institute. The other authors have nothing to disclose.

REFERENCES

1. Alicic RZ, Rooney MT, Tuttle KR. Diabetic Kidney Disease: Challenges, Progress, and Possibilities. Clin J Am Soc Nephrol CJASN 2017;12(12):2032–45.
2. Koye DN, Magliano DJ, Nelson RG, et al. The Global Epidemiology of Diabetes and Kidney Disease. Adv Chronic Kidney Dis 2018;25(2):121–32.

3. de Boer IH, Rue TC, Hall YN, et al. Temporal trends in the prevalence of diabetic kidney disease in the United States. JAMA 2011;305(24):2532–9.
4. Rabkin R. Diabetic nephropathy. Clin Cornerstone 2003;5(2):1–11.
5. Molitch ME, DeFronzo RA, Franz MJ, et al. Nephropathy in diabetes. Diabetes Care 2004;27(Suppl 1):S79–83.
6. Afkarian M, Sachs MC, Kestenbaum B, et al. Kidney Disease and Increased Mortality Risk in Type 2 Diabetes. J Am Soc Nephrol 2013;24(2):302–8.
7. McQueen RB, Farahbakhshian S, Bell KF, et al. Economic burden of comorbid chronic kidney disease and diabetes. J Med Econ 2017;20(6):585–91.
8. Mogensen CE. Microalbuminuria predicts clinical proteinuria and early mortality in maturity-onset diabetes. N Engl J Med 1984;310(6):356–60.
9. de Boer IH, Afkarian M, Rue TC, et al. Renal outcomes in patients with type 1 diabetes and macroalbuminuria. J Am Soc Nephrol JASN 2014;25(10):2342–50.
10. Adler AI, Stevens RJ, Manley SE, et al. Development and progression of nephropathy in type 2 diabetes: the United Kingdom Prospective Diabetes Study (UKPDS 64). Kidney Int 2003;63(1):225–32.
11. Lee GSL. Retarding the progression of diabetic nephropathy in type 2 diabetes mellitus: focus on hypertension and proteinuria. Ann Acad Med Singapore 2005;34(1):24–30.
12. Gheith O, Farouk N, Nampoory N, et al. Diabetic kidney disease: world wide difference of prevalence and risk factors. J Nephropharmacology 2016;5(1):49–56.
13. DeFronzo RA, Reeves WB, Awad AS. Pathophysiology of diabetic kidney disease: impact of SGLT2 inhibitors. Nat Rev Nephrol 2021;17(5):319–34.
14. Diabetes Control, Complications Trial Research Group, Nathan DM, Genuth S, Lachin J, et al. The effect of intensive treatment of diabetes on the development and progression of long-term complications in insulin-dependent diabetes mellitus. N Engl J Med 1993;329(14):977–86.
15. Stratton IM. Association of glycaemia with macrovascular and microvascular complications of type 2 diabetes (UKPDS 35): prospective observational study. BMJ 2000;321(7258):405–12.
16. de Boer IH, Caramori ML, Chan JC, et al. KDIGO 2020 clinical practice guideline for diabetes management in chronic kidney disease. Kidney Int 2020;98(4): S1–15.
17. Parving HH, Andersen AR, Smidt UM, et al. Early aggressive antihypertensive treatment reduces rate of decline in kidney function in diabetic nephropathy. Lancet Lond Engl 1983;1(8335):1175–9.
18. Patney V, Whaley-Connell A, Bakris G. Hypertension Management in Diabetic Kidney Disease. Diabetes Spectr Publ Am Diabetes Assoc 2015;28(3):175–80.
19. 2017 ACC/AHA/AAPA/ABC/ACPM/AGS/APhA/ASH/ASPC/NMA/PCNA Guideline for the Prevention, Detection, Evaluation, and Management of High Blood Pressure in Adults: A Report of the American College of Cardiology/American Heart Association Task Force on Clinical Practice Guidelines. J Am Coll Cardiol 2018; 71:e127–248.
20. American Diabetes Association. 11. Microvascular Complications and Foot Care: Standards of Medical Care in Diabetes—2019. Diabetes Care 2019; 42(Supplement_1):S124–38.
21. Kawanami D, Matoba K, Utsunomiya K. Dyslipidemia in diabetic nephropathy. Ren Replace Ther 2016;2(1):16.
22. Teles F, Machado FG, Ventura BH, et al. Regression of glomerular injury by losartan in experimental diabetic nephropathy. Kidney Int 2009;75(1):72–9.

23. Momoniat T, Ilyas D, Bhandari S. ACE inhibitors and ARBs: Managing potassium and renal function. Cleve Clin J Med 2019;86(9):601–7.
24. Brenner BM, Cooper ME, De Zeeuw D, et al. Effects of losartan on renal and cardiovascular outcomes in patients with type 2 diabetes and nephropathy. N Engl J Med 2001;345(12):861–9.
25. Parving HH, Lehnert H, Brochner-Mortensen J, et al. For the IRbesartan MicroAlbuminuria Type 2 Diabetes Mellitus in Hypertensive Patients (IRMA2) Study Group. The effect of irbesartan on the development of diabetic nephropathy in patients with Type 2 diabetes. N Engl J Med 2001;345:870–8.
26. Viberti G, Wheeldon NM. Microalbuminuria reduction with valsartan in patients with type 2 diabetes mellitus: a blood pressure–independent effect. Circulation 2002;106(6):672–8.
27. Barnett AH, Bain SC, Bouter P, et al. Angiotensin-Receptor Blockade versus Converting–Enzyme Inhibition in Type 2 Diabetes and Nephropathy. N Engl J Med 2004;351(19):1952–61.
28. Mogensen CE, Neldam S, Tikkanen I, et al. Randomised controlled trial of dual blockade of renin-angiotensin system in patients with hypertension, microalbuminuria, and non-insulin dependent diabetes: the candesartan and lisinopril microalbuminuria (CALM) study. BMJ 2000;321(7274):1440–4.
29. Ontarget Investigators. Telmisartan, ramipril, or both in patients at high risk for vascular events. N Engl J Med 2008;358(15):1547–59.
30. Fried LF, Emanuele N, Zhang JH, et al. Combined Angiotensin Inhibition for the Treatment of Diabetic Nephropathy. N Engl J Med 2013;369(20):1892–903.
31. KDIGO 2022 Clinical practice guideline for diabetes management in chronic kidney disease. 2022. Available at: https://kdigo.org/wp-content/uploads/2022/03/KDIGO-2022-Diabetes-Management-GL_Public-Review-draft_1Mar2022.pdf; https://kdigo.org/wp-content/uploads/2022/03/KDIGO-2022-Diabetes-Management-GL_Public-Review-draft_1Mar2022.pdf.
32. Clements JN. Development and Current Role of Sodium Glucose Cotransporter Inhibition in Cardiorenal Metabolic Syndrome. J Cardiovasc Pharmacol 2022;79(5):593–604. https://doi.org/10.1097/FJC.0000000000001248.
33. Taliercio JJ, Thomas G, Nakhoul GN, et al. SGLT-2 inhibitors: A new era in managing diabetic kidney disease starts now. Cleve Clin J Med 2021;88(1):59–63. https://doi.org/10.3949/ccjm.88a.20190.
34. Wanner C, Inzucchi SE, Lachin JM, et al. Empagliflozin and Progression of Kidney Disease in Type 2 Diabetes. N Engl J Med 2016;375(4):323–34. https://doi.org/10.1056/NEJMoa1515920.
35. Packer M, Anker SD, Butler J, et al. Cardiovascular and Renal Outcomes with Empagliflozin in Heart Failure. N Engl J Med 2020;383(15):1413–24. https://doi.org/10.1056/NEJMoa2022190.
36. Neal B, Perkovic V, Mahaffey KW, et al. Canagliflozin and Cardiovascular and Renal Events in Type 2 Diabetes. N Engl J Med 2017;377(7):644–57. https://doi.org/10.1056/NEJMoa1611925.
37. Wiviott SD, Raz I, Bonaca MP, et al. Dapagliflozin and Cardiovascular Outcomes in Type 2 Diabetes. N Engl J Med 2019;380(4):347–57. https://doi.org/10.1056/NEJMoa1812389.
38. Nelinson DS, Sosa JM, Chilton RJ. SGLT2 inhibitors: a narrative review of efficacy and safety. J Osteopath Med 2021;121(2):229–39.
39. Diabetes KDIGO (KDIGO), Work Group. Diabetes in CKD. 2020. Available at: https://kdigo.org/guidelines/diabetes-ckd/. Accessed June 26, 2022.

40. Nevola R, Alfano M, Pafundi PC, et al. Cardiorenal Impact of SGLT-2 Inhibitors: A Conceptual Revolution in The Management of Type 2 Diabetes, Heart Failure and Chronic Kidney Disease. Rev Cardiovasc Med 2022;23(3):0106.
41. Maruyama T, Takashima H, Oguma H, et al. Canagliflozin Improves Erythropoiesis in Diabetes Patients with Anemia of Chronic Kidney Disease. Diabetes Technol Ther 2019;21(12):713–20.
42. Mima A. Mitochondria-targeted drugs for diabetic kidney disease. Heliyon 2022; 8(2):e08878.
43. Liu H, Sridhar VS, Lovblom LE, et al. Markers of Kidney Injury, Inflammation, and Fibrosis Associated With Ertugliflozin in Patients With CKD and Diabetes. Kidney Int Reports 2021;6(8):2095–104.
44. Oluwo O, Scialla JJ. Uric Acid and CKD Progression Matures with Lessons for CKD Risk Factor Discovery. Clin J Am Soc Nephrol 2021;16(3):476–8.
45. Bailey CJ. Uric acid and the cardio-renal effects of SGLT2 inhibitors. Diabetes Obes Metab 2019;21(6):1291–8.
46. Ray EC, Boyd-Shiwarski CR, Liu P, et al. SGLT2 Inhibitors for Treatment of Refractory Hypomagnesemia: A Case Report of 3 Patients. Kidney Med 2020;2(3): 359–64.
47. Sakaguchi Y. The emerging role of magnesium in CKD. Clin Exp Nephrol 2022; 26(5):379–84.
48. Harmacek D, Pruijm M, Burnier M, et al. Empagliflozin Changes Urine Supersaturation by Decreasing pH and Increasing Citrate. J Am Soc Nephrol 2022;33(6): 1073–5.
49. Barrera-Chimal J, Jaisser F. Pathophysiologic mechanisms in diabetic kidney disease: A focus on current and future therapeutic targets. Diabetes Obes Metab 2020;22(S1):16–31.
50. Veneti S, Tziomalos K. The Role of Finerenone in the Management of Diabetic Nephropathy. Diabetes Ther 2021;12(7):1791–7. https://doi.org/10.1007/s13300-021-01085-z.
51. González-Blázquez R, Somoza B, Gil-Ortega M, et al. Finerenone Attenuates Endothelial Dysfunction and Albuminuria in a Chronic Kidney Disease Model by a Reduction in Oxidative Stress. Front Pharmacol 2018;9. https://doi.org/10.3389/fphar.2018.01131.
52. Lattenist L, Lechner SM, Messaoudi S, et al. Nonsteroidal Mineralocorticoid Receptor Antagonist Finerenone Protects Against Acute Kidney Injury-Mediated Chronic Kidney Disease: Role of Oxidative Stress. Hypertens (Dallas, Tex 1979) 2017;69(5):870–8.
53. Barrera-Chimal J, Estrela GR, Lechner SM, et al. The myeloid mineralocorticoid receptor controls inflammatory and fibrotic responses after renal injury via macrophage interleukin-4 receptor signaling. Kidney Int 2018;93(6):1344–55.
54. Bakris GL, Agarwal R, Chan JC, et al. Effect of Finerenone on Albuminuria in Patients With Diabetic Nephropathy: A Randomized Clinical Trial. JAMA 2015; 314(9):884–94.
55. Katayama S, Yamada D, Nakayama M, et al. A randomized controlled study of finerenone versus placebo in Japanese patients with type 2 diabetes mellitus and diabetic nephropathy. J Diabetes Complications 2017;31(4):758–65.
56. Bakris GL, Agarwal R, Anker SD, et al. Effect of Finerenone on Chronic Kidney Disease Outcomes in Type 2 Diabetes. N Engl J Med 2020;383(23):2219–29.
57. Pitt B, Filippatos G, Agarwal R, et al. Cardiovascular Events with Finerenone in Kidney Disease and Type 2 Diabetes. N Engl J Med 2021;385(24):2252–63. https://doi.org/10.1056/NEJMoa2110956.

58. Daza-Arnedo R, Rico-Fontalvo J-E, Pájaro-Galvis N, et al. Dipeptidyl Peptidase-4 Inhibitors and Diabetic Kidney Disease: A Narrative Review. Kidney Med 2021; 3(6):1065–73. https://doi.org/10.1016/j.xkme.2021.07.007.

59. Tanaka T, Higashijima Y, Wada T, et al. The potential for renoprotection with incretin-based drugs. Kidney Int 2014;86(4):701–11. https://doi.org/10.1038/ki. 2014.236.

60. Chen Y-T, Wallace CG, Yang C-C, et al. DPP-4 enzyme deficiency protects kidney from acute ischemia-reperfusion injury: role for remote intermittent bowel ischemia-reperfusion preconditioning. Oncotarget 2017;8(33):54821–37. https:// doi.org/10.18632/oncotarget.18962.

61. Mosenzon O, Leibowitz G, Bhatt DL, et al. Effect of Saxagliptin on Renal Outcomes in the SAVOR-TIMI 53 Trial. Diabetes Care 2017;40(1):69–76. https://doi. org/10.2337/dc16-0621.

62. Cornel JH, Bakris GL, Stevens SR, et al. Effect of Sitagliptin on Kidney Function and Respective Cardiovascular Outcomes in Type 2 Diabetes: Outcomes From TECOS. Diabetes Care 2016;39(12):2304–10. https://doi.org/10.2337/dc16-1415.

63. Rosenstock J, Perkovic V, Johansen OE, et al. Effect of Linagliptin vs Placebo on Major Cardiovascular Events in Adults With Type 2 Diabetes and High Cardiovascular and Renal Risk. JAMA 2019;321(1):69. https://doi.org/10.1001/jama.2018. 18269.

64. Groop P-H, Cooper ME, Perkovic V, et al. Linagliptin Lowers Albuminuria on Top of Recommended Standard Treatment in Patients With Type 2 Diabetes and Renal Dysfunction. Diabetes Care 2013;36(11):3460–8. https://doi.org/10.2337/ dc13-0323.

65. Zinman B, Wanner C, Lachin JM, et al. Empagliflozin, Cardiovascular Outcomes, and Mortality in Type 2 Diabetes. N Engl J Med 2015;373(22):2117–28.

66. Perkovic V, Jardine MJ, Neal B, et al. Canagliflozin and Renal Outcomes in Type 2 Diabetes and Nephropathy. N Engl J Med 2019;380(24):2295–306. https://doi. org/10.1056/NEJMoa1811744.

67. Cannon CP, Pratley R, Dagogo-Jack S, et al. Cardiovascular Outcomes with Ertugliflozin in Type 2 Diabetes. N Engl J Med 2020;383(15):1425–35. https://doi.org/ 10.1056/NEJMoa2004967.

68. Heerspink HJL, Stefánsson BV, Correa-Rotter R, et al. Dapagliflozin in Patients with Chronic Kidney Disease. N Engl J Med 2020. https://doi.org/10.1056/ nejmoa2024816.

69. EMPA-KIDNEY Collaborative Group. Design, recruitment, and baseline characteristics of the EMPA-KIDNEY trial. Nephrol Dial Transpl 2022;37(7):1317–29. https://doi.org/10.1093/ndt/gfac040.

70. Fioretto P, Steffes MW, Sutherland DER, et al. Reversal of Lesions of Diabetic Nephropathy after Pancreas Transplantation. N Engl J Med 1998;339(2):69–75.

71. Gu YY, Liu XS, Huang XR, et al. Diverse Role of TGF-β in Kidney Disease. Front Cell Dev Biol 2020;8:123.

72. RamachandraRao SP, Zhu Y, Ravasi T, et al. Pirfenidone Is Renoprotective in Diabetic Kidney Disease. J Am Soc Nephrol 2009;20(8):1765–75.

73. Sharma K, Ix JH, Mathew AV, et al. Pirfenidone for Diabetic Nephropathy. J Am Soc Nephrol 2011;22(6):1144–51.

74. Effect of Pirfenidone on Glomerular Filtration Rate and Albuminuria in Patients With Diabetic Nephropathy. Available at: Https://Clinicaltrials.Gov/Ct2/Show/ Study/NCT02689778.

75. Kohan DE, Barton M. Endothelin and endothelin antagonists in chronic kidney disease. Kidney Int 2014;86(5):896–904.

76. Waijer SW, Gansevoort RT, Bakris GL, et al. The Effect of Atrasentan on Kidney and Heart Failure Outcomes by Baseline Albuminuria and Kidney Function: A *Post Hoc* Analysis of the SONAR Randomized Trial. Clin J Am Soc Nephrol 2021;16(12):1824–32.

77. Bhattacharjee N, Barma S, Konwar N, et al. Mechanistic insight of diabetic nephropathy and its pharmacotherapeutic targets: An update. Eur J Pharmacol 2016;791:8–24.

78. Tuttle KR, Bakris GL, Toto RD, et al. The effect of ruboxistaurin on nephropathy in type 2 diabetes. Diabetes care 2005;28(11):2686–90.

79. Dou Jourde-Chiche. Endothelial Toxicity of High Glucose and its by-Products in Diabetic Kidney Disease. Toxins 2019;11(10):578.

80. Gregório PC, Favretto G, Sassaki GL, et al. Sevelamer reduces endothelial inflammatory response to advanced glycation end products. Clin Kidney J 2018; 11(1):89–98.

81. Brosius FC, Tuttle KR, Kretzler M. JAK inhibition in the treatment of diabetic kidney disease. Diabetologia 2016;59(8):1624–7.

82. Tuttle KR, Brosius FC, Adler SG, et al. JAK1/JAK2 inhibition by baricitinib in diabetic kidney disease: results from a Phase 2 randomized controlled clinical trial. Nephrol Dial Transpl 2018;33(11):1950–9.

83. Sakkas LI, Mavropoulos A, Bogdanos DP. Phosphodiesterase 4 Inhibitors in Immune-mediated Diseases: Mode of Action, Clinical Applications, Current and Future Perspectives. Curr Med Chem 2017;24(28). Available at: http://www.eurekaselect.com/152777/article [Internet]. [cited 2022 Jun 22].

84. Shan D, Wu HM, Yuan QY, et al. Pentoxifylline for diabetic kidney disease. Cochrane Kidney and Transplant Group, editor. Cochrane Database Syst Rev 2012. Available at: https://doi.wiley.com/10.1002/14651858.CD006800.pub2 [Internet]. [cited 2022 Jun 22].

85. Navarro-González JF, Mora-Fernández C, Muros de Fuentes M, et al. Effect of Pentoxifylline on Renal Function and Urinary Albumin Excretion in Patients with Diabetic Kidney Disease: The PREDIAN Trial. J Am Soc Nephrol 2015;26(1): 220–9.

86. Lee WC, Chen HC, Wang CY, et al. Cilostazol Ameliorates Nephropathy in Type 1 Diabetic Rats Involving Improvement in Oxidative Stress and Regulation of TGF-β and NF-κB. Biosci Biotechnol Biochem 2010;74(7):1355–61.

87. Gnudi L, Coward RJM, Long DA. Diabetic Nephropathy: Perspective on Novel Molecular Mechanisms. Trends Endocrinol Metab 2016;27(11):820–30.

88. Chian CW, Lee YS, Lee YJ, et al. Cilostazol ameliorates diabetic nephropathy by inhibiting high glucose- induced apoptosis. Korean J Physiol Pharmacol 2020; 24(5):403–12.

89. Tang WH, Lin FH, Lee CH, et al. Cilostazol effectively attenuates deterioration of albuminuria in patients with type 2 diabetes: a randomized, placebo-controlled trial. Endocrine 2014;45(2):293–301.

90. Possible Role of Roflumilast in Diabetic Nephropathy. ClinicalTrials.gov identifier: NCT04755946. 2021. Available at: https://clinicaltrials.gov/ct2/show/NCT04755946.

91. Saitoh M. Mammalian thioredoxin is a direct inhibitor of apoptosis signal-regulating kinase (ASK) 1. EMBO J 1998;17(9):2596–606.

92. Chertow GM, Pergola PE, Chen F, et al. Effects of Selonsertib in Patients with Diabetic Kidney Disease. J Am Soc Nephrol 2019;30(10):1980–90.

93. Yin H, Ru H, Yu L, et al. Targeting of Rho Kinase Ameliorates Impairment of Diabetic Endothelial Function in Intrarenal Artery. Int J Mol Sci 2013;14(10): 20282–98.

94. Gojo A, Utsunomiya K, Taniguchi K, et al. The Rho-kinase inhibitor, fasudil, attenuates diabetic nephropathy in streptozotocin-induced diabetic rats. Eur J Pharmacol 2007;568(1–3):242–7.

95. Targeting Leukotrienes in Kidney Disease. ClinicalTrials.gov Identifier: NCT05362474. 2022. Available at: https://clinicaltrials.gov/ct2/show/NCT05362474.

96. Boustany-Kari CM, Harrison PC, Chen H, et al. A Soluble Guanylate Cyclase Activator Inhibits the Progression of Diabetic Nephropathy in the ZSF1 Rat. J Pharmacol Exp Ther 2016;356(3):712–9.

97. A Study to Test the Effect of Different Doses of BI 685509 on Kidney Function in People With Diabetic Kidney Disease. ClinicalTrials.gov Identifier: NCT04750577. 2022. Available at: https://clinicaltrials.gov/ct2/show/NCT04750577.

Nagging Pain and Foot Ulcers Can be Treated into Remission

Craig B. Frey, DPM, AACFAS[a,1,*], Richard Park, DPM[b,1],
Rachel Robinson, DPM[b,2], Courtney Yoder, DPM[b,2]

KEYWORDS

- Wound • Amputation • Ulcer • Neuropathy • Diabetes • Foot • Graft • Flap

KEY POINTS

- Diabetic foot ulcers require a multidisciplinary approach and standards of care must be met before or in conjunction with advanced therapy.
- Standards of wound care are focused on infection management, moisture balance, offloading, perfusion, edema control, and debridement.
- Advanced treatment of diabetic ulcerations may consist of modalities such as biological skin cell substitutes, auto-grafting, flaps, and hyperbaric oxygen treatment.
- Neuropathic pain associated with diabetes can be debilitating and treatments exist beyond medical symptomatic management.
- Certain advancements in treatments for diabetic neuropathy may consist of nerve stimulation, nerve decompression, or physical therapy.

For many years, diabetes has been considered a major global health crisis. It is estimated that roughly over half a billion people worldwide are living with diabetes. This includes the millions of individuals who are underdiagnosed. In the United States alone, roughly 51 million adults suffer from diabetes.[1] Out of that number, 25% are unaware that they have diabetes. This global health crisis has placed a significant burden on the health care system, exhausting resources, and requiring an estimated $1 trillion in health care costs annually.[1] It is expected that the annual cost will continue to grow. Diabetes is widely known to cause significant damage to multiple organ systems

[a] University Hospitals Podiatric Medicine and Surgery, University Hospitals Advanced Limb Salvage and Reconstruction, 11100 Euclid Avenue, Cleveland, OH 44106, USA; [b] University Hospitals Podiatric Medicine and Surgery, 11100 Euclid Avenue, Cleveland, OH 44106, USA
[1] Present address: 13207 Ravenna Rd, Chardon, OH 44024
[2] 33790 Bainbridge Rd. Suite: 201, Solon, OH 44139.
* Corresponding author. 33790 Bainbridge Rd. Suite: 201, Solon, OH 44139.
E-mail address: Craig.frey@uhhospitals.org
Twitter: @craigbfrey (C.B.F.)

Endocrinol Metab Clin N Am 52 (2023) 119–133
https://doi.org/10.1016/j.ecl.2022.09.003
0889-8529/23/© 2022 Elsevier Inc. All rights reserved.

within the body including the cardiovascular system, renal system, endocrine system, nervous system, and visual acuity. An increase in complex lower limb wounds has been reported, resulting in an increased risk of lower limb amputation.[1] The 5 year mortality rate after non-traumatic lower extremity limb amputation in a patient with diabetes ranges from 40% to 50%. A higher mortality rate is directly correlated with an ascending or more proximal level of amputation relative to the lower extremity. An increase in age and body habitus also increase the mortality rate over 5 years with literature supporting a mortality rate of close to 100% within 5 years following amputation.[2] Preventive medicine remains paramount for reducing morbidity and mortality in the diabetic patient population.

Poorly managed diabetes can give rise to several long-term negative effects on the lower extremity. A common and detrimental pedal complication of diabetes is the development of a wound, which may lead to multiple hospitalizations that could require surgical intervention and possible amputation. Multiple wound care modalities have been explored to aid in the treatment of diabetic pedal wounds, and certain evidence-based algorithms dedicated to the prevention and treatment of lower extremity diabetic ulcerations have been studied and adopted in standard practice to prevent lower limb amputation.[2,3]

To better understand how diabetes affects the body, one must properly delineate and understand how diabetes alters the body on a cellular level. Type 1 diabetes is thought to result from an immune-regulated or mediated destruction of pancreatic β cells. These cells are responsible for insulin production. The destruction of these specific pancreatic cells has been shown to increase the number of inflammatory markers in the patient's serum. Early diagnosis is often accompanied by hallmark symptoms of polyuria, polydipsia, polyphagia, and hyperglycemia at an early age. This polygenetic disorder requires exogenous insulin to allow proper uptake of serum glucose into the tissue to be used for energy.[4] Type 2 diabetes is viewed as a multi-organ system disorder where the regulation of endogenous insulin and hepatic glucose release is no longer functioning properly. Research has looked at multiple factors, such as hormonal imbalance, skeletal muscle reuptake of glucose, testosterone imbalance, overproduction of glucose in the liver, underexcretion of glucose in the kidney as well as the role of catecholamines and lipolysis as potential contributing factors to form a complex multimodal approach to the treatment of this type of diabetes. Both type 1 and type 2 diabetes have been shown to cause devastating alterations and damage to end-organ function and overall life expectancy if left untreated or not appropriately managed.[5]

As a result of the multisystem impact of diabetes, wound prevalence and delayed healing, as well as pain, present a significant challenge to the health care provider. The neuropathic and immunocompromised complications of diabetes have led to the need for a multifaceted approach to lower limb preservation and direct care.[6] Regarding diabetic wounds, it has been shown that patients with diabetes have an altered wound healing cycle because of an inability to properly regulate the normal stages of wound healing, specifically the inflammatory and remodeling phases. During the normal inflammatory phase, the genetic regulation of pro-inflammatory markers is altered and macrophage dysfunction persists and has a direct negative impact on wound healing[7,8] (**Table 1**).

The purpose of this article is to discuss how diabetes affects the patient's pain and wound healing, the multiple modalities for the treatment of wounds, and the ability to properly achieve remission of diabetic wounds and pain by establishing a multidisciplinary approach that consists of both conservative and surgical treatment of limb preservation.

Table 1
Stages of wound healing

Hemostasis	Inflammatory	Proliferative	Remodeling
• Outpouring of lymphatic and blood • Hemostasis achieved • Damaged endothelial lining causes arterial vasoconstriction which results in the aggregation of platelets • This vasoconstriction is quickly followed by vasodilation which allows the influx of white cells and more thrombocytes • Typically combined with the inflammatory phase	• AKA substrate phase, lag phase • 1–7 d • Begins with hemostasis and chemotaxis • Release of cytokines and mediators • Agents such as PDGF and transforming growth factor attract fibroblasts and enhance the division and multiplication of fibroblasts • Other mediators such as serotonin and histamine released promote cellular permeability • Inflammatory cells (neutrophils, monocytes, endothelial cells) adhere to fibrin scaffold. Neutrophils allow phagocytosis of cellular debris and bacteria	• AKA fibroblastic phase, repair phase, granulation phase • Previously known to occur 5–20 but new research suggests that it is ongoing all the time in the background • Fibroblasts lay down collagen and glycosaminoglycans causing wound contraction and stabilization • Reepithelialization starts to occur with the migration of cells from the wound periphery • Neovascularization occurs via angiogenesis and vasculogenesis	• AKA maturation phase • Starts around week 3 and can last up to 12 mo • Excess collagen degrades and wound contraction also begins to peak • Wound contraction occurs to a much greater extent in secondary healing than in primary healing. The maximal tensile strength of the incision wound occurs after about 11–14 wk. • Resulting scar will have about 80% of tensile strength

Data from Ref. [9].

DIABETIC ULCERS

Traditionally, diabetic ulcers are thought to be present on the plantar aspect of the foot because of an underlying neurologic deficit.[10] Although this is the most common location for ulceration in patients with diabetes, it is important to note that diabetes can serve as a major impediment to healing for many different types of ulcerations. Other non-neuropathic traditional ulcerations may include venous, arterial, traumatic, and inflammatory etiologies.[11–13] As a result, to heal diabetic ulceration and prevent a recurrence, a systematic approach is ideal.

When addressing ulceration within a patient with diabetes, the standard of care must first be addressed. At a minimum, five criteria should be evaluated and assessed on every diabetic patient who presents with ulceration. These five criteria are effective offloading, moisture balance, infection control, perfusion assessment, edema control, and debridement of nonviable tissue. Although we have several advanced modalities, a lack of understanding and attention to these key mitigating factors will yield poor initial and long-term results.

Offloading

Historically, surgical shoes or walking boots have been used to offload ulcerations as they provide a flat and sturdy sole preventing motion within specific joints in the foot and ankle that may result in increased pressure areas. However, this approach has proven to be minimally effective.[14–16] In an acute wound setting, customized offloading inserts for the patient that evenly disperse pressure and offload the area of concern would be a better alternative. While it is noted that customized inserts may not be the ideal option during an acute wound, they serve as an excellent option for the prevention or recurrence of ulcerations.[17] Patients with diabetes who have experienced ulceration in their lifetime should be fitted for a customized insert and shoe on an annual basis. Total contact casts, when appropriate, have become the standard of care to offload neuropathic plantar foot ulcerations. These casts have evolved over the years to allow for easy application and the ability to ambulate with an attached boot. Total contact casts improve compliance, as they are not removable, like many other devices.

Local Wound Care and Dressings

Diabetic ulcers may present with little to no drainage or with very heavy exudate based on the wound etiology. Dry diabetic ulcers associated with gangrene are traditionally kept dry and as clean as possible, often with betadine or iodine to prevent infection. These patients may undergo an amputation if the wounds become infected or appropriate blood flow has been reestablished to the extremity down to the level of demarcation and a biomechanically functional level. If the patient presents with "wet" gangrene, which is defined as an active infection, immediate surgical debridement and amputation of the infected necrotic tissue is necessary. In general, a commonly used adage, "if it's wet make it dry and if it's dry, make it wet" is pertinent to many diabetic ulcerations and is an effective methodology for initial treatment. There are numerous wound care products available to assist in adding moisture or controlling drainage in the wound and peri-wound[18] (Table 2).

Infection Management

Most diabetic ulcerations present with some degree of contamination or colonization. This has been well described in the literature and is often referred to as biofilm. It is a complex structure of microbiome that has different bacterial colonies or a single type

Table 2
Wound care dressings

Dressing Agent	Primary Function	Generic Options
Film	Permeable to air and water vapor which allows a moist environment	Bioclusive (Systagenix) Opsite (Smith & Nephew) Tegaderm (3M)
Foam	Similar to foam and ability to cushion wounds and is, thus, useful over wounds with overlying bony prominences	Aquacel Foam (ConvaTec) Allevyn (Smith & Nephew) Mepilex (Molnlycke) HydroFera Blue (HydroFera)
Hydrocolloid	Flat occlusive dressing that is virtually impermeable to water vapor and air; upon contact with wound exudates, dressing produces gel which promotes a moist environment as well as mild cushioning to wound and autolytic debridement	Duoderm (ConvaTec) Nuderm (Systagenix) Tegasorb (3M)
Hydrofiber	Composed of sodium carboxymethylcellulose, which may be 3x as absorbent as alginate; forms a gel upon contact with wound exudate similar to hydrocolloid	Aquacel (ConvaTec)
Hydrogel	High water content and has the ability of rehydrating and maintaining a moist environment; thus, best applied to dry wounds	2nd skin (Spenco Medical, Ltd) Carrasyn (Carrington Laboratories) Flexigel (Smith & Nephew)
Alginate	Highly absorbable; capable of absorbing 15–20x its weight of fluid	Algisite (Smith & Nephew) SeaSorb (Coloplast) Sorbsan (UDL Laboratories)

Data from Ref. [56].

of cells in a group; it adheres to the surface.[19] A major impediment to healing in the presence of biofilm is quorum sensing, which effectively averts native leukocytes from adequate breakdown and elimination of pathologic bacteria. Biofilm has been shown to return to a wound within 18 to 24 hours following debridement and is best treated with routine mechanical and enzymatic debridement. The initial and serial routine cultures are performed to test the wound for pathologic bacteria, which may require systemic antibiosis. Most diabetic ulcers are polymicrobial and may consist of both aerobic and anaerobic organisms[20–22] (**Box 1**).

Tissue cultures are preferred over swabs for superior analysis. False negatives may be encountered, specifically when patients are currently on antibiotics. This is true for both superficial wound soft tissue and bone cultures. Continued routine cultures that yield potentially false negatives can be addressed through polymerase chain reaction (PCR) testing. While PCR testing will provide a genetic profile of the organisms within the soft tissue or bone, be cautioned that not all organisms that show up on a PCR test are pathologic. Bone infection (osteomyelitis) is traditionally treated with surgical debridement with or without intravenous antibiotics. Oral antibiotics with high levels of bone penetration may be used, at times, instead of intravenous antibiotics[23] (**Table 3**).

> **Box 1**
> **Most common pathogens in diabetic foot ulcers**
>
> *Staphylococcus aureus*
>
> Beta-hemolytic streptococci (groups A, B, and others)
>
> *Pseudomonas aeruginosa*
>
> Klebsiella species
>
> Anaerobic organisms
> • Bacteroides species
> • Clostridium species
> • Peptococcus and Peptostreptococcus species
>
> *Data from Ref.* [57].

Arterial and Venous Evaluation

A full and thorough arterial evaluation is mandatory for all patients with diabetes. Patients with diabetes with ulcerations may present with macrovascular or microvascular disease or a combination of both. Palpation of the pedal, popliteal, and femoral pulses are necessary to perform in all patients with diabetes, regardless of the presence of ulcerations. The most common location for arteriosclerosis or stenosis in the lower extremity is at the trifurcation of the popliteal artery and the posterior tibial artery, anterior tibial artery, and peroneal artery.[29,30] Non-invasive vascular studies, such as ankle–brachial index (ABI), pulse volume recording (PVR), and arterial ultrasound should be considered in patients suspicious of underlying vascular disease. The authors favor PVR studies as these will provide segmental pressures along with Doppler waveforms, which help circumvent unreliable readings in patients with non-compressible arteries. PVR studies will also provide information on perfusion down to the level of the toes, unlike ABIs or arterial ultrasounds. This is important in patients with the tibial and pedal disease, as the former two studies offer limited data. Computed tomographic angiography studies also serve an important role

Table 3
Antibiotic penetration into bone and joint tissues

Antibiotic	Average Cancellous Bone Concentration (Ugram/mL)	Average Cortical Bone (Ugram/mL)	Average Joint (Micro Gram/mL)
2/0.2 g IV amoxicillin/ clavulanate[24]	27.8/2.5	37.4/3.6	NA
4/0.5 g IV Piperacillin/ Tazobactam[25]	40.5/detectable	35.5/detectable	69.9/7.7
2 g IV Cefazolin[26]	75.4	Detectable	112.2
600 mg IV Clindamycin[27]	6.9		2
15 mg/kg IV Vancomyci[28]	4.4	2.1	NA

Osteomyelitis is conventionally treated with 6 wk of intravenous antibiotics, followed by a course of oral antibiotics for 2–4 wk.

when assessing inflow disease (proximal to the popliteal fossa and knee) and provide rapid and reliable information for the vascular surgeon.

Lower extremity edema and ulcerations are often synonymous with venous stasis ulcerations. It is important to respect the notion that edema inhibits healing, regardless of the underlying etiology, and may be from venous insufficiency, trauma, wound chronicity, or many other factors.[31] The standard of care has routinely focused on compression and elevation to account for lower extremity edema. Although this is often appropriate, a comprehensive evaluation of the patient is needed to determine the underlying cause of edema and to treat many diabetic wounds. The causative influence behind lower extremity edema may include valvular incompetence, venous obstructive disease, congestive heart failure, renal disease, and other pathologies. Compression and elevation in many of these patients may not be sufficient to heal diabetic ulcerations and prevent a recurrence.

Advanced Wound Care

Advanced wound care has evolved over the years. Currently, some of our most advanced therapies include biological skin cell substitutes, hyperbaric oxygen therapy, autologous stem cell therapy, skin grafting and flaps, and numerous other modalities. It is important to note that advanced treatment does not supplement the aforementioned standards of care. It is incorporated as an adjunctive therapy.[32]

Biological grafts are classified as skin cell substitutes and range from bovine collagen to placental or umbilical amnion. There are three specific components that may be incorporated into certain skin cell substitutes: an extracellular matrix, growth factors, and mesenchymal stem cells. Not every product has all three components, and each constituent varies. For example, some biological grafts may be composed of certain growth factors that support anti-inflammatory purposes (such as IL-1, IL-4, IL-10, and IL-11), whereas others may promote endothelial healing (such as platelet derived growth factor [PDGF] and vascular endotheial growth factor [VEGF]).[33] On the basis of the etiology, wound bed, and size of the wound, the selection of the grafts may vary from patient to patient. Hyperbaric oxygen treatment is not exactly a new concept. The notion of hyperbaric oxygen was first discovered in the 1600s, but evolved in medicine in the 1900s. Today, there are 13 approved diagnoses for medical use with numerous other illnesses currently being studied to determine the medical benefit of hyperbaric oxygen therapy. Diabetic foot ulcers assigned a "Wagner grade 3" or higher are appropriate for hyperbaric oxygen. These wounds have underlying osteomyelitis and/or gangrene. Hyperbaric oxygen helps to treat and eradicate osteomyelitis, in conjunction with surgical debridement, if possible, and systemic antibiotic therapy.[34] Although gangrene is not reversible, hyperbaric oxygen therapy can prevent the spread of gangrene by maintaining viability in the tissues adjacent to the injured tissue. Another common indication for hyperbaric oxygen treatment is the preparation or preservation of a skin graft or flap. It is important to note that except for cyanide poisoning, carbon monoxide poisoning, or decompression sickness, hyperbaric oxygen is used as adjunctive therapy in conjunction with numerous other modalities, not as a primary treatment and cure of disease.[35]

Skin and Soft Tissue Grafting and Flaps

Depending on the quality, location, sometimes size, and overall control of the patient's underlying pertinent and applicable comorbidities, skin grafting or flaps may be appropriate. The usage of autologous tissue is superior to biologics for numerous reasons. Autologous grafting allows for the transfer of a patient's tissue to a separate or adjacent site in the body and allows the recipient site to "accept" the tissue and potentially heal a wound via quicker means. The autologous tissue will also result in less scarring compared with wounds healing by second intention.[36] This is important because the restoration of native tissue, as opposed to scarred tissue, helps with the prevention of recurrence. Although skin grafting is a powerful and beneficial procedure, not all patients are candidates. A major impediment to the success of skin grafts is the presence of any arterial and venous disease, pressure, and motion. Another variable to consider is donor site morbidity. An additional wound is created to harvest or transfer tissue and an increased risk exists to heal the new wound, as well as any associated pain.[37] A common location to harvest a skin graft is the thigh, which often has adequate perfusion, and any pain typically lasts for approximately 3 to 10 days.

Numerous types of flaps can be performed in the lower extremity for a diabetic foot ulcer (**Table 4**). For more complex wounds, advanced flaps, including adipofascial, muscle, free flaps, and many others, may be used. These flaps are often performed in patients who are at a very high risk of amputation in the imminent future. These types of flaps are often used to help cover large deficits with or without osteomyelitis. An important consideration in these flaps, as mentioned before when performing a skin graft, is arterial perfusion, venous congestion, pressure, and motion. As a result, patients are often placed in an external fixator to allow for early and frequent evaluation of flap viability and to prevent any motion or direct pressure on the flap.[38] Furthermore, the use of an advanced flap routinely requires multiple surgical procedures. An assessment and understating of the patient's American Society of Anesthesiologists (ASA) classification are important to consider and discuss in advance with the patient. Although the failure of advanced flaps in the patients with diabetes may result in proximal amputation, it is crucial to note that these patients initially present at an extremely high risk of amputation. As previously discussed, the mortality rate of a diabetic patient who undergoes a proximal amputation is alarmingly high and, therefore, if appropriate, limb salvage should be considered in this patient population and a risk–benefit discussion with the patient is essential.[39]

Although healing ulcerations in a patient with diabetes is an arduous and challenging undertaking, advancements in therapies have immensely improved outcomes. However, initial attentiveness and prevention of recurrence are as important as active

Table 4
Treatment based on ulcer location

Foot Ulceration Location	Treatment
Distal tip of toes	Percutaneous flexor tenotomy
Medial Hallux IPJ	Midstep plantar fascia release
Sub 1st MPJ	Peroneus longus lengthening/tenotomy or peroneus longus to brevis tenodesis
Sub Lesser MPJ	Metatarsal head resection ± Gastrocnemius recession/Achilles tenotomy
Rocker Bottom Collapsed Midfoot	Charcot reconstruction with local wound care
5th Metatarsal base	Split tibialis anterior tendon transfer/Tibialis anterior tendon transfer
Posterior Heel	Offloading and floating heels

Adapted from Liette MD, Crisologo PA, Johnson LJ, Henning JA, Rodriguez-Collazo ER, Masadeh S. A Surgical Approach to Location-specific Neuropathic Foot Ulceration. Clin Podiatr Med Surg. 2021;38(1):31-53.

treatment and healing of open ulceration. This requires a multidisciplinary approach with numerous specialties, and routine evaluation and management are paramount.

DIABETIC NEUROPATHY

It is thought that the most common complication of diabetes is peripheral neuropathy. Approximately 50% of patients with diabetes will develop neuropathy, with the most of those patients having type 2 diabetes mellitus.[40] A typical presentation of diabetic peripheral neuropathy (DPN) is the symmetric stocking and glove pattern that affects the lower extremity, followed by the upper extremity. These patients will present with numbness, tingling, and burning sensations as the most common complaints. There is a pro-inflammatory component of DPN, where metabolic stressors damage the neuronal cells and lead to pain and paresthesia.[41]

Diabetic neuropathy can increase the risk of falls, chronic pain, and lead to both decreased mobility and quality of life. These patients also are more likely to be chronic users of opioid medications, which may result in abuse and other significant medical complications. Advanced imaging and electrodiagnostic studies are frequently ordered in these patients, which subsequently drives up the overall health care costs of DPN. The overall annual health care costs associated with DPN are an estimated $10 billion in the United States.[40,42,43] Several treatment modalities have been explored and developed to help these patients and to decrease the overall financial burden on the health care system, though with varying degrees of success. Discussion and referral to proper specialists for these treatments help to prevent gaps in care. The goal of this section is to briefly review common modalities to treat painful diabetic neuropathy.

Physical Activity

DPN was formerly a contraindication for any physical training because of concerns of injury to insensate feet along with impaired healing rates and increased risk for vascular compromise. However, this antiquated notion has evolved given research that shows physical activity is low risk for patients with DPN and without foot deformities.[44] It is well established that aerobic exercise improves overall fitness, glycemic control, and insulin sensitivity. Historically, physical activity was discouraged because of the risk of neuropathic wounds and Charcot deformity, limiting patients with DPN to low-impact forms of fitness. In 2008, Lemaster and colleagues concluded that there was not an increase in neuropathic ulcerations for a cohort of patients with DPN who were subjected to weight-bearing activities, leading to a change in mindset for physical activities for these patients.[45]

Recent studies in animal models have shown that exercise is effective at reducing inflammation and oxidative stress and restoring neurotrophin levels while preventing damage to nerve myelin and possibly improving nerve regeneration. Beneficial effects of exercise on animal models with diabetes include enhanced nerve regeneration and improved electrical functioning.[46] In addition, studies of patients with DPN who underwent regular physical activity showed a decrease in overall fatigue, decreased pain, improved nerve conduction velocity, and improvements in balance, gait, and mobility.[47]

These practices should be initiated and closely followed by someone from the multi-specialty care team and the patient should be evaluated for risks and potential complications of greater activity. In general, patients and their care teams should develop a patient-specific regimen for exercise including flexibility, aerobic exercises, resistance training, and training specific to ADLs. A key component of the care team is the role of

Table 5
Diabetic foot examination

Basic Pedal Examination	Risk Factors of Ulceration
Vascular	Absence of or weakened dorsalis pedis or posterior tibial pulses Sluggish capillary refill time Lack of pedal hair growth Localized edema
Neurologic	Lack of vibratory sensation Loss of protective sensation Absent Achilles reflex
Dermatologic	History of previous ulceration site Pre-ulcerative lesion or irritated skin Macerated tissue Thickened hyperkeratotic tissue Thickened or dystrophic nails Skin fissures Xerotic skin
Musculoskeletal	General foot morphology (Pes planus vs pes cavus) Amputations Muscle weakness or limited joint range of motion Inappropriate shoe gear both inside and outside the household

physical and occupational therapists. However, providers should also have basic exercises on hand and local community center information handouts for patients. Regular basic pedal examinations (**Table 5**) should be implemented during this therapy, and patients educated on daily foot checks for the signs and symptoms of problems that may occur due to increased activity, such as neuropathic ulcerations or infections. The authors suggest patients buy a handheld mirror to check their feet daily for changes, have someone in their household regularly check them, and check their shoes and socks when donning and doffing them to lessen the chance of new wound formation and infection.

Oral and Topical Treatments

First-line oral treatments for neuropathic pain are commonly prescribed by many providers and can include pregabalin, gabapentin, and duloxetine. These therapies have shown satisfactory pain relief in 30% to 40% of patients and have systemic side effects, both potentially positive and negative.[48] Tramadol and other strong opioids have been shown to provide short-term pain relief for DPN, but the risk of overdosing and abuse is high, which is why these opioids tend to be second- and third-line treatments. The most common side effects of these drugs are well known, including sedation, nausea, constipation, and drug–drug interactions.[41]

Vitamins and other supplements for neuropathic pain have also shown benefits to patients in some trials. B complex, vitamin C, and vitamin E are beneficial for overall nerve health, especially in the setting of nerve injury. A combination of these vitamins has demonstrated a decrease in oxidative stresses on nerves, although most of these studies have been performed on animal models.[49–51] Nesbit and colleagues also detailed the efficacy of alpha-lipoic acid (ALA) through the review of six randomized controlled study (RCTs), where they found ALA was more effective than placebo at lowering the pain related to DPN.

Another unconventional method of treating DPN is cannabis use, which is becoming more popular among the general public in both recreational and medicinal forms. Both inhaled cannabis and topical cannabinoidal (CBD) have been studied recently in trials of patients suffering from painful DPN. Xu and colleagues (2020) found, in their small cohort, a significant reduction in neuropathic pain and paresthesia when using CBD oil topically and found this to be well tolerated by patients.[52] A small 2015 RCT was able to show a dose-dependent relationship between inhaled tetrahydrocannabinol (THC) concentration and painful DPN, but a revisit of the study in 2020 found that there was an ideal concentration dose where the pain was most decreased, which was found to be 16 to 31 ng/mL.[53] The most common adverse effects of cannabis use during the trial were euphoria and somnolence.[53]

Two of the most common topical treatments include lidocaine and capsaicin patches. Varying concentrations and applications of lidocaine are well tolerated and have shown short-term pain relief, but this is not maintained in the long term.[54] Capsaicin patches, typically provided in 8% dosages, have been proven to provide rapid desensitization with better longer lasting results than lidocaine, but also have the risk of causing dermatitis and burns to the tissue, and can be difficult for patients to apply.[41] Other topicals such as phenytoin, diclofenac, ketamine, and baclofen have proven effective in small trials.[55] There is less risk for overdosing and polypharmacy interactions when implementing a topical therapy as there is less systemic absorption of the drug. There is hope that topical and compounded topical medications may lessen the systemic burden on these patients and the health care system, although there is a paucity of studies on this topic.

Spinal and Peripheral Nerve Surgeries

It has been determined that spinal cord stimulation can improve symptoms of painful DPN and improve the function of life. In 1996, it was suggested as a last resort treatment of DPN. van Beek and colleagues found in their study that the pain scores of their patients decreased within the first year after implantation, and this was again seen at a 5 year follow-up. Pain scores for their patient cohort were statistically significant and less than they were before implantation, with a pain reduction of >50% during the day in 47% of patients after 3 years. They deemed that 86% of their patients had treatment success after 1 year and 55% after 5 years. The study concluded that there was a decrease in pain for the patients over the 5 year follow-up period compared with baseline, with the most of the patients still using their devices regularly.[58,59]

In 1992, Dellon published his findings on performing peripheral nerve releases on patients suffering from painful DPN. He theorized that there were common places of localized nerve entrapments in the lower extremity that showed improvement in symptoms after surgical release in approximately 80% of patients, which he proved was upheld in a follow-up article in 2008. These entrapments were common from either prior trauma or the stiffening of tissues from diabetes. The entrapments are either diagnosed clinically with a positive Tinel's sign or with a positive electromyography and nerve conduction velocity study noting latency in signal conduction at a common entrapment location, notably the common peroneal nerve around the fibular neck or the tibial nerve at the tarsal tunnel. These releases were noted to decrease pain, improve conduction, and prevent falls and neuropathic ulcerations.[60–62]

SUMMARY

Diabetes is an expensive global pandemic that weighs heavily on our health care systems and our patients. Some of the most common diabetes-associated pathologies treated included painful diabetic neuropathy and chronic wounds. With a multispeciality team approach and early interventions, the patient's quality of life and activities of daily living can improve, and diabetic ulcerations and pain can be treated into remission.

CLINICS CARE POINTS

- In the United States alone roughly 51 million adults suffer from diabetes and 25% of these people are unaware they have diabetes.
- The 5 year mortality rate after non-traumatic lower extremity limb amputation in patients with diabetes ranges from 40% to 50%.
- Most diabetic ulcers are polymicrobial and may consist of both aerobic and anaerobic organisms.
- During the normal inflammatory phase, the genetic regulation of pro-inflammatory markers is altered and macrophage dysfunction persists and has a directly negative impact on wound healing.

DISCLOSURE

The authors have nothing to disclose.

REFERENCES

1. International Diabetes Federation, IDF diabetes atlas. 10th edition. https://diabetesatlas.org/. Accessed 15 March 2022.
2. Thorud JC, Plemmons B, Buckley CJ, et al. Mortality after nontraumatic major amputation among patients with diabetes and peripheral vascular disease: a systematic review. J Foot Ankle Surg 2016;55(3):591-9.
3. Meloni M, Izzo V, Vainieri E, et al. Management of negative pressure wound therapy in the treatment of diabetic foot ulcers. World J Orthopedics 2015;6(4):387.
4. Atkinson MA, Eisenbarth GS, Michels AW. Type 1 diabetes. Lancet 2014;383(9911):69-82.
5. Brunton S. Pathophysiology of type 2 diabetes: the evolution of our understanding. J Fam Pract 2016;65(4 Suppl):0416.
6. Hong JP, Oh TS. An algorithm for limb salvage for diabetic foot ulcers. Clin Plast Surg 2012;39(3):341-52.
7. Boniakowski AE, Kimball AS, Jacobs BN, et al. Macrophage-mediated inflammation in normal and diabetic wound healing. J Immunol 2017;199(1):17-24.
8. Rafehi H, El-Osta A, Karagiannis TC. Genetic and epigenetic events in diabetic wound healing. Int Wound J 2011;8(1):12-21.
9. Wallace HA, Basehore BM, Zito PM. Wound Healing Phases. [Updated 2021 Nov 15]. In: StatPearls [Internet]. Treasure Island (FL): StatPearls Publishing; 2022 Jan-. Available from: https://www.ncbi.nlm.nih.gov/books/NBK470443/
10. Leese GP, Reid F, Green V, et al. Stratification of foot ulcer risk in patients with diabetes: a population-based study. Int J Clin Pract 2006;60(5):541-5.
11. Dinh TL, Veves A. A review of the mechanisms implicated in the pathogenesis of the diabetic foot. Int J Low Extrem Wounds 2005;4(3):154-9.
12. Boulton AJ. The pathway to foot ulceration in diabetes. Med Clin North Am 2013;97(5):775-90.

13. Baltzis D, Eleftheriadou I, Veves A. Pathogenesis and treatment of impaired wound healing in diabetes mellitus: new insights. Adv Ther 2014;31(8):817–36.

14. Fleischli JG, Lavery LA, Vela SA, et al. William J. Stickel Bronze Award. Comparison of strategies for reducing pressure at the site of neuropathic ulcers. J Am Podiatr Med Assoc 1997;87(10):466–72.

15. Armstrong DG, Stacpoole-Shea S. Total contact casts and removable cast walkers. Mitigation of plantar heel pressure. J Am Podiatr Med Assoc 1999;89(1):50–3. PMID: 9926687.

16. Frigg A, Pagenstert G, Schäfer D, et al. Recurrence and prevention of diabetic foot ulcers after total contact casting. Foot Ankle Int 2007;28(1):64–9.

17. Rizzo L, Tedeschi A, Fallani E, et al. Custom-made orthesis and shoes in a structured follow-up program reduces the incidence of neuropathic ulcers in high-risk diabetic foot patients. Int J Low Extrem Wounds 2012;11(1):59–64.

18. Broussard KC, Powers JG. Wound dressings: selecting the most appropriate type. Am J Clin Dermatol 2013;14(6):449–59.

19. Sharma D, Misba L, Khan AU. Antibiotics versus biofilm: an emerging battleground in microbial communities. Antimicrob Resist Infect Control 2019;8:76.

20. Lipsky BA, Senneville É, Abbas ZG, et al. International Working Group on the Diabetic Foot (IWGDF). Guidelines on the diagnosis and treatment of foot infection in persons with diabetes (IWGDF 2019 update). Diabetes Metab Res Rev 2020;36(Suppl 1):e3280.

21. Banu A, Noorul Hassan MM, Rajkumar J, et al. Spectrum of bacteria associated with diabetic foot ulcer and biofilm formation: A prospective study. Australas Med J 2015;8(9):280–5.

22. Al Ayed MY, Ababneh M, Alwin Robert A, et al. Common Pathogens and Antibiotic Sensitivity Profiles of Infected Diabetic Foot Ulcers in Saudi Arabia. Int J Low Extrem Wounds 2018;17(3):161–8.

23. Thabit AK, Fatani DF, Bamakhrama MS, et al. Antibiotic penetration into bone and joints: An updated review. Int J Infect Dis 2019;81:128–36.

24. Weismeier K, Adam D, Heilmann HD, et al. Penetration of amoxicillin/clavulanate into human bone. J Antimicrob Chemother 1989;24(Suppl B):93–100.

25. Incavo SJ, Ronchetti PJ, Choi JH, et al. Penetration of piperacillin-tazobactam into cancellous and cortical bone tissues. Antimicrob Agents Chemother 1994;38:905–7.

26. Yamada K, Matsumoto K, Tokimura F, et al. Are bone and serum cefazolin concentrations adequate for antimicrobial prophylaxis? Clin Orthop Relat Res 2011;469:3486–94.

27. Mueller SC, Henkel K-O, Neumann J, et al. Perioperative antibiotic prophylaxis in maxillofacial surgery: penetration of clindamycin into various tissues. J Craniomaxillofac Surg 1999;27:172–6.

28. Graziani AL, Lawson LA, Gibson GA, et al. Vancomycin concentrations in infected and noninfected human bone. Antimicrob Agents Chemother 1988;32:1320–2.

29. Kallero KS, Bergqvist D, Cederholm C, et al. Late mortality and morbidity after arterial reconstruction: the influence of arteriosclerosis in the popliteal artery trifurcation. J Vasc Surg 1985;2:541–6.

30. Weitz JI, Byrne J, Clagett GP, et al. Diagnosis and treatment of chronic arterial insufficiency of the lower extremities: A critical review. Circulation 1996;94(11):3026–49.

31. Burian EA, Karlsmark T, Nørregaard S, et al. Wounds in chronic leg oedema. Int Wound J 2022;19(2):411–25.

32. Gottrup F, Holstein P, Jørgensen B, et al. A new concept of a multidisciplinary wound healing center and a national expert function of wound healing. Arch Surg 2001;136(7):765–72.

33. Dai C, Shih S, Khachemoune A. Skin substitutes for acute and chronic wound healing: an updated review. J Dermatolog Treat 2020;31(6):639–48.

34. Savvidou OD, Kaspiris A, Bolia IK, et al. Effectiveness of Hyperbaric Oxygen Therapy for the Management of Chronic Osteomyelitis: A Systematic Review of the Literature. Orthopedics 2018;41(4):193–9.

35. Nik Hisamuddin NAR, Wan Mohd Zahiruddin WN, Mohd Yazid B, Rahmah S. Use of hyperbaric oxygen therapy (HBOT) in chronic diabetic wound - A randomised trial. Med J Malaysia 2019;74(5):418–24.

36. Yi JW, Kim JK. Prospective randomized comparison of scar appearances between cograft of acellular dermal matrix with autologous split-thickness skin and autologous split-thickness skin graft alone for full-thickness skin defects of the extremities. Plast Reconstr Surg 2015;135(3):609e–16e.

37. Herskovitz I, Hughes OB, Macquhae F, et al. Epidermal skin grafting. Int Wound J 2016;13(Suppl 3):52–6.

38. Clemens MW, Attinger CE. Functional reconstruction of the diabetic foot. Semin Plast Surg 2010;24(1):43–56.

39. Klaphake S, de Leur K, Mulder PG, et al. Mortality after major amputation in elderly patients with critical limb ischemia. Clin Interv Aging 2017;12:1985–92.

40. Feldman EL, Callaghan BC, Pop-Busui R, et al. Diabetic neuropathy. Nat Rev Dis primers 2019;5(1):1–18.

41. Kopsky DJ, Hesselink JMK. Topical phenytoin for the treatment of neuropathic pain. J Pain Res 2017;10:469.

42. Callaghan BC, Price RS, Chen KS, et al. The importance of rare subtypes in diagnosis and treatment of peripheral neuropathy: a review. JAMA Neurol 2015;72:1510–8.

43. Smith AG, Živković S. The hidden costs of painful diabetic neuropathy revealed. Neurol Clin Pract 2020;10(1):3–4.

44. Kluding PM, Bareiss SK, Hastings M, et al. Physical training and activity in people with diabetic peripheral neuropathy: paradigm shift. Phys Ther 2017;97(1):31–43.

45. LeMaster JW, Mueller MJ, Reiber GE, et al. Effect of Weight-Bearing Activity on Foot Ulcer Incidence in People With Diabetic Peripheral Neuropathy: Feet First Randomized Controlled Trial. Phys Ther 2008;88(11):1385–98.

46. Verge VM, Andreassen CS, Arnason TG, et al. Mechanisms of disease: role of neurotrophins in diabetes and diabetic neuropathy. Handb Clin Neurol 2014;126:443–60.

47. Yoo M, D'Silva LJ, Martin K, et al. Pilot study of exercise therapy on painful diabetic peripheral neuropathy. Pain Med 2015;16:1482–9.

48. Hansson PT, Attal N, Baron R, et al. Toward a definition of pharmacoresistant neuropathic pain. Eur J Pain 2009;13(5):439–40.

49. Camarena V, Wang G. The epigenetic role of vitamin C in health and disease. Cell Mol Life Sci 2016;73(8):1645–58.

50. Tütüncü NB, Bayraktar M, Varli K. Reversal of defective nerve conduction with vitamin E supplementation in type 2 diabetes: a preliminary study. Diabetes care 1998;21(11):1915–8.

51. Apostolopoulou K, Konstantinou D, Alataki R, et al. Ischemia–reperfusion injury of sciatic nerve in rats: Protective role of combination of vitamin C with E and tissue plasminogen activator. Neurochem Res 2018;43(3):650–8.

52. Xu DH, Cullen BD, Tang M, et al. The effectiveness of topical cannabidiol oil in symptomatic relief of peripheral neuropathy of the lower extremities. Curr Pharm Biotechnol 2020;21(5):390–402.
53. Wallace MS, Marcotte TD, Atkinson JH, et al. A secondary analysis from a randomized trial on the effect of plasma tetrahydrocannabinol levels on pain reduction in painful diabetic peripheral neuropathy. J Pain 2020;21(11–12):1175–86.
54. Sommer C, Cruccu G. Topical treatment of peripheral neuropathic pain: applying the evidence. J Pain Symptom Manage 2017;53(3):614–29.
55. Cline AE, Turrentine JE. Compounded topical analgesics for chronic pain. Dermatitis 2016;27(5):263–71.
56. Sood A, Granick MS, Tomaselli NL. Wound Dressings and Comparative Effectiveness Data. Adv Wound Care (New Rochelle). 2014;3(8):511-529. doi:10.1089/wound.2012.0401
57. Matheson EM, Bragg SW, Blackwelder RS. Diabetes-Related Foot Infections: Diagnosis and Treatment. Am Fam Physician. 2021;104(4):386-394.
58. van Beek M, Geurts JW, Slangen R, et al. Severity of neuropathy is associated with long-term spinal cord stimulation outcome in painful diabetic peripheral neuropathy: five-year follow-up of a prospective two-center clinical trial. Diabetes Care 2018;41(1):32–8.
59. Amato Nesbit S, Sharma R, Waldfogel JM, et al. Non-pharmacologic treatments for symptoms of diabetic peripheral neuropathy: a systematic review. Curr Med Res Opin 2019;35(1):15–25.
60. Dellon AL. Treatment of symptomatic diabetic neuropathy by surgical decompression of multiple peripheral nerves. Plast Reconstr Surg 1992;89(4):689–97.
61. Dellon AL. The Dellon approach to neurolysis in the neuropathy patient with chronic nerve compression. Handchir Mikrochir Plast Chir 2008;40(06):351–60.
62. Rodriguez-Collazo ER, Masadeh S. Orthoplastic techniques for lower extremity reconstruction Part 1, An issue of clinics in podiatric medicine and surgery. In: Rodriguez-Collazo ER, Masadeh S, editors. E-Book, vol. 37. Chicago, IL: Elsevier Health Sciences; 2020.

Ameliorating Cardiovascular Risk in Patients with Type 2 Diabetes

Issam Motairek, MD, Sadeer Al-Kindi, MD*

KEYWORDS

• Cardiovascular disease • Type 2 diabetes mellitus • Risk factors

KEY POINTS

• Ameliorating cardiovascular disease in patients with diabetes requires a tight risk-factor control, including that of lipids, blood pressure, and glycemia. Complete amelioration of traditional risk factors in type 2 diabetes can lead to significantly improved outcomes.
• Lifestyle interventions that focus on diet, exercise, and smoking cessation are essential components of comprehensive cardiovascular risk reduction.
• Nontraditional risk factors, such as social and environmental determinants of health, play a significant role in cardiovascular morbidity and mortality in patients with diabetes.

INTRODUCTION

Cardiovascular disease (CVD) remains the main cause of mortality and morbidity in patients with type 2 diabetes (T2D). People with T2D are 2 to 4 times more likely to experience cardiovascular events and mortality, owing to traditional and residual CVD risk factors.[1] Ameliorating CVD risk in patients with T2D requires comprehensive cardiovascular risk reduction with multiple risk factor control, including, but not limited to, blood pressure (BP), lipids, glycemia, and lifestyle modifications. Emerging data also support the role of residual CVD risk from inflammation, environmental exposures, socioeconomic status, and neighborhood effects (**Fig. 1**). While large retrospective studies suggest that multiple risk factor control in T2D can ameliorate CVD risk, only a small fraction of patients with T2D in the real world achieve optimal CVD risk reduction. In this review, we summarize the evidence for comprehensive CVD risk reduction in T2D for each risk factor.

University Hospitals Harrington Heart and Vascular Institute, Case Western Reserve University School of Medicine, 11100 Euclid Avenue, Cleveland, OH 44106, USA
* Corresponding author. University Hospitals Harrington Heart and Vascular Institute, Case Western Reserve University School of Medicine, 11100 Euclid Avenue, Cleveland, OH 44106.
E-mail address: Sadeer.Al-Kindi@UHhospitals.org

Endocrinol Metab Clin N Am 52 (2023) 135–147
https://doi.org/10.1016/j.ecl.2022.07.002
0889-8529/23/© 2022 Elsevier Inc. All rights reserved.

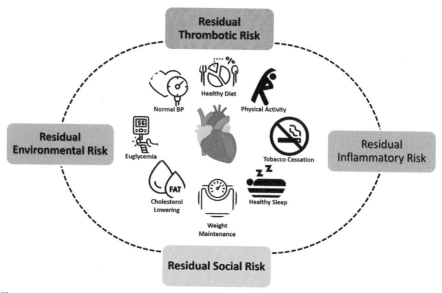

Fig. 1. Comprehensive cardiovascular risk reduction in T2D.

LIPID CONTROL

Dyslipidemia in T2D is not limited to high low-density lipoprotein (LDL), but also includes low high-density lipoprotein (HDL) levels, high triglyceride (TG) and TG-rich remnant lipoproteins, as well as increased levels of LDL and Apo B lipoproteins.[2] LDL in diabetes is more likely to be smaller particles and more atherogenic because of increased glycation and oxidation in patients with T2D.[3] In fact, among all risk factors, LDL cholesterol was the best predictor for myocardial infarction (MI) in the United Kingdom Prospective Diabetes Study (UKPDS), with a 57% increased risk for every 1 mmol/L increase of LDL.[4]

Because of the strong causal relationship between LDL cholesterol concentrations and CVD outcomes, statins have been the cornerstone of treatment in the primary and secondary prevention of cardiovascular events in patients with T2D. The protective effects of statins transcend to a lower risk in patients without a history of CVD and patients without high levels of cholesterol.[5]

Many studies have demonstrated the importance of LDL control in patients with T2D. In a meta-analysis of 18,686 patients with T2D, there was a 13% reduction in CVD mortality per 1 mmol/L (39 mg/dL) reduction in LDL, which was comparable to the observed reductions in patients without T2D. Further, statins led to similar proportional effects irrespective of a history of vascular disease and other baseline characteristics.[6]

Intensive lowering of LDL cholesterol is needed in patients with T2D and pre-existing atherosclerotic CVD (ASCVD) given the elevated baseline risk. A meta-analysis including 4351 patients with T2D comparing the efficacy of standard (moderate-intensity statins) and intensive statin treatment (high-intensity statins) in the secondary prevention of cardiovascular events demonstrated a 15% decrease in standard therapy compared with placebo, while intensive therapy added a 9% reduction in CVD events.[7] The American Diabetes Association (ADA) guidelines recommend moderate-intensity statin therapy in any patient age 40 to 75 years without CVD risk, age 20 to 39 years with any CVD risk factors, and initiating high-intensity statins in patients with established CVD.[8] The 2018 multisocietal lipid guidelines recommend moderate-intensity statin initiation in T2D (40–75 years of age) with an option to upgrade to high-intensity statins in patients 50 to 75 years of age with multiple risk factors.[9]

An appropriate target for LDL-C would be 70 mg/dl, which can be achieved by statins with or without ezetimibe. The IMProved Reduction of Outcomes: The Vytorin Efficacy International Trial (IMPROVE-IT) showed that the addition of ezetimibe to statins can decrease LDL-C and CVD risk when compared to statins alone (27% of patients had T2D).[10] Evidence from large randomized controlled trials also showed that proprotein convertase subtilisin/kexin type 9 inhibitors (PCSK9i) have comparable efficacy in lowering LDL-C and reducing cardiovascular risk in patients with T2D versus those without, implying a role in secondary prevention in this group.[11]

Two recent large RCTs with conflicting results addressed whether triglyceridemia is causal in CVD. The REDUCE-IT trial[12] randomized 8179 patients with established ASCVD or T2D and other risk factors who were on statins and had fasting TG levels between 135 and 499 mg/dL to 4 g of icosapent ethyl or mineral oil (placebo) and followed them for the primary endpoint, which was a composite of CV death, nonfatal MI, nonfatal stroke, coronary revascularization, or unstable angina. Patients receiving icosapent ethyl (58% with T2D) had significantly lower rates of the composite CV outcome [hazard ratio (HR) 0.75; 95% confidence interval (CI), 0.68–0.83] without significant heterogeneity by diabetes status. The STRENGTH trial[13] randomized 13,078 statin-treated participants with high cardiovascular risk, hypertriglyceridemia, and low levels of HDL-C (70% with T2D) to 4 g/d of omega-3 carboxylic acid versus corn oil (placebo) and followed them for a composite measure of cardiovascular events. The trial was halted prematurely because of low probability of benefit with omega-3 carboxylic acid (HR 0.99; 95% CI, 0.90–1.09). Based on these findings, the benefits of icosapent ethyl in statin-treated patients with T2D with residual hyperglyceridemia remain to be elucidated.

BLOOD PRESSURE CONTROL

Hypertension is common in patients with T2D, which is a strong risk factor for microvascular (retinopathy, nephropathy, and neuropathy) and macrovascular (MI and strokes) complications.[14] Societal guidelines recommend weight loss, salt restriction, healthy diet, and exercise to treat hypertension in T2D.[8] The UKPDS trial and the Hypertension Optimal Treatment trial showed decreased cardiovascular risk in patients with diabetes and hypertension who were on antihypertensive therapy.[15] The Action to Control Cardiovascular Risk in Diabetes (ACCORD) trial[16] examined whether an intensive systolic BP (SBP) target less than 120 mm Hg would decrease CV risk compared with a standard BP (SBP 130–140 mm Hg). Intensive SBP control did not show a significant decrease in the composite major adverse cardiovascular events. However, it did show a significant decrease in stroke, outweighed by serious side effects, such as hypotension, renal failure, and arrhythmias.

Recent meta-analyses compared the cardiovascular risk of intensive versus standard BP control and also identified appropriate targets. A meta-analysis of 73,738 patients with T2D showed that antihypertensive treatment significantly reduces cardiovascular risk in patients with an SBP greater than 140 mm Hg but increases cardiovascular mortality in patients with an SBP of less than 140 mm Hg.[17]

Current guidelines recommend initiating and titrating antihypertensive medication for BP greater than 140/90 mm Hg in most patients with T2D[8] (**Table 1**). This should

Table 1
Current recommendations on cardiovascular disease risk factor control in diabetes

Risk factors	Recommendations	Levels of Evidence
Cholesterol control	For patients with diabetes aged 40–75 y without atherosclerotic cardiovascular disease, use moderate-intensity statin therapy in addiction to lifestyle therapy	ADA: A; ACC/AHA: I ADA: B; ACC/AHA Class II
	In patients with diabetes at higher risk, especially those with multiple atherosclerotic cardiovascular disease risk factors or aged 50–70 y, it is reasonable to use high-intensity therapy	ADA: A
	For patients all the ages with diabetes and atherosclerotic cardiovascular disease, high-intensity statin therapy should be added to lifestyle therapy	
Blood pressure	Treat to a blood pressure target of <140/90 mm Hg for most patients with diabetes	ADA: A ADA: B
	For individuals with diabetes and hypertension at higher cardiovascular risk (existing atherosclerotic cardiovascular disease [ASCVD] or 10-y ASCVD risk ≥15%), a blood pressure target of <130/80 mm Hg may be appropriate, if it can be safely attained	
Glycemic control	An A1C goal for many nonpregnant adults of <7% (53 mmol/mol) without significant hypoglycemia is appropriate	ADA: A ADA: B ADA: B
	On the basis of provider judgment and patient preference, achievement of lower A1C levels than the goal of 7% may be acceptable and even beneficial if it can be achieved safely without significant hypoglycemia or the other adverse effect of treatment	
	Less stringent A1C goals (such as <8% [64 mmol/mol]) may be appropriate for patients with limited life expectancy or where the harms of treatment are greater than the benefits.	
Antiplatelet agent	Use aspirin therapy (75–162 mm/d) as a secondary prevention strategy in those with diabetes and a history of atherosclerotic cardiovascular disease	ADA: A; ACC/AHA: I

be supplemented with lifestyle modifications, such as diet and exercise. Patients with BP greater than 160/100 mm Hg may benefit from combination antihypertensive therapy. Lower targets, such as SBP less than 130 mm Hg, may be appropriate for younger patients with diabetes and other cardiovascular risk factors or a history of cerebrovascular disease, with the assumption that lower targets can be achieved safely.[18] Angiotensin-converting-enzyme inhibitors or angiotensin-receptor blockers may be the preferred medication in patients with diabetes and hypertension because of their kidney-protective properties.[19]

GLYCEMIA

Glycemia in T2D is an important risk factor for CVD morbidity and mortality. Multiple studies have demonstrated that tight glycemic control can decrease microvascular complications. The UKPDS study showed a 25% reduction in the microvascular endpoint in the intensive group compared with the conventional group.[20] A follow-up study to determine the relationship between exposure to glycemia and cardiovascular events in patients with diabetes demonstrated that a 1% reduction in HbA1c was associated with a 37% reduction in microvascular complications.[21]

The evidence regarding the effects of glycemic control on macrovascular complications is mixed. Earlier studies found a trend toward reduced macrovascular risk that was not apparent until long-term follow-up. For example, the UKPDS and the Diabetes Control and Complications Trial initially did not show significant reductions in CV events.[22] However, in both of these trials, a 10-year follow-up showed a reduced risk of cardiovascular events, highlighting the importance of early intensive glycemic control in building a metabolic memory, allowing for long-term rather than short-term CVD protection.[22]

Because of the uncertainty about whether intensive glycemic control can decrease CVD in patients with diabetes, several long-term clinical trials were launched, including ADVANCE, Veterans Affairs Diabetes Trial (VADT), and ACCORD. These trials compared CVD events in the intensive glucose control group (HbA1c < 7%) with the standard glucose control group (HbA1c levels ≥ 7%). All three major trials have demonstrated that intensive glucose control did not reduce cardiovascular events in patients with T2D.[23–25] They did, however, show some benefit for microvascular events, but this was overshadowed by higher rates of weight gain and hypoglycemia.

In the primary and secondary prevention of microvascular and macrovascular complications of diabetes, the ADA, American College of Cardiology, and American Heart Association recommend an HbA1c goal of less than 7%[8] (see **Table 1**). In patients with a decreased life expectancy, extensive comorbidities, or a high risk of hypoglycemia, target levels of HbA1c > 7% may be reasonable.

NEW ANTIHYPERGLYCEMIC AGENTS

Improvement in glycemic control has only recently been associated with tangible macrovascular and heart failure benefits with the introduction of newer antihyperglycemic agents. The introduction of SGLT-2i sodium-glucose cotransporter-2 inhibitors (SGLT-2i) and the glucagon-like peptide-1 receptor agonists (GLP-1RA) created a paradigm shift in how clinicians perceive CVD risk reduction in patients with diabetes, shifting from target-based to agent-based approaches.

SGLT-2i decreases blood glucose by reducing glucose reabsorption in the kidney tubules. A recent meta-analysis of 46,969 patients showed that SGLT-2i inhibitors were associated with a 10% reduction in major adverse CV events. It also showed that risk reductions in hospitalizations for heart failure were significantly reduced in a manner consistent across various trials, in contrast to significant heterogeneity in risk reductions for cardiovascular deaths.[26]

GLP-1RAs activate their receptors in the pancreas, leading to increased insulin release, reducing glucagon release, decreasing gastric emptying, and increasing appetite. GLP-1RAs have been shown to improve glycemic control with a low risk of hypoglycemia. A meta-analysis of over 56,000 participants with T2D demonstrated that patients on GLP-1 agonists had a 12% relative risk reduction in major adverse cardiovascular events, particularly cardiovascular death.[27]

MINERALOCORTICOIDS

Mineralocorticoid receptor antagonists (MRAs) play a major role in inhibiting the renin–angiotensin–aldosterone system and have established indications in heart failure. Prior studies suggest MRAs have renal benefit in T2D, particularly in patients with diabetic nephropathy.[28] The interest in studying the cardiovascular benefits of MRAs has been renewed with the development of nonsteroidal MRAs (finerenone). In two large placebo-controlled trials of finerinone in diabetic nephropathy patients (FIGARIO-DKD and FIDELIO-DKD), the composite cardiovascular outcome (nonfatal MI, nonfatal stroke, heart failure hospitalization, or cardiovascular death) was reduced by 14% (HR, 0.86; 95% CI, 0.75-0.99) and 13% (HR, 0.87; 95% CI, 0.76-0.98), respectively.[29,30] Accordingly, finerenone has received Food and Drug Administration approval to reduce renal and cardiovascular events in patients with diabetic nephropathy.[31]

MULTIFACTORIAL RISK REDUCTION IN DIABETES

Most randomized trials discussed the effect of an isolated risk factor intervention on cardiovascular outcomes in patients with diabetes. The extent to which multifactorial risk-factor modification mitigates CVD is uncertain. A cohort study of 271,174 patients with T2D and control of their CVD risk factors [glycemia (HbA1c), LDL-C, albuminuria, smoking, and hypertension] showed little to no excess risk of death, MI, or stroke compared with patients without T2D.[32] Therefore, it is often thought that complete amelioration of traditional risk factors in T2D can lead to significantly improved outcomes.

ANTIPLATELET AND ANTICOAGULATION

While T2D has been considered to be a coronary artery disease risk equivalent, there is significant heterogeneity in this risk. Aspirin has been previously recommended to reduce CVD risk in patients with T2D. More recent studies have highlighted the bleeding risk of low-dose aspirin. In the A Study of Cardiovascular Events iN Diabetes (ASCEND) trial, 15,480 patients with T2D but no established ASCVD were randomized to low-dose aspirin (100 mg/d) versus placebo and followed for composite cardiovascular events and major bleeding events. At a follow-up of 7.4 years, the CVD composite outcome was reduced with aspirin (HR, 0.88; 95% CI, 0.79–0.97; $P = .01$), which was counterbalanced by increased major bleeding risk (HR, 1.29; 95% CI, 1.09–1.52; $P = .003$).[33] It is important to note that ASCEND included patients with T2D but without established ASCVD, and, therefore, aspirin remains indicated for patients with established ASCVD (see **Table 1**). Low-dose anticoagulation has also shown a role in reducing risk in patients with ASCVD and T2D. In patients with polyvascular disease (38% with T2D), the addition of low-dose rivaroxaban (2.5 mg twice daily) to low-dose aspirin (100 mg daily) led to a significant reduction of major adverse cardiovascular events (HR, 0.76; 95% CI, 0.66–0.86) without significant increases in intracranial or fatal bleeding and without differences between patients with or without T2D.[34]

RESIDUAL INFLAMMATORY RISK AND THE ROLE OF ANTI-INFLAMMATORY THERAPIES

Studies suggest that patients with T2D and residual inflammatory risk are at a higher risk of major adverse cardiovascular events.[35] The Anti-inflammatory Therapy with Canakinumab for Atherosclerotic Disease (CANTOS) trial randomized 10,061 patients with prior MI (40% with T2D) and evidence of systemic inflammation (high-sensitivity c-reactive protein $\geq$ 2 mg/L) to canakinumab (interleukin-1β inhibitor) with different doses (50–300 mg subcutaneously every 3 months) versus placebo and showed a reduction of major adverse cardiovascular events (HR, 0.83; 95% CI, 0.73–0.95) with the 150 mg dose, at the expense of an increased risk of fatal infections.[36,37] Accordingly, given limited evidence, routine use of anti-inflammatory therapy in patients with T2D and residual inflammatory risk is not warranted.

LIFESTYLE CHANGES AND DIET COUNSELING

The main pillars of lifestyle modification in patients with diabetes include diet, exercise, and smoking cessation. Some trials have targeted lifestyle intervention as a whole, while others have targeted individual measures. The Look AHEAD trial (Action for Health and Diabetes) randomized over 5000 patients with diabetes into intensive lifestyle intervention versus usual care. The lifestyle intervention included caloric restriction, meal replacement products, and at least 175 minutes of moderate-intensity physical activity per week. Although lifestyle intervention did not decrease the rate of CVD events, it was associated with decreased weight, improved glycemic control of HbA1c, and decreased requirements for antihypertensives, lipid-, and glucose-lowering therapies, which might have confounded the results relative to cardiovascular events.[38]

Patients with diabetes should be referred to a registered dietitian who has knowledge and experience in managing T2D-specific nutritional therapy. In fact, nutritional therapy with a registered dietician is associated with up to a 2% decrease in HbA1c levels.[39] Although the ultimate diet chosen may differ by nutrient composition, it should create a caloric deficit sufficient for weight reduction in patients who are overweight and have diabetes. Weight loss of more than 5% that is sustained can improve CVD risk factors, including glycemia, BP, and lipid control in patients with T2D.[40] Nutritional therapy and meal planning should be personalized and consider food availability, preference, and health status. There are, however, key diets that have been associated with decreased cardiovascular risk, including the Mediterranean diet, Dietary Approaches to Stop Hypertension (DASH) diet, and plant-based diet.[41,42] Exercise has been associated with better glucose control and reduced cardiovascular risk factors. Structured exercise interventions lasting more than 8 weeks have been associated with a 0.66% reduction in HbA1c in patients with T2D irrespective of a significant body mass index change.[43] The ADA recommends at least 150 minutes of moderate-vigorous intensity exercise per week, spread over 3 days with no more than 2 consecutive days without exercise.[43] Physical activity should be tailored for the patient according to health status, exercise capacity, age, and associated comorbidities.[43]

Sleep disturbances are highly prevalent in patients with T2D, with frequent nocturnal awakening, and have been associated with T2D self-care.[44] Several sleep parameters (eg, sleep duration, variability, subjective sleep quality) have been linked to poor glycemia. Sleep duration has also been linked to the risk of T2D, with the lowest risk seen in people who sleep 7 to 8 hours, and both longer and shorter sleep durations are associated with higher risk (U-shaped relationship).[45] The 2022 ADA Standards of Medical Care in Diabetes recommends assessment of sleep duration and obstructive sleep apnea as part of comprehensive medical care in T2D.[46]

SMOKING

The totality of evidence suggests that tobacco smoking leads to CVD, especially in patients with diabetes.[43] Thus, it is essential that clinicians assess tobacco use and encourage cessation when possible. Pharmacologic therapy has been effective in helping patients with diabetes quit smoking.[47] Motivational interviewing is an evidence-based approach for tobacco cessation and should be performed by a trained clinician with patients with T2D.[43]

SOCIAL AND ENVIRONMENTAL DETERMINANTS OF CARDIOVASCULAR DISEASE IN TYPE 2 DIABETES

Social determinants of health (SDOH) have been implicated in T2D. Some studies have found that patients with lower socioeconomic status are at an increased risk for developing T2D.[48] Various SDOH domains are associated with CVD risk in patients with T2D, even in regions with free access to medical care.[49] This is further complicated by disparities in the utilization of medications with cardiovascular benefits (eg, GLP-1RA, SGLT-2i), which will likely worsen these outcome gaps.

There is still a gap in the literature describing the impact of SDOH interventions on diabetes-related outcomes.[48] In a meta-analysis of 1874 patients with diabetes, health-literacy-sensitive diabetes management interventions were associated with modest but significant decreases in HbA1c levels.[50] Use of community health workers can also lead to improved glycemic control in certain community-based settings and may help reduce CVD risk disparities in T2D.[51]

A robust body of literature links environmental factors to health, including in patients with T2D. A meta-analysis of 462,220 participants showed that exposure to green space was associated with a significant reduction of T2D incidence (OR, 0.72: 95% CI, 0.61–0.85).[52] Toxic environmental exposures have been associated with diabetes incidence, prevalence, and outcomes.[48] Studies exploring the effects of environmental interventions on CVD outcomes in T2D are scarce owing to the limited control of individuals over environmental agents. A recent meta-analysis of 604 patients showed a 4 mm Hg reduction in SBP following the insertion of a home particulate matter filter.[53] Some studies have also described a decreased burden of disease associated with reduced pollution levels. A study of 2132 US counties found that reducing particulate matter (2.5 microns) from 1990 to 2010 resulted in a 5.7% decrease in CVD mortality.[54]

PERSONALIZED CARDIOVASCULAR DISEASE RISK REDUCTION IN TYPE 2 DIABETES

Studies have shown that the CVD risk posed by T2D is heterogeneous.[55] Given the expansion of preventive therapies in T2D, it is important to characterize CVD risk early on to facilitate therapeutic interventions in high-risk patients and defer expensive therapeutics in low-risk patients. This approach may also provide a solution for medical inertia by focusing on a high-risk subset of the overall cohort of T2D patients with novel and costly intensive interventions. Individualized risk reduction approaches require precision diagnostics and precision care delivery. Recent advances in imaging, genomics, proteomics, and artificial intelligence approaches now allow for improved predictive accuracy for CVD risk in T2D. For example, imaging modalities (eg, coronary artery calcium scoring) can improve ASCVD prediction in patients with T2D and reclassify patients' risk compared with risk-factor based probabilistic scores.[56] Data-driven machine learning approaches can identify novel T2D phenotypes with a differential risk of complications,[57] which may be helpful for CVD risk prediction. Integrative approaches that combine imaging, proteomics, lipidomics, genomics, and social/environmental factors may provide more refined estimates of cardiovascular risk and, subsequently, can lead to improved utilization of intensive preventive strategies and reduce cardiovascular risk in high-risk individuals with T2D.

DIABETES REMISSION AND CARDIOVASCULAR DISEASE

Patients living with T2D may experience improvements in glycemia with medical interventions, lifestyle changes, or even spontaneously. These improvements might persist thereafter, even after discontinuation of pharmacologic therapy. A consensus report termed this phenomenon "remission," with HbA1c < 6.5% measures at least 3 months after stopping glucose-lowering drugs as the diagnostic criterion.[58]

Limited evidence exists to examine the relationship between T2D remission and CVD risk. A cohort study of 60,287 people with T2D showed that remission was associated with reduced CVD events, including risk of micro- and macro-vascular complications. This association was not modified by pre-existing CVD, body mass index, diabetes duration, and HbA1c levels.[59] Because diagnosis of remission relies on biochemical criteria of lower glucose levels, the findings of this study are consistent with a few meta-analyses reporting the association between intensive glucose control and lower CVD risk.

SUMMARY

CVD remains the most common cause of mortality in patients with diabetes. Cardiovascular risk amelioration requires comprehensive assessment and targeting of traditional (BP, lipid, and glycemia) and nontraditional (social and environmental determinants of health) risk factors as well as appropriate lifestyle modifications (diet, exercise, and smoking cessation). Complete risk factor reduction may provide a potentiated benefit. Risk reduction strategies should be personalized and tailored to individuals, taking into consideration health status, comorbidities, and the ability to achieve target goals safely.

CLINIC CARE POINTS

- A comprehensive multifaceted approach is warranted to ameliorate cardiovascular risk in patients with diabetes, including traditional and nontraditional risk factors.
- Lifestyle modifications, including appropriate diet, exercise, and smoking cessation, are essential.
- Risk reduction should be done safely, taking into consideration the patient's medical history and current health status.
- Newer antihyperglycemic therapies, such as SGLT-2i inhibitors and GLP-1RA, may offer significant cardiovascular protective properties.

FUNDING

This work was partly funded by the National Institute on Minority Health and Health Disparities (P50MD017351-01).

DISCLOSURE

The authors have nothing to disclose.

REFERENCES

1. Rawshani A, Rawshani A, Franzén S, et al. Mortality and Cardiovascular Disease in Type 1 and Type 2 Diabetes. N Engl J Med 2017;376(15):1407–18.
2. Lazarte J, Hegele RA. Dyslipidemia Management in Adults With Diabetes. Can J Diabetes 2020;44(1):53–60.

3. Rana JS, Liu JY, Moffet HH, et al. Metabolic Dyslipidemia and Risk of Coronary Heart Disease in 28,318 Adults With Diabetes Mellitus and Low-Density Lipoprotein Cholesterol <100 mg/dl. Am J Cardiol 2015;116(11):1700–4.

4. Turner RC, Millns H, Neil HaW, et al. Risk factors for coronary artery disease in non-insulin dependent diabetes mellitus: United Kingdom prospective diabetes study (UKPDS: 23). BMJ 1998;316(7134):823–8.

5. Colhoun HM, Betteridge DJ, Durrington PN, et al. Primary prevention of cardiovascular disease with atorvastatin in type 2 diabetes in the Collaborative Atorvastatin Diabetes Study (CARDS): multicentre randomised placebo-controlled trial. Lancet Lond Engl 2004;364(9435):685–96.

6. Kearney PM, Blackwell L, Collins R, et al, Cholesterol Treatment Trialists' (CTT) Collaborators. Efficacy of cholesterol-lowering therapy in 18,686 people with diabetes in 14 randomised trials of statins: a meta-analysis. Lancet Lond Engl 2008; 371(9607):117–25.

7. Vries FM de, Kolthof J, Postma MJ, et al. Efficacy of Standard and Intensive Statin Treatment for the Secondary Prevention of Cardiovascular and Cerebrovascular Events in Diabetes Patients: A Meta-Analysis. PLOS ONE 2014;9(11):e111247.

8. American Diabetes Association Professional Practice Committee. Cardiovascular Disease and Risk Management: Standards of Medical Care in Diabetes—2022. Diabetes Care 2021;45(Supplement_1):S144–74.

9. Grundy SM, Stone NJ, Bailey AL, et al. 2018 AHA/ACC/AACVPR/AAPA/ABC/ACPM/ADA/AGS/APhA/ASPC/NLA/PCNA Guideline on the Management of Blood Cholesterol. J Am Coll Cardiol 2019;73(24):e285–350.

10. Cannon CP, Blazing MA, Giugliano RP, et al. Ezetimibe Added to Statin Therapy after Acute Coronary Syndromes. N Engl J Med 2015;372(25):2387–97.

11. Sabatine MS, Leiter LA, Wiviott SD, et al. Cardiovascular safety and efficacy of the PCSK9 inhibitor evolocumab in patients with and without diabetes and the effect of evolocumab on glycaemia and risk of new-onset diabetes: a prespecified analysis of the FOURIER randomised controlled trial. Lancet Diabetes Endocrinol 2017;5(12):941–50.

12. Bhatt DL, Steg PG, Miller M, et al. Cardiovascular Risk Reduction with Icosapent Ethyl for Hypertriglyceridemia. N Engl J Med 2019;380(1):11–22.

13. Nicholls SJ, Lincoff AM, Garcia M, et al. Effect of High-Dose Omega-3 Fatty Acids vs Corn Oil on Major Adverse Cardiovascular Events in Patients at High Cardiovascular Risk: The STRENGTH Randomized Clinical Trial. JAMA 2020;324(22): 2268–80.

14. de Boer IH, Bangalore S, Benetos A, et al. Diabetes and Hypertension: A Position Statement by the American Diabetes Association. Diabetes Care 2017;40(9): 1273–84.

15. 38 Collaborators UKPDS. Tight blood pressure control and risk of macrovascular and microvascular complications in type 2 diabetes. BMJ 1998;317(7160): 703–13.

16. The Action to Control Cardiovascular Risk in Diabetes Study Group. Effects of Intensive Blood-Pressure Control in Type 2 Diabetes Mellitus. N Engl J Med 2010;362(17):1575–85.

17. Brunström M, Carlberg B. Effect of antihypertensive treatment at different blood pressure levels in patients with diabetes mellitus: systematic review and meta-analyses. BMJ 2016;352:i717.

18. Newman JD, Schwartzbard AZ, Weintraub HS, et al. Primary Prevention of Cardiovascular Disease in Diabetes Mellitus. J Am Coll Cardiol 2017;70(7):883–93.

19. Standards of Medical Care in Diabetes—2016 Abridged for Primary Care Providers. Clin Diabetes Publ Am Diabetes Assoc 2016;34(1):3–21.
20. 33 Collaborators UKPDS. Intensive blood-glucose control with sulphonylureas or insulin compared with conventional treatment and risk of complications in patients with type 2 diabetes. Lancet 1998;352(9131):837–53.
21. Stratton IM, Adler AI, Neil HA, et al. Association of glycaemia with macrovascular and microvascular complications of type 2 diabetes (UKPDS 35): prospective observational study. BMJ 2000;321(7258):405–12.
22. Brown A, Reynolds LR, Bruemmer D. Intensive glycemic control and cardiovascular disease: an update. Nat Rev Cardiol 2010;7(7):369–75.
23. Duckworth W, Abraira C, Moritz T, et al. Glucose Control and Vascular Complications in Veterans with Type 2 Diabetes. N Engl J Med 2009;360(2):129–39.
24. The Action to Control Cardiovascular Risk in Diabetes Study Group. Effects of Intensive Glucose Lowering in Type 2 Diabetes. N Engl J Med 2008;358(24):2545–59.
25. Patel A, MacMahon S, Chalmers J, et al, ADVANCE Collaborative Group. Intensive Blood Glucose Control and Vascular Outcomes in Patients with Type 2 Diabetes. N Engl J Med 2008;358(24):2560–72.
26. McGuire DK, Shih WJ, Cosentino F, et al. Association of SGLT2 Inhibitors With Cardiovascular and Kidney Outcomes in Patients With Type 2 Diabetes: A Meta-analysis. JAMA Cardiol 2021;6(2):148–58.
27. Kristensen SL, Rørth R, Jhund PS, et al. Cardiovascular, mortality, and kidney outcomes with GLP-1 receptor agonists in patients with type 2 diabetes: a systematic review and meta-analysis of cardiovascular outcome trials. Lancet Diabetes Endocrinol 2019;7(10):776–85.
28. Schjoedt KJ, Rossing K, Juhl TR, et al. Beneficial impact of spironolactone in diabetic nephropathy. Kidney Int 2005;68(6):2829–36.
29. Bakris GL, Agarwal R, Anker SD, et al. Effect of Finerenone on Chronic Kidney Disease Outcomes in Type 2 Diabetes. N Engl J Med 2020;383(23):2219–29.
30. Pitt B, Filippatos G, Agarwal R, et al. Cardiovascular Events with Finerenone in Kidney Disease and Type 2 Diabetes. N Engl J Med 2021;385(24):2252–63.
31. Frampton JE. Finerenone: First Approval. Drugs 2021;81(15):1787–94.
32. Rawshani A, Rawshani A, Franzén S, et al. Risk Factors, Mortality, and Cardiovascular Outcomes in Patients with Type 2 Diabetes. N Engl J Med 2018;379(7):633–44.
33. The ASCEND Study Collaborative Group. Effects of Aspirin for Primary Prevention in Persons with Diabetes Mellitus. N Engl J Med 2018;379(16):1529–39.
34. Eikelboom JW, Connolly SJ, Bosch J, et al. Rivaroxaban with or without Aspirin in Stable Cardiovascular Disease. N Engl J Med 2017;377(14):1319–30.
35. Sharif S, Van der Graaf Y, Cramer MJ, et al. Low-grade inflammation as a risk factor for cardiovascular events and all-cause mortality in patients with type 2 diabetes. Cardiovasc Diabetol 2021;20(1):220.
36. Ridker PM, Everett BM, Thuren T, et al. Antiinflammatory Therapy with Canakinumab for Atherosclerotic Disease. N Engl J Med 2017;377(12):1119–31.
37. Tardif JC, Kouz S, Waters DD, et al. Efficacy and Safety of Low-Dose Colchicine after Myocardial Infarction. N Engl J Med 2019;381(26):2497–505.
38. Wing RR, Bolin P, Brancati FL, et al, Look AHEAD Research Group. Cardiovascular effects of intensive lifestyle intervention in type 2 diabetes. N Engl J Med 2013;369(2):145–54.
39. Franz MJ, MacLeod J, Evert A, et al. Academy of Nutrition and Dietetics Nutrition Practice Guideline for Type 1 and Type 2 Diabetes in Adults: Systematic Review

of Evidence for Medical Nutrition Therapy Effectiveness and Recommendations for Integration into the Nutrition Care Process. J Acad Nutr Diet 2017;117(10): 1659–79.

40. Franz MJ, Boucher JL, Rutten-Ramos S, et al. Lifestyle weight-loss intervention outcomes in overweight and obese adults with type 2 diabetes: a systematic review and meta-analysis of randomized clinical trials. J Acad Nutr Diet 2015; 115(9):1447–63.

41. Estruch R, Ros E, Salas-Salvadó J, et al. Primary Prevention of Cardiovascular Disease with a Mediterranean Diet Supplemented with Extra-Virgin Olive Oil or Nuts. N Engl J Med 2018;378(25):e34.

42. Siervo M, Lara J, Chowdhury S, et al. Effects of the Dietary Approach to Stop Hypertension (DASH) diet on cardiovascular risk factors: a systematic review and meta-analysis. Br J Nutr 2015;113(1):1–15.

43. American Diabetes Association Professional Practice Committee. 5. Facilitating Behavior Change and Well-being to Improve Health Outcomes: Standards of Medical Care in Diabetes—2022. Diabetes Care 2021;45(Supplement_1): S60–82.

44. Zhu B, Quinn L, Kapella MC, et al. Relationship between sleep disturbance and self-care in adults with type 2 diabetes. Acta Diabetol 2018;55(9):963–70.

45. Shan Z, Ma H, Xie M, et al. Sleep Duration and Risk of Type 2 Diabetes: A Meta-analysis of Prospective Studies. Diabetes Care 2015;38(3):529–37.

46. 4. Comprehensive Medical Evaluation and Assessment of Comorbidities: Standards of Medical Care in Diabetes-2022. - Abstract - Europe PMC. Available at: https://europepmc.org/article/med/34964869. Accessed July 1, 2022.

47. Tonstad S, Lawrence D. Varenicline in smokers with diabetes: A pooled analysis of 15 randomized, placebo-controlled studies of varenicline. J Diabetes Investig 2017;8(1):93–100.

48. Hill-Briggs F, Adler NE, Berkowitz SA, et al. Social Determinants of Health and Diabetes: A Scientific Review. Diabetes Care 2020;44(1):258–79.

49. Falkentoft AC, Zareini B, Andersen J, et al. Socioeconomic position and first-time major cardiovascular event in patients with type 2 diabetes: a Danish nationwide cohort study. Eur J Prev Cardiol 2022;28(16):1819–28.

50. Kim SH, Lee A. Health-Literacy-Sensitive Diabetes Self-Management Interventions: A Systematic Review and Meta-Analysis. Worldviews Evid Based Nurs 2016;13(4):324–33.

51. Palmas W, March D, Darakjy S, et al. Community Health Worker Interventions to Improve Glycemic Control in People with Diabetes: A Systematic Review and Meta-Analysis. J Gen Intern Med 2015;30(7):1004–12.

52. Twohig-Bennett C, Jones A. The health benefits of the great outdoors: A systematic review and meta-analysis of greenspace exposure and health outcomes. Environ Res 2018;166:628–37.

53. Walzer D, Gordon T, Thorpe L, et al. Effects of Home Particulate Air Filtration on Blood Pressure. Hypertension 2020;76(1):44–50. https://doi.org/10.1161/HYPERTENSIONAHA.119.14456.

54. Peterson GCL, Hogrefe C, Corrigan AE, et al. Impact of Reductions in Emissions from Major Source Sectors on Fine Particulate Matter-Related Cardiovascular Mortality. Environ Health Perspect 2020;128(1):17005.

55. Sarkar S, Orimoloye OA, Nass CM, et al. Cardiovascular Risk Heterogeneity in Adults with Diabetes: Selective Use of Coronary Artery Calcium in Statin Use Decision-making. J Gen Intern Med 2019;34(11):2643–7.

56. Malik S, Zhao Y, Budoff M, et al. Coronary Artery Calcium Score for Long-term Risk Classification in Individuals With Type 2 Diabetes and Metabolic Syndrome From the Multi-Ethnic Study of Atherosclerosis. JAMA Cardiol 2017;2(12): 1332–40.
57. Ahlqvist E, Storm P, Käräjämäki A, et al. Novel subgroups of adult-onset diabetes and their association with outcomes: a data-driven cluster analysis of six variables. Lancet Diabetes Endocrinol 2018;6(5):361–9.
58. Riddle MC, Cefalu WT, Evans PH, et al. Consensus Report: Definition and Interpretation of Remission in Type 2 Diabetes. Diabetes Care 2021;44(10):2438–44.
59. Hounkpatin H, Stuart B, Farmer A, et al. Association of type 2 diabetes remission and risk of cardiovascular disease in pre-defined subgroups. Endocrinol Diabetes Metab 2021;4(3):e00280.

Nonalcoholic Fatty Liver Disease

Scott Isaacs, MD[a,b,*]

KEYWORDS

- NAFLD • NASH • Steatohepatitis • Cirrhosis • Metabolic syndrome
- Type 2 diabetes • Obesity • FIB-4

KEY POINTS

- Management of nonalcoholic fatty liver disease (NAFLD) is essential for type 2 diabetes (T2D) remission because there is shared pathophysiology of insulin resistance and lipotoxicity.
- NAFLD has two subtypes: nonprogressive, NAFL and progressive, nonalcoholic steatohepatitis (NASH) that can advance to fibrosis, cirrhosis, and hepatocellular carcinoma.
- The leading cause of mortality in persons with NAFLD is atherosclerotic cardiovascular disease, followed by cancer and liver disease.
- The goal in NAFLD diagnosis is to determine who has progressive NAFLD and assess risk for clinically significant fibrosis.
- Treatments aimed at preventing advanced liver disease (ie, weight loss, medications) can also lead to T2D remission.

INTRODUCTION

The diagnosis and treatment of nonalcoholic fatty liver disease (NAFLD) is an essential component of type 2 diabetes (T2D) remission. NAFLD prevalence has risen over the last five decades paralleling obesity and T2D. T2D and NAFLD share common pathophysiology mediated through insulin resistance and lipotoxicity. NAFLD is the leading cause of chronic liver disease globally commonly associated with visceral adiposity, dysglycemia, atherogenic dyslipidemia, and hypertension. NAFLD is a hypernym that includes the entire spectrum of fatty liver disease from simple steatosis to progressive steatosis with inflammation, fibrosis, cirrhosis, and hepatocellular carcinoma (HCC). The diagnosis of NAFLD is made by excluding significant alcohol use or secondary causes of hepatic steatosis and/or elevated aminotransferases (**Box 1**).[1–3] NAFLD has two subtypes: the nonprogressive form—nonalcoholic fatty liver (NAFL)—and the progressive form—nonalcoholic steatohepatitis (NASH). NAFL or

[a] Emory University School of Medicine, 775 Johnson Ferry Rad. NE, Atlanta, GA 30342, USA;
[b] Atlanta, GA, USA
* 775 Johnson Ferry Rd. NE, Atlanta, GA 30342
E-mail address: drisaacs@atlantaendocrine.com
Twitter: @scottisaacsmd (S.I.)

Endocrinol Metab Clin N Am 52 (2023) 149–164
https://doi.org/10.1016/j.ecl.2022.06.007
0889-8529/23/© 2022 Elsevier Inc. All rights reserved.

endo.theclinics.com

Box 1
Secondary causes of hepatic steatosis and/or elevated aminotransferases

Secondary Causes of Hepatic Steatosis
- Excessive alcohol consumption[a]
  - >21 drinks/week (men)
  - >14 drinks/week (women)
- Hepatitis C (genotype 3)
- Lipodystrophy (congenital or acquired)
- Acute weight loss (bariatric surgery, starvation)
- Malnutrition
- Parenteral nutrition
- Abetalipoproteinemia
- Reye's syndrome
- Pregnancy associated
  - HELLP syndrome
  - Acute fatty liver of pregnancy
- Medications (eg, corticosteroids, mipomersen, lomitapide, amiodarone, methotrexate, tamoxifen, valproate, antiretroviral medicines)
- Rare causes: autoimmune hepatitis, Alpha-1 antitrypsin deficiency, Wilson syndrome, other

Additional Causes of Elevated Aminotransferases
- Medications, vitamins, supplements
- Viral hepatitis (A, B, C)
- Endocrine disorders (hyper- or hypothyroidism, Cushing syndrome, hypogonadism, growth hormone deficiency, Addison's disease, other)
- Hemochromatosis
- Autoimmune hepatitis
- Primary biliary cholangitis
- Alpha-1 antitrypsin deficiency
- Budd–Chiari syndrome
- Mass lesions

Laboratory Evaluation
- Hepatitis C
  - HCV antibody with reflex testing HCV RNA
- Additional tests to consider:
  - Hepatitis B: HBsAg, HBsAb, HBcAb
  - ANA
  - AMA
  - ASMA
  - Immunoglobulins
  - Ferritin
  - A1AT

The diagnosis of NAFLD is made by excluding significant alcohol use or secondary causes of hepatic steatosis and/or elevated aminotransferases. Liver ultrasound is not required to diagnose hepatic steatosis in high-risk patients (eg, T2D, obesity, metabolic syndrome) after ruling out secondary causes of liver disease.

[a]A standard alcoholic drink is 12 ounces of regular beer, 5 ounces of wine, or 1.5 ounces of distilled spirits (∼14 g of pure alcohol).

Abbreviations: A1AT, alpha-1 antitrypsin; AMA, antimitochondrial antibodies; ANA, antinuclear antibodies; ASMA, antismooth muscle antibodies; HBcAb, hepatitis B core antibody; HBsAb, hepatitis B surface antigen; HBsAg, hepatitis B surface antigen; HCV, hepatitis C virus; HELLP, Hemolysis, elevated liver enzymes, and low platelet count.

Data from Refs.[2,3]

simple steatosis is defined histologically as hepatic triglyceride accumulation in > 5% of hepatocytes, mild or no inflammation, and no evidence of hepatocyte injury. NASH entails progressive liver injury with steatosis, significant lobular inflammation, liver cell swelling and degeneration (ballooning), and hepatocyte necrosis. Early NASH can progress to fibrotic NASH, cirrhosis, and HCC although the process is not always linear, and HCC can develop in the absence of fibrosis or cirrhosis. Fibrosis is staged F0–F4 based on histologic criteria with stage ≥F2 considered clinically significant fibrosis (**Fig. 1** and **Tables 1** and **2**). The risk of liver-related mortality increases exponentially with increasing fibrosis stage.[3-5]

Lean Nonalcoholic Fatty Liver Disease

The definition of lean NAFLD is the presence of hepatic steatosis with a body mass index (BMI) < 25 kg/m^2 or < 23 kg/m^2 in Asian populations. The prevalence of lean NAFLD is 10%–40% with the highest rates in Asian populations. The term "lean" may be misleading because the definition is based solely on BMI. Most patients with lean NAFLD have "metabolic obesity" with increased visceral fat, insulin resistance, and components of the metabolic syndrome. The development of lean NAFLD also stems from a lipodystrophic state with insufficient adipocyte storage capacity. Patients with inherited or acquired lipodystrophy represent the most extreme form of lean NAFLD with minimal to no subcutaneous fat and severe hepatic steatosis.[5]

Metabolic-Associated Fatty Liver Disease

Since the term NASH was first coined by Ludwig and colleagues[6] in 1980, the nomenclature using the word "nonalcoholic" has remained the same. Metabolic-associated fatty liver disease (MAFLD) has been proposed as an overarching term to replace the NAFLD because it better reflects the complex and disparate pathogenesis resulting in different NAFLD phenotypes. From a patient's perspective, the term "NAFLD" may trivialize the condition and is pejorative. The term "nonalcoholic" is not appropriate for children, presuming alcohol-related liver disease is not typically seen in the pediatric population. Currently, MAFLD is not an official term, although it is used informally.[7]

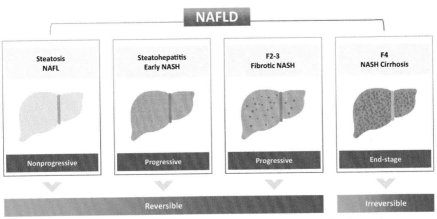

Fig. 1. The spectrum of nonalcoholic fatty liver disease. NAFLD includes the entire spectrum of fatty liver disease from the NAFL to progressive steatosis (NASH) with associated inflammation and fibrosis, which can lead to cirrhosis, and HCC.

Table 1 Stages of fibrosis		
F0	No Fibrosis	
F1	Mild fibrosis	(Perisinusoidal or Periportal fibrosis)
F2	Moderate fibrosis	(Perisinusoidal and Portal/Periportal fibrosis)
F3	Precirrhosis	(Bridging fibrosis)
F4	Cirrhosis	

Fibrosis is staged F0–F4 based on histologic criteria with stage $\geq$F2 considered clinically significant fibrosis.

Adapted from Cusi K, Isaacs S, Barb D, et al. American Association of Clinical Endocrinology Clinical Practice Guideline for the Diagnosis and Management of Nonalcoholic Fatty Liver Disease in Primary Care and Endocrinology Clinical Settings: Co-Sponsored by the American Association for the Study of Liver Diseases (AASLD). Endocr Pract. 2022;28(5):528-562.

NATURAL HISTORY OF NONALCOHOLIC FATTY LIVER DISEASE

The transition from NAFL to NASH is nonlinear and can be highly variable and dynamic. The trajectory of progression is influenced by an interaction of genetics, epigenetics, environment, lifestyle, microbiota, and cardiometabolic risk factors, such as T2D, hypertension, and dyslipidemia. Persons with NAFL experience slow progression, advancing one fibrosis stage in approximately 14 years. Those with NASH typically have faster progression, advancing one fibrosis stage in 7 years. However, approximately one in five persons with NASH is rapid progressor, advancing to cirrhosis in 10 years. Predictors of rapid progression have not been fully elucidated, but include higher alanine aminotransferase (ALT) levels, presence of T2D (especially if poorly controlled), family history of cirrhosis, and genetic susceptibility.

Approximately, 20%–30% of persons with NAFLD have NASH, and of those, about 20%–30% will progress to cirrhosis over the next 30–40 years. Rates of NASH-related HCC have been increasing over the past decade. People with advanced fibrosis or cirrhosis have an approximately 1.5%–2% risk of developing HCC per year. Therefore, patients with advanced fibrosis or NASH cirrhosis should be screened for HCC every 6 months by ultrasound (US) with or without alpha-fetoprotein measurement.

Table 2 Effect of diabetes medications on nonalcoholic fatty liver disease			
Medication	Hepatic Steatosis	Steatohepatitis	Fibrosis
Pioglitazone	Decreased	Decreased	Decreased
GLP-1 RA	Decreased	Decreased	Unknown
SGLT2 inhibitors	Decreased	Unknown	Unknown
DPP-IV inhibitors	Unchanged	Unknown	Unknown
Metformin	Unchanged	Neutral	Unknown
Insulin	Decreased	Neutral	Unknown

T2D medications and their efficacy for the treatment of hepatic steatosis, steatohepatitis, and fibrosis.

Adapted from Cusi K, Isaacs S, Barb D, et al. American Association of Clinical Endocrinology Clinical Practice Guideline for the Diagnosis and Management of Nonalcoholic Fatty Liver Disease in Primary Care and Endocrinology Clinical Settings: Co-Sponsored by the American Association for the Study of Liver Diseases (AASLD). Endocr Pract. 2022;28(5):528-562.

Progression to HCC occurs in persons with noncirrhotic NAFLD at rates higher than other types of chronic liver disease.[8]

The leading cause of mortality in persons with NAFLD is atherosclerotic cardiovascular disease (ASCVD), followed by cancer and liver disease. The risk of all-cause, liver-related, and cardiovascular mortality is increased with all stages of NAFLD and is highest with advanced fibrosis. ASCVD risk may be increased as high as 10-fold in NAFLD, regardless of fibrosis stage when compared to those without NAFLD. Stage 2 fibrosis is the tipping point where liver-related mortality begins to increase exponentially with the increasing fibrosis stage.[9] When cirrhosis develops, the liver disease becomes the most common cause of mortality. NASH is now the second most common indication for liver transplants and is expected to surpass viral hepatitis as the leading indication within the next 10 years.[4,10,11]

EPIDEMIOLOGY OF NONALCOHOLIC FATTY LIVER DISEASE

25% of the worldwide population is estimated to have NAFLD. The prevalence varies among the different geographic areas of the world. The highest rates of NAFLD are in the Middle East and South America, and the lowest in Africa. The prevalence of NAFLD in the United States increased from 20% in 1988–1994 to 32% in 2012–2016. Currently, 80–100 million persons in the United States have NAFLD. Further, NAFLD is more common in the Hispanic population and less common in the African-American population. The increasing rates of NAFLD are also observed in children and adolescents in the United States and globally, including in Europe, China, India, and other areas. In a recent prospective evaluation of the prevalence of NAFL and NASH in a large middle-aged US cohort, it was found that 38% had NAFL, 14% had NASH, and 6% had significant liver fibrosis.[4,5,8,12,13]

NONALCOHOLIC FATTY LIVER DISEASE AND TYPE 2 DIABETES

The prevalence of NAFLD in T2D is as high as 90% when assessed with sensitive methods of detecting steatosis, such as controlled attenuation parameter (CAP) or MRI techniques. Earlier studies underestimated the prevalence of hepatic steatosis in T2D because they used less sensitive screening with US or transaminase levels.[1] NAFLD causes hepatic insulin resistance and hyperglycemia, which increases the risk of developing T2D by more than twofold and makes diabetes more difficult to control. The prevalence of NASH in T2D is from 30% to 40%, which is two- to three-fold the prevalence in the general population. Those with NASH have a higher risk of developing T2D, which is further enhanced in persons with advanced liver fibrosis.[1,5,14–16]

Having T2D doubles the risk of hepatic steatosis. T2D is the leading predictor of liver-related morbidity and mortality while also increasing the risk of ASCVD. T2D doubles the risk of both cirrhosis and HCC. Patients with T2D plus additional components of the metabolic syndrome have a fivefold increased risk of HCC and having a BMI > 35 kg/m^2 quadruples the risk. Central adiposity independent of BMI heightens the risk for HCC, revealing the importance of assessing waist circumference as a metabolic risk factor for HCC.[1,15,17]

COMORBIDITIES ASSOCIATED WITH NONALCOHOLIC FATTY LIVER DISEASE

The risk of ASCVD goes up with increasing severity of NAFLD although patients at lower risk for fibrosis remain at high risk for ASCVD. In a prospective observational study, the risk for cardiovascular events was 4.5 times greater in patients with a Fibrosis-4 Index (FIB-4) > 2.67 compared to those with an FIB-4 ≤ 2.67.[18] Other cardiac manifestations include an increased risk for early heart failure, atrial fibrillation, and ventricular arrhythmias. NAFLD is associated with an increased risk for comorbidities, including sarcopenia, gallstone disease, chronic kidney disease, obstructive sleep apnea, polycystic ovary syndrome, osteoarthritis, and extrahepatic malignancies (stomach, pancreas, and lung).[8] Although a normal liver contains fat, hepatic steatosis (>5% liver fat) is considered "ectopic" fat. Similar pathophysiology leads to ectopic fat in other organs: muscle (myosteatosis), heart (pericardial fat), vasculature (perivascular fat), pancreas (nonalcoholic fatty pancreatic disease), and kidney (fatty kidney disease).[5] Associations between NAFLD and other endocrinopathies have been reported, including type 1 diabetes, growth hormone deficiency, hypogonadism, and hypothyroidism. However, these appear to be mainly due to insulin resistance and visceral adiposity, in some cases, a result of the underlying endocrinopathy.[1]

PATHOPHYSIOLOGY OF NONALCOHOLIC FATTY LIVER DISEASE

The complex and disparate pathogenesis of NAFLD is influenced by an interaction of multiple factors. The result is insufficient adipocyte storage capacity, offloading of free fatty acids into the circulation, and ectopic accumulation of fat (**Fig. 2**).[4,19]

Calorie Excess

Excess calories from any source are the building blocks for NAFLD. High-calorie diets, particularly overconsumption of fructose, fuel hepatic steatosis. Fructose is especially pathogenic because it induces hepatic insulin resistance and de novo lipogenesis. Major sources of fructose include high fructose corn syrup and table sugar (sucrose is 50% fructose and 50% glucose). Insufficient physical activity affects energy balance and increases risk for NAFLD independent of BMI.

Insulin Resistance

The insulin resistance phenotype with central obesity (increased visceral fat and less gluteofemoral fat) and decreased muscle mass, contributes to the development of NAFLD and the risk for fibrosis. Insulin resistance induces lipotoxicity, disrupts lipid

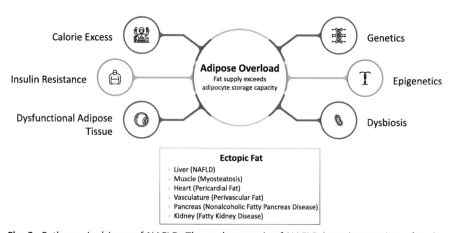

Fig. 2. Pathogenic drivers of NAFLD. The pathogenesis of NAFLD is an interaction of multiple factors that lead to overwhelming adipocyte storage capacity resulting in ectopic accumulation of fat in the liver and other organs, such as muscle, heart, vasculature, pancreas, and kidney.

metabolism, and causes systemic inflammation, increased proinflammatory cyto-kines, increased hepatokines, decreased adiponectin levels, oxidative stress, mito-chondrial dysfunction, and endothelial dysfunction. Hyperglycemia increases de novo lipogenesis. The common pathophysiology of insulin resistance leading to T2D and NAFLD is reciprocally harmful, leading to more severe disease and comorbidities.

Dysfunctional Adipose Tissue

Adipose tissue biology plays a critical role in the development of NAFLD by deter-mining adipocyte storage capacity. There is a spectrum of lipodystrophic states from mild to severe. Adipose tissue dysfunction predominates as a pathogenic contributor in lean NAFLD, especially in Asian populations. The gene variant trans-membrane 6 superfamily member 2 (TM6SF2) (related to lipid metabolism in hepato-cyte Golgi) is associated with lean NAFLD. Patients with inherited or acquired lipodystrophy represent the most severe manifestation of insufficient adipocyte stor-age capacity with minimal to no subcutaneous fat and severe ectopic fat accumulation in the liver and other organs.

Genetics

Genetics affect the entire spectrum of NAFLD including body weight, appetite, insulin resistance, adipocyte biology, steatosis, development of fibrosis, cirrhosis, and HCC. Several genetic risk variants related to hepatic lipid metabolism are associated with NAFLD. The most studied is patatin-like phospholipase domain-containing 3 (PNPLA3), which regulates hepatocyte lipid droplet remodeling. The PNPLA3 rs738409 (C>G) gene polymorphism increases the risk for progression cirrhosis and HCC and is more prevalent in Hispanic populations. Other genes associated with NAFLD include TM6SF2, MBOAT7, and GCKR. The HSD17B13 gene variant is thought to be protective.

Epigenetics

Epigenetic factors associated with the development of NAFLD include intrauterine exposure to a high-fat diet, intrauterine growth retardation, and accelerated fetal growth.

Dysbiosis

Alterations in gut-microbiome-bile acids lead to a decrease in microbial diversity with a shift toward more Gram-negative microbes. NAFLD has been associated with higher Enterobacteriaceae, *Streptococcus*, and *Velonella* and lower Faecalibacterium, *Rumi-noccus*, and *Lactobacillus*.

DIAGNOSIS OF NONALCOHOLIC FATTY LIVER DISEASE

Most persons with NAFLD are asymptomatic or have nonspecific complaints, such as fatigue or vague right upper quadrant pain. An imaging study is not necessary for routine clinical diagnosis, although many cases are discovered incidentally with US, computed tomography (CT), or MRI. A firm or nodular liver and/or splenomegaly may be detected on physical examination, which can indicate advanced liver disease. There may be elevations in serum aminotransferases where ALT is usually higher than serum aspartate aminotransferase (AST). However, aminotransferases are normal in 70% of persons with NAFLD and should not be used alone for diagnosis. In advanced fibrosis, the ratio of AST to ALT may reverse with higher AST levels. A decreased platelet count may occur because of splenic sequestration and decreased hepatic

---

Box 2
Clinical features of advanced liver disease

Physical Examination:
  Ascites
  Asterixis
  Caput medusae
  Clubbing
  Dupuytren's contracture
  Epigastric vascular murmur
  Gynecomastia
  Jaundice
  Nodular liver
  Palmer erythema
  Spider angiomata
  Splenomegaly
  White nails

Laboratory:
  Elevated AST/ALT ratio
  Elevated PT/INR
  Low albumin
  Low platelets

A significant number of patients with liver fibrosis is asymptomatic or have nonspecific complaints. Clinical assessment of NAFLD includes physical examination and laboratory evaluation for signs of advanced liver disease.

Data from Kanwal F, Shubrook JH, Adams LA, et al. Clinical Care Pathway for the Risk Stratification and Management of Patients With Nonalcoholic Fatty Liver Disease. Gastroenterology. 2021;161(5):1657-1669.

---

production of thrombopoietin. As liver disease progresses, there may be evidence of hepatic synthetic dysfunction with decreased serum albumin and increased prothrombin time (**Box 2**).[1,4]

Imaging to detect hepatic steatosis includes US, CT, MRI, and CAP. The two most sensitive methods to detect steatosis are proton magnetic resonance spectroscopy (^{1}H-MRS) and LiverMultiScan MRI-proton density fat fraction (PDFF) (MRI-PDFF) mainly used in research settings. Because NAFLD is extremely common, the diagnostic challenge is not assessing liver fat, but rather the risk for significant fibrosis, which represents the burden of clinical disease. High-risk groups that should be screened for NAFLD include those who have overweight or obesity, T2D, or components of the metabolic syndrome (**Box 3**). Patients with persistently elevated AST or ALT > 30 IU/L for more than 6 months or those with hepatic steatosis on any imaging modality should also be considered high risk. Patients have a higher risk for cirrhosis with T2D or prediabetes, age > 50, BMI >40 kg/m^2, increasing number of metabolic risk factors, or a family history of NASH.[1,20]

The best initial screening test is FIB-4, which is a simple score calculated using a person's age, AST, ALT, and platelet count (**Box 4**). FIB-4 is the most validated test among many others studied to this end. FIB-4 can predict changes over time in hepatic fibrosis and allows risk stratification for future liver-related morbidity and mortality. Patients with a FIB-4 < 1.3 are considered low risk and those with FIB-4 $\geq$ 2.67 are at high risk for clinically significant fibrosis. A FIB-4 between 1.3 and 2.67 is the indeterminate risk where additional noninvasive testing can be done to further assess risk. Those at low risk should have the FIB-4 repeated every year and focus on traditional cardiometabolic risk reduction. Those at high risk should be referred to a liver

---

Box 3
Components of the metabolic syndrome (NCEP ATP III)

Waist Circumference
> >40 inches in men
> >35 inches in women

Triglycerides ≥150 mg/dL

HDL-Cholesterol
> <40 mg/dL in men
> <50 mg/dL in women

Blood pressure ≥130/≥85 mm Hg

Fasting glucose ≥100 mg/dL (prediabetes)

Components of the metabolic syndrome include increased blood pressure, dysglycemia, central adiposity, and low HDL cholesterol or high triglyceride levels. NAFLD is considered the hepatic manifestation of the metabolic syndrome. Having more components of the metabolic syndrome increases the risk of clinically significant liver fibrosis.

Adapted from Grundy SM, Cleeman JI, Daniels SR, et al. Diagnosis and management of the metabolic syndrome: an American Heart Association/National Heart, Lung, and Blood Institute Scientific Statement [published correction appears in Circulation. 2005 Oct 25;112(17):e297] [published correction appears in Circulation. 2005 Oct 25;112(17):e298]. Circulation. 2005;112(17):2735-2752.

---

specialist for management of liver disease, and continuing cardiometabolic disease management by the primary care or endocrinology team (**Fig. 3**).[1,2,5,11]

NONINVASIVE TESTS

For those with an indeterminate FIB-4, a second noninvasive test should be performed to increase predictive value. The sequential use of noninvasive tests (NITs) maintains sensitivity and specificity while enabling the classification of a larger proportion of patients. NITs to assess risk for fibrosis include serologic markers and imaging modalities (**Fig. 4**).[1,5,11]

Serologic Markers

Simple serologic markers
Simple serologic markers include NAFLD fibrosis score, AST/ALT ratio, and AST-to-Platelet Ratio Index (APRI) although none offer a clear advantage over FIB-4.

Box 4
The FIB-4 Index

FIB-4 = Age (years) × AST (U/L)/[PLT (10^9/L) × ALT ½ (U/L)

<1.3 Low risk

1.3–2.67 Indeterminate risk

≥2.67 High risk

Online calculator: https://www.mdcalc.com/fibrosis-4-fib-4-index-liver-fibrosis.

The FIB-4 index is calculated using a person's age, AST, ALT, and platelet count to assess risk for advanced fibrosis and future liver-related morbidity and mortality.

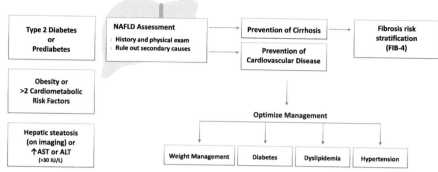

Fig. 3. High-Risk patients for the development of NAFLD. High-risk groups for NAFLD should be evaluated with history and physical exam. Secondary causes of hepatic steatosis should be ruled out. Screen patients with the FIB-4 index, which predicts risk for cirrhosis. Prevention of ASCVD includes weight management and optimizing treatments for diabetes, hypertension, and dyslipidemia. (*Adapted from* Cusi K, Isaacs S, Barb D, et al. American Association of Clinical Endocrinology Clinical Practice Guideline for the Diagnosis and Management of Nonalcoholic Fatty Liver Disease in Primary Care and Endocrinology Clinical Settings: Co-Sponsored by the American Association for the Study of Liver Diseases (AASLD). Endocr Pract. 2022;28(5):528-562.)

Complex serologic markers

Complex serologic markers include enhanced liver fibrosis (ELF), Fibrosure, NIS4 (NASHnext), and Pro-C3. The ELF test is a quantitative biomarker panel that has been approved by The United States Food and Drug Administration (FDA) in 2021 for prognostic risk assessment. The test combines three biomarkers involved in fibrosis and extracellular matrix turnover (hyaluronic acid, tissue inhibitors of metalloproteinase 1, and procollagen III N-terminal peptide). The ELF test estimates the rate of liver extracellular matrix metabolism reflecting the severity of liver fibrosis. An ELF score of <7.7 indicates low risk for fibrosis, a score of 7.7–9.8 indicates indeterminate or moderate risk, and a score of ≥9.8 is high risk. ELF score at baseline and change over time is associated with clinical outcomes and disease progression.

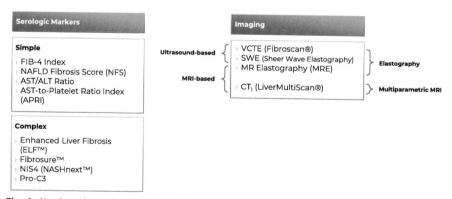

Fig. 4. Noninvasive tests to evaluate fibrosis risk. Noninvasive tests to assess risk for clinically significant fibrosis include serologic markers (simple and complex) and imaging modalities (ultrasound-based or MRI-based technologies).

Imaging Modalities

Vibration controlled transient elastography (Fibroscan®)

Vibration controlled transient elastography (VCTE) measures two parameters to assess liver fat and liver fibrosis. CAP, expressed in decibel per meter accurately quantifies liver fat and is correlated to liver steatosis. The liver stiffness measurement (LSM) is an indirect measurement of liver fibrosis based on elastography and is expressed in kilopascal (kPa). LSM < 8 kPa means the liver is soft and fibrosis risk is low. LSM > 12 kPa indicates a stiff liver with a high risk for fibrosis. LSM 8–12 kPa is considered indeterminate. Advantages of VCTE are that it is an inexpensive point of care test and is supported by a large body of literature. The disadvantage of VCTE is that it is less accurate in cases of mild fibrosis and in persons with a BMI > 40.

Shear wave elastography

Shear wave elastography is a liver stiffness assessment based on elastography and liver volume visualization. Ultrasound waves are pulsed into the liver to generate a shear wave that is measured by assessing tissue displacement. This test is newer and less well-validated.

Magnetic resonance elastography

MR elastography uses technology that combines MRI imaging with low-frequency vibrations to quantitatively assess the mechanical properties of tissues providing an indication of liver stiffness. MR elastography is expensive and has limited availability; so, it is ordered primarily by the liver specialist.

LiverMultiScan

LiverMultiScan is a multiparametric MRI to noninvasively quantify liver fat and assess disease activity. It uses standard MRI technology analyzed with proprietary software. Three parameters are assessed. The most useful of these is corrected T1 (cT1) imaging, which quantifies liver fibrosis and inflammation. The PDFF is a highly sensitive quantification of hepatic steatosis, and T2 assesses iron content of the liver. LiverMultiScan is not confounded by body habitus and is accurate at high BMI levels. LiverMultiScan was FDA approved in 2015 to detect early liver disease. The test is becoming increasingly available and is covered by most insurance payors.

Liver Biopsy

Liver biopsy remains the gold standard to establish a diagnosis of NASH, fibrosis, and cirrhosis and to rule out other causes of liver disease. Limitations are cost, risk of bleeding, pain, and sampling variability. Liver biopsy results vary with concordance rates < 70%. Although the trend has been moving away from doing liver biopsies, it can be considered when there is diagnostic doubt, suspicion of advanced liver disease, or a need to rule out other causes of liver disease. A liver biopsy can be performed at the same time as bariatric surgery when clinically indicated.

MANAGEMENT

Aggressive management of NAFLD plays a vital role in T2D remission by reducing hepatic insulin resistance and lipotoxicity. Currently, there are no FDA-approved medications available to treat NAFLD. Therefore, treatment must focus on weight loss by any means and medications with proven benefits in NAFLD (**Fig. 3**). These treatments not only improve NAFLD but can lead to T2D remission. Reduction in hepatic steatosis is seen with a minimum of 5% weight loss and even greater liver histologic and cardiometabolic improvements, including fibrosis resolution with a minimum of 10% weight loss. Management includes recommending minimal or abstinence from alcohol and vaccines for patients with chronic liver disease [Hepatitis A, Hepatitis B, Pneumococcal polysaccharide (PPSV23)].[1,2]

Limitations of the Literature

There are limitations of the current literature for NAFLD treatment modalities. Although many lifestyle studies have been published, sample sizes are small, and none have extended longer than 1 year. Randomized controlled trials to assess the efficacy of pioglitazone are from 2 years to 3 years and glucagon-like peptide 1 receptor agonists (GLP-1 RAs) for 1.5 years. Open-label trials with sodium-glucose cotransporter 2 (SGLT2) inhibitors have used noninvasive endpoints and have not been done with paired biopsies to assess the effect on liver histology.

NONPHARMACOLOGIC TREATMENT OPTIONS: LIFESTYLE MODIFICATION

Lifestyle modification is the cornerstone of any plan for T2D remission, weight management, and liver health. Although alcohol consumption is discouraged, drinking $\geq$ 2 cups of caffeinated coffee each day is recommended because it reduces the risk of liver fibrosis in several liver diseases, including NAFLD. Dietary guidance includes adherence to a low-calorie diet with restriction of saturated fat and sugar (especially fructose) and improved eating patterns (eg, Mediterranean diet, minimally processed whole foods). Even without weight loss, a better-quality dietary composition has been shown to improve liver histology. A structured weight loss program is preferred, when possible, tailored to the individual's lifestyle and personal preferences. Although the effect on weight is small, physical activity is a key component of lifestyle modification and overall cardiometabolic health. Exercise is critical for weight loss maintenance and has benefits on visceral fat and liver fat that are independent of weight loss. Liver benefits from exercise are from adherence and intensity rather than a specific type of exercise.[1,2,4,21]

PHARMACOLOGIC TREATMENT OPTIONS
Diabetes Medications

Several medications that can induce remission of T2D can also improve NAFLD. GLP-1 RAs, pioglitazone, and SGLT2 inhibitors are preferred for T2D patients who have NAFLD because of the reduction in hepatic steatosis and cardiovascular benefits. GLP-1 RA and pioglitazone have demonstrated benefits on liver histology. Pioglitazone improves insulin resistance, adipose tissue dysfunction, dyslipidemia, reduces the risk of ASCVD, and prevents the progression of prediabetes to T2D. Pioglitazone improves NASH in patients with or without diabetes. Side effects of pioglitazone include weight gain, edema, osteoporosis, heart failure, and bladder cancer. The clinical benefits of GLP-1 RAs include weight loss, diabetes control, reduction in CKD, and cardiovascular risk reduction. GLP-1 RA treatment reduces hepatic steatosis, ALT and AST levels, and improves liver histology, including resolution of NASH but not fibrosis. Side effects of GLP-1 RAs include gastrointestinal symptoms, nausea, and risk for pancreatitis or medullary thyroid carcinoma. SGLT2 inhibitors reduce hepatic steatosis by creating energy deficit through glycosuria that leads to weight loss and decreased de novo lipogenesis. Studies are limited and there is no evidence of benefit for steatohepatitis. SGLT2 inhibitors reduce ASCVD, heart failure, and chronic kidney disease. The most common side effects of SGLT2 inhibitors are genital yeast infections and increased urination. Severe side effects can be euglycemic diabetic ketoacidosis, and Fournier's gangrene. Although metformin has been shown to

Table 3
Antiobesity medications

Antiobesity Medication	Doses (Increase Dose as Clinically Indicated)	Potential Side Effects/Considerations
Approved for chronic use:		
Orlistat	60–120 mg TID	Steatorrhea, flatulence, fecal incontinence Must adhere to a low-fat diet
Phentermine/Topiramate-ER	Starting dose 3.75 mg/23 mg qd × 14 d Initial treatment dose 7.5 mg/46 mg qd Titration dose 11.25/69 mg qd × 14 d Maximum dose 15 mg/92 mg qd	Restlessness, insomnia, headache, dry mouth, tachycardia, BP elevation, paresthesia, dysgeusia, kidney stones, mood changes, mental clouding, blurred vision Avoid in pregnancy, uncontrolled hypertension or hyperthyroidism
Naltrexone-ER/Bupropion-ER	Starting dose one 8 mg/90 mg tablet qd Titrated to treatment dose 2 tablets bid (32 mg/360 mg daily)	Nausea, vomiting, constipation, headache, fatigue, mood changes, agitation, insomnia, blurred vision, dry mouth Avoid if history of seizure, uncontrolled hypertension, opioid use
Liraglutide	Starting dose 0.6 mg daily sc injection Titrate to maximum dose 3 mg/d	Nausea, vomiting, diarrhea, constipation, headache, fatigue, tachycardia, pancreatitis, gallbladder disease Avoid if history of MTC or MEN2
Semaglutide	Starting dose 0.25 mg weekly sc injection Titrate to maximum dose 2.4 mg/wk	Nausea, vomiting, diarrhea, constipation, headache, fatigue, tachycardia, pancreatitis, gallbladder disease Avoid if history of MTC or MEN2
Approved for short-term use:		
Phentermine	Low dose: 8 mg/d Maximum dose: 37.5 mg/d	Restlessness, insomnia, headache, dry mouth, tachycardia BP elevation. Avoid in ASCVD, uncontrolled hypertension

Antiobesity medications should be considered as an adjunct to lifestyle modification in NAFLD patients with BMI > 27 kg/m^2 (or > 25 kg/m^2 in Asian populations).

reduce the risk for HCC in patients with T2D, there is no evidence that metformin, acarbose, DPP-IV inhibitors, or insulin improve NAFLD, but these medications should be continued as needed for appropriate diabetes management (Table 3).[1,2,22–24]

Antiobesity Medications

Weight loss with any of the FDA-approved antiobesity medications can improve NAFLD and induce remission of T2D by reducing overall fat mass. Medications for the chronic treatment of obesity include phentermine/topiramate ER, naltrexone/bupropion ER, orlistat, liraglutide, and semaglutide. Antiobesity medications are approved for individuals with comorbidity of obesity and BMI > 27 kg/m^2. When combined with lifestyle modification, medication-assisted weight loss is 7%–18% at one year. Greater initial weight loss tends to result in better long-term outcomes. GLP-1 RAs are preferred weight loss agents because of the liver benefits previously discussed. Of the medications approved for obesity treatment, semaglutide has the best efficacy in attaining 10, 15, and even ≥20% weight loss in some patients **(Table 3)**.[1]

Statins

Statins are indicated for ASCVD risk reduction and are safe for patients with NAFLD. Some studies have shown that statins improve liver enzymes. However, there is not enough data to support the use of statins for specifically treating NAFLD.[25]

Vitamin E

Vitamin E 800 IU daily improves liver histology in nondiabetic adults with NASH. Risks include an increase in mortality, stroke, and prostate cancer risk. Vitamin E is not recommended in patients with T2D, NAFLD without a liver biopsy, NASH cirrhosis, or cryptogenic cirrhosis.[24]

BARIATRIC SURGERY

Bariatric surgery is highly effective for the remission of T2D and NAFLD because it can achieve the greatest amount of sustained weight loss. Bariatric surgery has been shown to improve or resolve steatosis, fibrosis, and reduction in risk of HCC. In addition, bariatric surgery improves other comorbidities, such as hypertension, sleep apnea, and atherogenic dyslipidemia, and reduces the risk of cardiovascular disease. In a recent study, bariatric surgery, compared with nonsurgical management, was associated with an 88% lower risk of major adverse liver outcomes and a 70% reduction in adverse cardiovascular events.[21,26]

SUMMARY

Owing to common pathophysiology, management of NAFLD is essential for T2D remission. NAFLD is the leading cause of chronic liver disease and is soon to be the most common indication for a liver transplant. Because symptoms are vague and liver enzyme levels are usually normal, many patients with clinically significant liver fibrosis remain undiagnosed. Patients at highest risk for progressive NAFLD are those having T2D, prediabetes, overweight or obesity, components of the metabolic syndrome, steatosis on any imaging study or persistently elevated AST or ALT > 30 IU/L. One should screen high-risk patients with FIB-4 followed by additional NITs as needed. NAFLD treatments parallel strategies for T2D remission, including optimization of weight, glucose, blood pressure, and lipids.

CLINICS CARE POINTS

- Nonalcoholic fatty liver disease (NAFLD) and type 2 diabetes (T2D) have a detrimental bidirectional relationship with shared pathophysiology where each condition exacerbates the other.
- Treating NAFLD reduces hepatic insulin resistance and lipotoxicity, which is necessary for T2D remission.
- NAFLD is a hypernym that includes the entire spectrum of fatty liver disease from simple steatosis to progressive steatosis with inflammation and fibrosis, which can lead to cirrhosis and hepatocellular carcinoma.
- T2D is the most important risk factor for advanced liver disease.
- The leading cause of mortality in persons with NAFLD is atherosclerotic cardiovascular disease, followed by cancer and liver disease.
- Stage 2 fibrosis is the tipping point where liver-related mortality begins to increase exponentially with the increasing fibrosis stage.
- The goal of NAFLD diagnosis is to determine which patients have progressive NAFLD, at risk for advanced liver disease.
- Individuals with high-risk NAFLD include T2D, prediabetes, obesity or overweight, metabolic syndrome, steatosis on any imaging study, or persistently elevated aspartate aminotransferase or alanine aminotransferase greater than 30 IU/L.
- High-risk individuals should be screened for fibrosis risk with Fibrosis-4 followed by additional noninvasive tests for indeterminate scores.
- Treatments for NAFLD also help with T2D remission and focus on weight loss by any means and medications with proven benefits.

DISCLOSURE

The author has nothing to disclose.

REFERENCES

1. Cusi K, Isaacs S, Barb D, et al. American association of clinical endocrinology (AACE) clinical practice guideline for the diagnosis and management of non-alcoholic fatty liver disease in primary care and endocrinology settings. Endocr Pract 2022;28(5):528–62.
2. Kanwal F, Shubrock J, Adams L, et al. Clinical care pathway for the risk stratification and management of patients with nonalcoholic fatty liver disease. Gastroenterology 2021;161(5):1657–69.
3. Chalasani N, Younossi Z, Lavine J, et al. The diagnosis and management of nonalcoholic fatty liver disease: practice guidance from the American association for the study of liver diseases. Hepatology 2018;67:328–57.
4. Diehl A, Day C. Cause, pathogenesis, and treatment of nonalcoholic steatohepatitis. N Engl J Med 2017;377(21):2063–72.
5. Younossi A, Henry L. Fatty liver through the ages: nonalcoholic steatohepatitis. Endocr Pract 2022;28(2):204–13.
6. Ludwig J, Viggiano T, McGill D, et al. Nonalcoholic steatohepatitis: mayo clinic experiences with a hitherto unnamed disease. Mayo Clin Proc 1980;55(7):434–8.
7. Eslam M, Sanyal A, George J, et al. MAFLD: a consensus-driven proposed nomenclature for metabolic associated fatty liver Disease. Gastroenterology 2020;158(7):1999–2014.e1.

8. Loomba R, Friedman S, Shulman G, et al. Mechanisms and disease consequences of nonalcoholic fatty liver disease. Cell 2021;184(10):2537–64.

9. Dulai P, Singh S, Patel J, et al. Increased risk of mortality by fibrosis stage in nonalcoholic fatty liver disease: systematic review and meta-analysis. Hepatology 2017;65(5):1557–65.

10. Simon T, Roelstraete B, Khalili H, et al. Mortality in biopsy-confirmed nonalcoholic fatty liver disease: results from a nationwide cohort. Gut 2021;70(7):1375–82.

11. Younossi Z, Corey K, Alkhouri N, et al. Clinical assessment for high-risk patients with non-alcoholic fatty liver disease in primary care and diabetology practices. Aliment Pharmacol Ther 2020;52(3):513–26.

12. Harrison S, Gawrieh S, Roberts K, et al. Prospective evaluation of the prevalence of non-alcoholic fatty liver disease and steatohepatitis in a large middle-aged US cohort. J Hepatol 2021;75(2):284–91.

13. Younossi Z, Golabi P, de Avila L, et al. The global epidemiology of NAFLD and NASH in patients with type 2 diabetes: a systematic review and meta-analysis. J Hepatol 2019;71(4):793–801.

14. Bril F, Cusi K. Management of Nonalcoholic fatty liver disease in patients with type 2 diabetes: a call to action. Diabetes Care 2017;40(3):419–30.

15. Cusi K. A Diabetologist's Perspective of Non-alcoholic Steatohepatitis (NASH): knowledge gaps and future directions. Liver Int 2020;40(Suppl 1):82–8.

16. Lomonaco H, Leiva E, Bril F, et al. Advanced liver fibrosis is common in patients with type 2 diabetes followed in the outpatient setting: the need for systematic screening. Diabetes Care 2021;44(2):399–406.

17. Cusi K. Time to include nonalcoholic steatohepatitis in the management of patients with type 2 diabetes. Diabetes Care 2020;43(2):275–9.

18. Baratta F, Pastori D, Angelico F, et al. Nonalcoholic fatty liver disease and fibrosis associated with increased risk of cardiovascular events in a prospective study. Clin Gastroenterol Hepatol 2020;18(10):2324–31.e4.

19. Khan R, Bril F, Cusi K, et al. Modulation of insulin resistance in nonalcoholic fatty liver disease. Hepatology 2019;70(2):711–24.

20. Grundy S, Cleeman J, Daniels S, et al. Diagnosis and management of the metabolic syndrome: an American Heart Association/National Heart, Lung, and Blood Institute scientific statement. Circulation 2005;112:2735–52.

21. Hannah W, Harrison S. Effect of weight loss, diet, exercise, and bariatric surgery on nonalcoholic fatty liver disease. Clin Liver Dis 2016;20(2):339–50.

22. Budd J, Cusi K. Role of agents for the treatment of diabetes in the management of nonalcoholic fatty liver disease. Curr Diab Rep 2020;20(11):59.

23. Chavez C, Cusi K, Kadiyala S. The emerging role of glucagon-like peptide-1 receptor agonists for the management of NAFLD. J Clin Endocrinol Metab 2022;107(1):29–38.

24. Sanyal A, Chalasani N, Kowdley K, et al. Pioglitazone, vitamin E, or placebo for nonalcoholic steatohepatitis. N Engl J Med 2010;362(18):1675–85.

25. Kargiotis K, Athyros V, Giouleme O, et al. Resolution of non-alcoholic steatohepatitis by rosuvastatin monotherapy in patients with metabolic syndrome. World J Gastroenterol 2015;21(25):7860–8.

26. Aminan A, Al-Kurd A, Wilson R, et al. Association of bariatric surgery with major adverse liver and cardiovascular outcomes in patients with biopsy-proven nonalcoholic steatohepatitis. JAMA 2021;326(20):2031–42.

Remission in Ketosis-Prone Diabetes

Nupur Kikani, MD[a], Ashok Balasubramanyam, MD[b],*

KEYWORDS

- Atypical diabetes • Remission • Diabetic ketoacidosis • Beta-cell • C-peptide
- Ketosis-prone diabetes • Autoantibodies • Insulin

KEY POINTS

- Ketosis-prone diabetes (KPD) is a heterogenous syndrome increasingly described in racial and ethnic groups worldwide and characterized by patients who present with diabetic ketoacidosis (DKA) but lack the typical characteristics of autoimmune type 1 diabetes (T1D).
- A large proportion of patients with the A-β+ form of KPD, especially those whose index episode of DKA does not have an identifiable precipitating factor (denoted "unprovoked A-β+ KPD"), have substantial beta-cell functional reserve and can attain insulin-free remission for prolonged periods of time.
- We propose criteria for insulin-free remission in patients with unprovoked A-β+ KPD to comprise: HbA1c <6.5% with a fasting C-peptide-to-glucose ratio of greater than 11 nmol/mmol ×100 at least 6 months after the index episode of DKA, and at least 3 consecutive months off insulin therapy.
- Following the declaration of insulin-free remission, clinical and biochemical surveillance should be performed routinely, with periodic measurements of HbA1c and C-peptide as well as standard monitoring for diabetic complications.

INTRODUCTION

Clinical heterogeneity within all forms of diabetes, and within type 2 diabetes (T2D) in particular, challenges our current classification systems, diagnostic categories, and treatment paradigms.[1] The emergence of atypical forms of diabetes that do not fit standard definitions of autoimmune type 1 diabetes (T1D) or T2D, with phenotypes ranging from severe insulin deficiency to severe insulin resistance including syndromic and monogenic forms, have given rise to the concept that diabetes includes a spectrum of etiologically different conditions leading to hyperglycemia.[1] Within this

a Department of Endocrine Neoplasia and Hormonal Disorders, University of Texas MD Anderson Cancer Center, Unit 1461, 1515 Holcombe Boulevard, Houston, TX 77030, USA; b Division of Diabetes, Endocrinology, and Metabolism, Baylor College of Medicine, BCM 179A, One Baylor Plaza, Houston, TX 77030, USA
* Corresponding author. ashokb@bcm.edu
E-mail address: ashokb@bcm.edu

Endocrinol Metab Clin N Am 52 (2023) 165–174
https://doi.org/10.1016/j.ecl.2022.06.005
0889-8529/23/© 2022 Elsevier Inc. All rights reserved.

Abbreviations	
KPD	Ketosis-prone diabetes

spectrum of "atypical" diabetes are conditions whose natural histories include periods of partial or complete remission. Understanding the characteristics and pathophysiology of these conditions could inform our understanding of the factors associated with remission in common forms of T2D.

Examples of partial remission can be found among heterogeneous forms of KPD, characterized by patients who present with DKA, often at the time of initial diabetes diagnosis, but lack the typical features or traditional biomarkers of autoimmune T1D.[2] This emerging group of conditions has been noted across different ethnic and racial populations including West African, South Asian, US Hispanic, South American, Native American, Middle Eastern, African American, and Afro-Caribbean populations.[3-19] A specific subgroup of patients with KPD have shown a unique propensity towards prolonged remission from insulin dependence following the index episode of DKA. In this review, we discuss the characteristics of the subgroups of KPD, define and interpret the concept of remission within the relevant subgroup, attempt to delineate predictors of remission, and present strategies for clinical monitoring during remission and relapse in KPD.

CHARACTERISTICS OF KETOSIS-PRONE DIABETES

Initially described in a smattering of case reports from West Africa and the Caribbean,[20,21] KPD is now widely recognized across ethnic and racial groups.[2-18] Based on quantitative measurements and longitudinal analysis, a prospectively validated 2x2 factorial classification scheme based on biomarkers of islet autoimmunity and beta-cell functional reserve defines distinct phenotypes of KPD.[22] This Aβ classification scheme uses islet cell autoantibody positivity or negativity and evidence-based cutoffs for beta-cell functional reserve to classify patients who present with DKA into four distinct KPD subgroups: A-β+ (antibody negative and beta-cell function present), A-β- (antibody negative and beta-cell function absent), A+β+ (antibody-positive and beta-cell function present), and A+β- (antibody-positive and beta-cell function absent).[22] Of the groups defined by this approach, the A-β+ and A-β- groups represent atypical forms of diabetes, as they present with DKA despite lacking the biomarkers that traditionally define autoimmune T1D.

Although community prevalence rates of the KPD subgroups cannot be defined in a rigorous epidemiologic manner given a bias in the ascertainment of the patients (after presentation to a hospital with DKA), their frequencies in a US adult, multiethnic, urban population appear to be: 50% A-β+, 20% A-β-, 20% A+β-, and 10% A+β+.[22] The two subgroups in which beta-cell function is absent (β-) are typically lean, have early onset of diabetes, and remain insulin-dependent.[22] The A+β-subgroup is synonymous with autoimmune T1D. Although clinical characteristics of the A-β- subgroup of KPD are similar to those of the A+β- subgroup, they lack islet cell autoantibodies and have lower frequencies of human leukocyte antigen (HLA) alleles associated with susceptibility to T1D.[22] Approximately 25% of those in the A-β- KPD subgroup have likely pathogenic variants in genes encoding hepatocyte nuclear factor-1α (HNF1α) and pancreas-duodenum homeobox-1 (PDX-1), which are essential transcription factors for beta-cell development and function.[23] Another 25% of patients with A-β- have T-cell reactivity to islet cell autoantigens despite lacking evidence for humoral autoimmunity in the form of the classic circulating T1D autoantibodies.[24]

In the β+ subgroups of KPD, patients are overweight or obese, with later onset of diabetes and significant beta-cell functional reserve.[22] Those with A+β+ KPD have a late-onset, slowly developing form of autoimmune diabetes, with a predilection to the DPD epitope-specific glutamic acid decarboxylase 65 autoantibody (GAD65-Ab) and a higher frequency of DPD-specific anti-idiotypic antibodies[25,26] than patients with autoimmune T1D, and coexpression of both high-risk and protective T1D HLA class II alleles.[22]

Patients with A-β+ KPD are phenotypically similar to patients with T2D, with the striking difference that they present with DKA. A-β+ KPD is unique amongst the four subgroups of KPD in that a significant proportion experience a kind of partial remission of diabetes, at least from insulin dependence. These patients can discontinue insulin therapy 1 to 2 months following the index DKA episode due to their substantial beta-cell functional reserve,[22] which remarkably is present even during an acute episode of DKA.[27] Approximately half of the patients with A-β+ KPD are able to maintain adequate glycemic control on oral medications (usually with metformin alone, and sometimes just with lifestyle management) for many years[2] indicating sustained preservation of their beta-cell function. The other half of patients with A-β+ KPD experience only a brief period of insulin independence after the index DKA episode followed by progressive beta-cell function decline and relapse to insulin dependence.[28] Analysis has shown that those who relapse quickly (usually in less than 1 year) to insulin dependence typically have a known precipitating cause of their index DKA, denoted "provoked" DKA. On the other hand, patients with A-β+ KPD who are able to maintain glycemic control without ketosis on oral agents alone for many years have "unprovoked" DKA (ie, their index DKA occurred in the absence of any clinically apparent stressor such as infection, trauma, or acute systemic decompensation). Unprovoked A-β+ KPD patients display male predominance, greater obesity, later age of onset, and lack of HLA class II T1D susceptibility alleles or T-cell reactivity to islet autoantigens.[24,28] Detailed plasma metabolomics and kinetic studies reveal that patients with unprovoked A-β+ KPD have defects in branch chain amino acid metabolism leading to excessive ketone production and defective ketone oxidation,[29] and in arginine/citrulline/glutamine metabolic pathways leading to blunted beta-cell responsiveness during sustained hyperglycemia.[29,30] Together, these defects result in a proclivity to developing ketoacidosis without a clinically identifiable precipitating factor.

DEFINITION AND INTERPRETATION OF REMISSION IN UNPROVOKED A-β+ KPD

Remission has been well described in patients with T2D resulting from short-term pharmacologic therapy[31–33] or significant changes in body weight loss and nutritional intake,[34,35] and most dramatically after bariatric surgery.[36–38] All of these interventions may result in the achievement of prolonged normoglycemia early in the course of T2D due to partial recovery of insulin secretion and sensitivity.[39]

The concept of remission was formally described by the American Diabetes Association (ADA) in their consensus guidelines in 2009 after recognizing the need for terminology describing improvement in glycemia among patients with T2D.[40] Remission is defined as "abatement or disappearance of the signs and symptoms" of diabetes.[40] Three categories of remission were proposed: partial, complete, and prolonged. Partial remission was defined as hyperglycemia below diagnostic thresholds for diabetes (HbA1c <6.5% (<48 mmol/mol) or fasting plasma glucose (FPG) level 100 to 125 mg/dL (5.6–6.9 mmol/L)) without glucose-lowering pharmacotherapy for at least 1 year. Complete remission was defined by the maintenance of normal glucose levels

(HbA1c "normal" and FPG <100 mg/dL (<5.6 mmol/L)) without pharmacotherapy for 1 year. Prolonged remission was defined as complete remission that persisted for 5 years or more without pharmacotherapy.[40]

An expert group was convened by the ADA in 2019 to refine the definition of remission in T2D and provide guidance for treatment and intervention.[41] The revised guidelines suggest that remission is not equivalent to the absence of evidence of disease. This concept reflects our understanding that the pathophysiology of the disease, including both deficiency of insulin and insulin resistance, is rarely fully normalized by any current interventions.[41–44] The group also proposed that a single definition of remission is optimal in lieu of the previous distinctions of partial, complete and prolonged remissions.[41] Our investigations into the pathophysiology of unprovoked A-β+ KPD also support the notion that key underlying metabolic defects (abnormal branch chain amino acid catabolism and mild elevation of serum beta-hydroxybutyrate level) persist even after the patients have achieved near-normoglycemia or normoglycemia without insulin therapy after the index DKA.[29]

In the context of KPD, we favor a definition that focuses specifically on prolonged remission from insulin dependence in patients with unprovoked A-β+ KPD following the index episode of DKA.[28] Defining this phenomenon by poorly characterized concepts such as a "honeymoon period" (as sometimes applied to patients early in the course of autoimmune T1D) is inappropriate and inadequate: first, this phenomenon occurs in patients who do not have the phenotype of T1D, but rather have substantial beta-cell function both during[27] and after[22] an episode of DKA; and second, the patients experience many months to years of near-normoglycemia without insulin. Remission in "usual" T2D is defined by the cessation of all glucose-lowering agents for a sufficient interval "to allow waning of the drug's effects and to assess the effect of the absence of drugs on HbA1c values.[41]" This absolute therapeutic criterion may be too stringent to define remission in patients with unprovoked A-β+ KPD, as physicians are reluctant to discontinue all pharmacotherapy in patients who have experienced an episode of DKA. A modified therapeutic definition of remission in A-β+ KPD as freedom from insulin therapy is meaningful in that it indicates sufficiently preserved capacity of their beta-cell function to overcome the metabolic limitations imposed by systemic insulin resistance and excessive generation of ketones. Moreover, as the Aβ classification system has been shown to have a high predictive value in regard to the capacity to become insulin-independent while maintaining excellent glycemic control,[45] patients classified as unprovoked A-β+ KPD can undergo a safe and practicable protocol to discontinue insulin therapy.

DIAGNOSIS OF REMISSION IN KPD

Riddle and colleagues proposed HbA1c less than 6.5% (48 mmol/mol) sustained for at least 3 months after discontinuing antihyperglycemic agents as criteria for the definition of remission in T2D.[41,46–48] Alternative defining criteria were explored, including measures of FPG, 2-hour plasma glucose level during an oral glucose tolerance test, and mean daily glucose measured by continuous glucose monitor (CGM). For patients in whom the HbA1c may not be accurate (eg, due to variant hemoglobins, disease states that impact erythrocyte survival, differing rates of glycation), 24-h mean glucose concentration by CGM and glucose management indicator (GMI, a calculated estimate of HbA1c from CGM data) were proposed as alternatives.[41,49,50] Continuous glucose monitoring is a valuable tool to identify patterns of glycemic variability[51,52] that may not be revealed by HbA1c measurements.[53,54] At least three FPG levels less than 126 mg/dL (7.0 mmol/L) could be used as an alternative criterion for remission.[41] The

2-h plasma glucose level following a 75 g oral glucose challenge was found to be sub-optimal in diagnosing remission of T2D.[41]

We propose modified criteria for remission in the context of KPD. We suggest criteria for insulin-free remission in unprovoked A-β+ KPD to comprise: HbA1c <6.5% (ADA cutoff for the diagnosis of diabetes[55]) with a fasting C-peptide-to-glucose ratio of greater than 11 nmol/mmol x100 at least 6 months after the index episode of DKA, and at least 3 consecutive months off insulin therapy.[56] These cutoffs are based on our published analysis of factors associated with successful insulin discontinuation in a cohort of 106 patients with "β+" KPD followed with repeated measurements of HbA1c, fasting glucose, fasting C-peptide measurements and insulin requirements for 915 ± 375 days.[56] This definition might represent "partial remission" as most patients who met the above criteria continued to receive oral glucose-lowering therapy (mainly metformin monotherapy).

PREDICTORS OF DIABETES REMISSION IN KPD

As described above, the majority of new-onset unprovoked patients with A-β+ KPD have sufficient beta-cell functional reserve to attain insulin-free remission.[22,28] Highly significant factors that predict successful insulin discontinuation with sustained glycemic control are the occurrence of unprovoked DKA at initial diagnosis of diabetes, a C-peptide-to-glucose ratio greater than 11 nmol/mmol x 100 and HbA1c <7% measured at least 6 months after the index DKA.[56]

HLA class II alleles associated with T1D also influence beta-cell functional status in patients with KPD.[57] Nalini and colleagues demonstrated that alleles associated with resistance to autoimmune T1D were present at a higher frequency among KPD subgroups with preserved beta-cell function. In particular, the resistance allele DQB1*0602 was more frequent in patients with β+ than patients with β- KPD suggesting a possible effect of this allele in protecting beta-cell function.[57] A follow-up study showed that among patients with A-β+ KPD, those with unprovoked DKA had a higher frequency of DQB1*0602, whereas those with provoked DKA had higher frequencies of the T1D susceptibility alleles DQB*0302 and DRB1*04.[28] Collectively, these data suggest that possession of the DQB1*0602 HLA class II allele and absence of T1D-associated susceptibility alleles are associated with prolonged preservation of beta-cell function and unprovoked A-β+ KPD status. Hence, HLA testing or possibly a T1D polygenic risk score could help in assessing the propensity to remission in patients with KPD.

FOLLOW-UP AND SURVEILLANCE DURING REMISSION

Routine surveillance is necessary to ensure that hyperglycemia or DKA does not recur in patients with KPD. Lifestyle modifications with an emphasis on weight reduction and a low-calorie diet should be recommended and remain an important pillar of therapy, regardless of remission status.[58] In addition to measurements of islet autoantibodies, fasting glucose levels and HbA1c, serum C-peptide measurements should be obtained 2 to 4 months after the index episode of DKA if the patient is clinically stable and near-normoglycemic. If the fasting C-peptide level is > 1 ng/mL (0.33 nmol/L) or the peak C-peptide level 5 to 10 minutes after intravenous administration of 1 mg glucagon is > 1.5 ng/mL (0.5 nmol/L), and all islet autoantibodies are negative, the patient may be designated "A-β+ KPD." Attempts to wean patients so designated off insulin may then be initiated.[2,22,59] We have established the following protocol: if the patient's fasting and premeal capillary blood glucose levels are consistently less than 130 mg/dL and bedtime glucose levels are less than 180 mg/dL, the total daily insulin dose is decreased by 50%.[58] The patient is monitored for hyperglycemia and ketosis. If capillary blood glucose levels rise above 200 mg/dL, an oral glucose-lowering drug such as metformin[58,59] is initiated. If glucose levels remain at goal at two consecutive visits, insulin is discontinued. If hyperglycemia recurs without ketosis, additional oral pharmacotherapy is initiated. If ketosis occurs at any point during a reduction in insulin doses, the insulin regimen is intensified and the patient is no longer considered a candidate for insulin discontinuation.

Long-term management should include frequent clinic follow-up and management of metabolic syndrome. Standards of diabetes care should be maintained in these patients. Patients with A-β+ may relapse to unprovoked hyperglycemia and ketosis 1 to 10 years after diagnosis, with a median time to relapse of about 4 years.[5,60] Predictors of early relapse to hyperglycemia and insulin include younger age at presentation with DKA, lower beta-cell function reserve, and higher HbA1c levels 1 year after the index DKA episode.[60] Thus, close monitoring for relapse is prudent in long-term management of patients with A-β+ KPD who have successfully discontinued insulin therapy. We recommend regular measurement of HbA1c every 3 months and periodic assessment of beta-cell reserve using C-peptide measurements within the first year of diagnosis.[58]

Progression of some chronic complications of diabetes may occur despite improvement in glycemic control in patients with all forms of diabetes.[61–63] Hence patients with KPD in insulin-free remission should continue to be monitored for retinopathy, renal function, neuropathy and blood pressure, lipid and weight control, based on the current guidelines.[41]

SUMMARY

The A-β+ subgroup of KPD provides unique insight into the concept of "remission" in diabetes. Despite initial presentation with DKA, these patients have substantial preservation of beta-cell function and the majority can discontinue insulin therapy, often maintaining remission for years. Measurements of C-peptide levels are essential to predict remission and guide the potential withdrawal of insulin. Research into etiologic factors suggest that in the future, HLA testing, polygenic risk score screening, or targeted metabolomics may assist in predicting the likelihood of insulin-free remission. Further studies into factors associated with metabolic improvement, duration of remission, and clinical markers of relapse are needed to help improve the predictability of this phenomenon. By developing tools to predict remission and relapse, we hope to guide patients with this phenotype of KPD safely toward remission and develop targeted treatment options for their atypical form of diabetes.

CLINICS CARE POINTS

- Patients with A-β+ KPD have sufficient beta-cell functional reserve to attain insulin-free remission. Factors that predict successful insulin discontinuation are the occurrence of unprovoked DKA at initial diagnosis of diabetes, a C-peptide-to-glucose ratio greater than 11 nmol/mmol x 100 and HbA1c <7% measured at least 6 months after the index DKA.

- Measurements of islet autoantibodies, fasting glucose levels, HbA1c and serum C-peptide should be obtained 2 to 4 months after the index episode of DKA. If the fasting C-peptide level is > 1 ng/mL (0.33 nmol/L) or the peak C-peptide level 5 to 10 minutes after intravenous administration of 1 mg glucagon is > 1.5 ng/mL (0.5 nmol/L), and all islet autoantibodies are negative, the patient may be designated "A-β+ KPD." Attempts to wean patients off insulin may then be initiated.

- If the patient's fasting and premeal capillary blood glucose levels are consistently less than 130 mg/dL and bedtime glucose levels are less than 180 mg/dL, the total daily insulin dose is decreased by 50%. The patient is monitored for hyperglycemia and ketosis. If capillary blood glucose levels rise above 200 mg/dL, an oral glucose-lowering drug is initiated. If glucose levels remain at goal at two consecutive visits, insulin is discontinued.

- If hyperglycemia recurs without ketosis, additional oral pharmacotherapy is added. If ketosis occurs at any point during a reduction in insulin doses, the insulin regimen is intensified and the patient is no longer considered a candidate for insulin discontinuation.

- Patients with A-β+ KPD who successfully discontinue insulin therapy may relapse to unprovoked hyperglycemia and ketosis. Predictors of early relapse include young age at presentation with DKA, lower beta-cell function reserve, and higher HbA1c levels 1 year after the index DKA episode. We recommend regular measurement of HbA1c every 3 months and periodic assessment of beta-cell reserve using C-peptide measurements within the first year of diagnosis to monitor for relapse.

DISCLOSURE

The authors have nothing to disclose

ACKNOWLEDGMENTS

Work in the authors' laboratory related to KPD has been supported by NIH grants R01 DK101411 (AB) and R01 DK104832 (AB) and by the Rutherford Chair Fund for Diabetes Research.

REFERENCES

1. Redondo MJ, Balasubramanyam A. Toward an Improved Classification of Type 2 Diabetes: Lessons From Research into the Heterogeneity of a Complex Disease. J Clin Endocrinol Metab 2021;106(12):e4822–33.
2. Balasubramanyam A, Nalini R, Hampe C, et al. Syndromes of ketosis-prone diabetes mellitus. Endocr Rev 2008;29(3):292–302.
3. Balasubramanyam A, Yajnik CS, Tandon N. Non-traditional forms of diabetes worldwide: implications for translational investigation. In: Translational Endocrinology & metabolism: type 2 diabetes Update, in Endocrine Society. Washington D.C: AC Powers; 2011. p. 43–67.
4. Balasubramanyam A, Zern JW, Hyman DJ, et al. New profiles of diabetic ketoacidosis: type 1 vs type 2 diabetes and the effect of ethnicity. Arch Intern Med 1999;159(19):2317–22.
5. Mauvais-Jarvis F, Sobngwi E, Porcher R, et al. Ketosis-prone type 2 diabetes in patients of sub-Saharan African origin: clinical pathophysiology and natural history of beta-cell dysfunction and insulin resistance. Diabetes 2004;53(3):645–53.
6. Gupta RD, Ramachandran R, Gangadhara P, et al. Clinical characteristics, beta-cell dysfunction and treatment outcomes in patients with A-beta+ Ketosis-Prone Diabetes (KPD): The first identified cohort amongst Asian Indians. J Diabetes Complications 2017;31(9):1401–7.
7. Umpierrez GE, Casals MM, Gebhart SP, et al. Diabetic ketoacidosis in obese African-Americans. Diabetes 1995;44(7):790–5.
8. Umpierrez GE, Woo W, Hagopian WA, et al. Immunogenetic analysis suggests different pathogenesis for obese and lean African-Americans with diabetic ketoacidosis. Diabetes Care 1999;22(9):1517–23.

9. Banerji MA. Impaired beta-cell and alpha-cell function in African-American children with type 2 diabetes mellitus–"Flatbush diabetes". J Pediatr Endocrinol Metab 2002;15(Suppl 1):493–501.

10. Banerji MA, Chaiken RL, Huey H, et al. GAD antibody negative NIDDM in adult black subjects with diabetic ketoacidosis and increased frequency of human leukocyte antigen DR3 and DR4. Flatbush diabetes. Diabetes 1994;43(6):741–5.

11. Aizawa T, Katakura M, Taguchi N, et al. Ketoacidosis-onset noninsulin dependent diabetes in Japanese subjects. Am J Med Sci 1995;310(5):198–201.

12. Jabbar A, Farooqui K, Habib A, et al. Clinical characteristics and outcomes of diabetic ketoacidosis in Pakistani adults with Type 2 diabetes mellitus. Diabet Med 2004;21(8):920–3.

13. Kim MK, Lee SH, Kim JH, et al. Clinical characteristics of Korean patients with new-onset diabetes presenting with diabetic ketoacidosis. Diabetes Res Clin Pract 2009;85(1):e8–11.

14. Tan KC, Mackay IR, Zimmet PZ, et al. Metabolic and immunologic features of Chinese patients with atypical diabetes mellitus. Diabetes Care 2000;23(3):335–8.

15. Pinto ME, Villena JE, Villena AE. Diabetic ketoacidosis in Peruvian patients with type 2 diabetes mellitus. Endocr Pract 2008;14(4):442–6.

16. Wilson C, Krakoff J, Gohdes D. Ketoacidosis in Apache Indians with non-insulin-dependent diabetes mellitus. Arch Intern Med 1997;157(18):2098–100.

17. Pitteloud N, Philippe J. Characteristics of Caucasian type 2 diabetic patients during ketoacidosis and at follow-up. Schweiz Med Wochenschr 2000;130(16):576–82.

18. Westphal SA. The occurrence of diabetic ketoacidosis in non-insulin-dependent diabetes and newly diagnosed diabetic adults. Am J Med 1996;101(1):19–24.

19. Ramos-Roman MA, Pinero-Pilona A, Adams-Huet B, et al. Comparison of type 1, type 2, and atypical ketosis-prone diabetes at 4 years of diabetes duration. J Diabetes Complications 2006;20(3):137–44.

20. Dodu SR. Diabetes in the tropics. Br Med J 1967;2(5554):747–50.

21. Oli JM. Remittant diabetes mellitus in Nigeria. Trop Geogr Med 1978;30(1):57–62.

22. Maldonado M, Hampe CS, Gaur LK, et al. Ketosis-prone diabetes: dissection of a heterogeneous syndrome using an immunogenetic and beta-cell functional classification, prospective analysis, and clinical outcomes. J Clin Endocrinol Metab 2003;88(11):5090–8.

23. Haaland WC, Scaduto DI, Maldonado MR, et al. A-beta-subtype of ketosis-prone diabetes is not predominantly a monogenic diabetic syndrome. Diabetes Care 2009;32(5):873–7.

24. Brooks-Worrell BM, Iyer D, Coraza I, et al. Islet-specific T-cell responses and proinflammatory monocytes define subtypes of autoantibody-negative ketosis-prone diabetes. Diabetes Care 2013;36(12):4098–103.

25. Oak S, Gaur LK, Radtke J, et al. Masked and overt autoantibodies specific to the DPD epitope of 65-kDa glutamate decarboxylase (GAD65-DPD) are associated with preserved beta-cell functional reserve in ketosis-prone diabetes. J Clin Endocrinol Metab 2014;99(6):E1040–4.

26. Hampe CS, Nalini R, Maldonado MR, et al. Association of amino-terminal-specific antiglutamate decarboxylase (GAD65) autoantibodies with beta-cell functional reserve and a milder clinical phenotype in patients with GAD65 antibodies and ketosis-prone diabetes mellitus. J Clin Endocrinol Metab 2007;92(2):462–7.

27. Jahoor F, Hsu JW, Mehta PB, et al. Metabolomics profiling of patients with A(-) beta(+) Ketosis-Prone Diabetes during diabetic ketoacidosis. Diabetes 2021;70(8):1898–909.

28. Nalini R, Ozer K, Maldonado M, et al. Presence or absence of a known diabetic ketoacidosis precipitant defines distinct syndromes of "A-beta+" ketosis-prone diabetes based on long-term beta-cell function, human leukocyte antigen class II alleles, and sex predilection. Metabolism 2010;59(10):1448–55.

29. Patel SG, Hsu JW, Jahoor F, et al. Pathogenesis of A(-)beta(+) ketosis-prone diabetes. Diabetes 2013;62(3):912–22.

30. Mulukutla SN, Hsu JW, Gaba R, et al. Arginine Metabolism Is Altered in Adults with A-beta + Ketosis-Prone Diabetes. J Nutr 2018;148(2):185–93.

31. McInnes N, Smith A, Otto R, et al. Piloting a Remission Strategy in Type 2 Diabetes: Results of a Randomized Controlled Trial. J Clin Endocrinol Metab 2017; 102(5):1596–605.

32. Kramer CK, Zinman B, Retnakaran R. Short-term intensive insulin therapy in type 2 diabetes mellitus: a systematic review and meta-analysis. Lancet Diabetes Endocrinol 2013;1(1):28–34.

33. Kramer CK, Zinman B, Choi H, et al. Predictors of sustained drug-free diabetes remission over 48 weeks following short-term intensive insulin therapy in early type 2 diabetes. BMJ Open Diabetes Res Care 2016;4(1):e000270.

34. Gregg EW, Chen H, Wagenknecht LE, et al. Association of an intensive lifestyle intervention with remission of type 2 diabetes. JAMA 2012;308(23):2489–96.

35. Lean ME, Leslie WS, Barnes AC, et al. Primary care-led weight management for remission of type 2 diabetes (DiRECT): an open-label, cluster-randomised trial. Lancet 2018;391(10120):541–51.

36. Rubino F, Nathan DM, Eckel RH, et al. Metabolic Surgery in the Treatment Algorithm for Type 2 Diabetes: A Joint Statement by International Diabetes Organizations. Surg Obes Relat Dis 2016;12(6):1144–62.

37. Schauer PR, Bhatt DL, Kirwan JP, et al. Bariatric Surgery versus Intensive Medical Therapy for Diabetes - 5-Year Outcomes. N Engl J Med 2017;376(7):641–51.

38. Mingrone G, Panunzi S, Gaetano AD, et al. Metabolic surgery versus conventional medical therapy in patients with type 2 diabetes: 10-year follow-up of an open-label, single-centre, randomised controlled trial. Lancet 2021;397(10271): 293–304.

39. White MG, Shaw JA, Taylor R. Type 2 Diabetes: The Pathologic Basis of Reversible beta-Cell Dysfunction. Diabetes Care 2016;39(11):2080–8.

40. Buse JB, Caprio S, Cefalu WT, et al. How do we define cure of diabetes? Diabetes Care 2009;32(11):2133–5.

41. Riddle MC, Cefalu WT, Evans PH, et al. Consensus report: Definition and interpretation of remission in type 2 diabetes. Diabet Med 2022;39(3):e14669.

42. Lim EL, Hollingsworth KG, Aribisala BS, et al. Reversal of type 2 diabetes: normalisation of beta cell function in association with decreased pancreas and liver triacylglycerol. Diabetologia 2011;54(10):2506–14.

43. Taylor R, Al-Mrabeh A, Zhyzhneuskaya S, et al. Remission of Human Type 2 Diabetes Requires Decrease in Liver and Pancreas Fat Content but Is Dependent upon Capacity for beta Cell Recovery. Cell Metab 2018;28(4):547–556 e3.

44. Camastra S, Manco M, Mari A, et al. Beta-cell function in severely obese type 2 diabetic patients: long-term effects of bariatric surgery. Diabetes Care 2007; 30(4):1002–4.

45. Balasubramanyam A, Garza G, Rodriguez L, et al. Accuracy and predictive value of classification schemes for ketosis-prone diabetes. Diabetes Care 2006;29(12): 2575–9.

46. Jeppsson JO, Kobold U, Barr J, et al. Approved IFCC reference method for the measurement of HbA1c in human blood. Clin Chem Lab Med 2002;40(1):78–89.

47. Consensus C. Consensus statement on the worldwide standardization of the hemoglobin A1C measurement: the American Diabetes Association, European Association for the Study of Diabetes, International Federation of Clinical Chemistry and Laboratory Medicine, and the International Diabetes Federation. Diabetes Care 2007;30(9):2399–400.

48. Eur AcTG. EurA1c: The European HbA1c Trial to Investigate the Performance of HbA1c Assays in 2166 Laboratories across 17 Countries and 24 Manufacturers by Use of the IFCC Model for Quality Targets. Clin Chem 2018;64(8):1183–92.

49. Bergenstal RM, Beck RW, Close KL, et al. Glucose Management Indicator (GMI): A New Term for Estimating A1C From Continuous Glucose Monitoring. Diabetes Care 2018;41(11):2275–80.

50. Danne T, Nimri R, Battelino T, et al. International Consensus on Use of Continuous Glucose Monitoring. Diabetes Care 2017;40(12):1631–40.

51. Whyte MB, Joy M, Hinton W, et al. Early and ongoing stable glycaemic control is associated with a reduction in major adverse cardiovascular events in people with type 2 diabetes: A primary care cohort study. Diabetes Obes Metab 2022; 24(7):1310–8.

52. Wang T, Zhang X, Liu J. Long-Term Glycemic Variability and Risk of Cardiovascular Events in Type 2 Diabetes: A Meta-Analysis. Horm Metab Res 2022;54(2): 84–93.

53. Shah VN, DuBose SN, Li Z, et al. Continuous Glucose Monitoring Profiles in Healthy Nondiabetic Participants: A Multicenter Prospective Study. J Clin Endocrinol Metab 2019;104(10):4356–64.

54. Beck RW, Connor CG, Mullen DM, et al. The Fallacy of Average: How Using HbA1c Alone to Assess Glycemic Control Can Be Misleading. Diabetes Care 2017;40(8):994–9.

55. American Diabetes Association Professional Practice C, Draznin B, Aroda VR, et al. 6. Glycemic Targets: Standards of Medical Care in Diabetes-2022. Diabetes Care 2022;45(Suppl 1):S83–96.

56. Maldonado MR, Otiniano ME, Cheema F, et al. Factors associated with insulin discontinuation in subjects with ketosis-prone diabetes but preserved beta-cell function. Diabet Med 2005;22(12):1744–50.

57. Nalini R, Gaur LK, Maldonado M, et al. HLA class II alleles specify phenotypes of ketosis-prone diabetes. Diabetes Care 2008;31(6):1195–200.

58. Gaba R, Mehta P, Balasubramanyam A. Evaluation and management of ketosis-prone diabetes. Expert Rev Endocrinol Metab 2019;14(1):43–8.

59. Vellanki P, Smiley DD, Stefanovski D, et al. Randomized Controlled Study of Metformin and Sitagliptin on Long-term Normoglycemia Remission in African American Patients With Hyperglycemic Crises. Diabetes Care 2016;39(11):1948–55.

60. Gaba R, Gambhire D, Uy N, et al. Factors associated with early relapse to insulin dependence in unprovoked A-beta+ ketosis-prone diabetes. J Diabetes Complications 2015;29(7):918–22.

61. The Diabetes Control and Complications Trial Research Group. Early worsening of diabetic retinopathy in the Diabetes Control and Complications Trial. Arch Ophthalmol 1998;116(7):874–86.

62. Arun CS, Pandit R, Taylor R. Long-term progression of retinopathy after initiation of insulin therapy in Type 2 diabetes: an observational study. Diabetologia 2004; 47(8):1380–4.

63. Ceriello A. The emerging challenge in diabetes: the "metabolic memory. Vascul Pharmacol 2012;57(5–6):133–8.

What Is a Honeymoon in Type 1, Can It Go into Remission?

Anuradha Viswanathan, MBBS[a],*, Jamie R. Wood, MD[b],
Betul A. Hatipoglu, MD[c]

KEYWORDS

• Honeymoon • Remission • T1D • Type 1 diabetes

KEY POINTS

• Many children go into honeymoon phase a few weeks to months after diagnosis of type 1 diabetes.
• Exogenous insulin requirement is significantly reduced while optimal control of blood glucose is maintained during the honeymoon phase.
• The honeymoon phase is thought to result from improved β-cell functioning leading to more endogenous insulin production.
• Type 1 diabetes is a waxing and waning autoimmune process. Improved β-cell functioning is attributed to β-cell rest and increased ability to secrete insulin in residual β cells following exogenous insulin initiation. In addition, there is some β-cell regeneration because of reduction in autoimmune β-cell loss.
• Even a small amount of residual β-cell function is associated with better prognosis, with less risk for severe hypoglycemia and less microvascular complications.

INTRODUCTION

Type 1 diabetes (T1D) is a chronic autoimmune disorder in which β-cell destruction occurs leading to the body's inability to make adequate insulin.[1,2] According to the SEARCH study, the incidence rates of T1D increased in the United States by an estimated 1.4% per year in children and young adults younger than 20 years of age from 2002 to 2012.[3] Genetic and environmental risk factors play a role in this disease.[4] Several markers of autoimmunity, such as insulin antibody, insulinoma-associated

[a] Section for Pediatric Endocrinology, Cleveland Clinic Children's, 9500 Euclid Avenue, R Building- R-3, Cleveland, OH 44195, USA; [b] University Hospitals Cleveland Medical Center, Rainbow Babies and Children's Hospital, Case Western Reserve University, 11100 Euclid Avenue, Cleveland, OH 44106, USA; [c] University Hospitals Cleveland Medical Center, Case Western Reserve University, 11100 Euclid Avenue, Cleveland, OH 44106, USA
* Corresponding author.
E-mail address: viswana2@ccf.org

Endocrinol Metab Clin N Am 52 (2023) 175–185
https://doi.org/10.1016/j.ecl.2022.08.001
0889-8529/23/© 2022 Elsevier Inc. All rights reserved.

antigen-2 antibody, islet cell antibody, zinc transporter 8 antibody, and glutamic acid decarboxylase 65 antibody, have been discovered.[5] The autoimmune process seems to vary by individual with generally a greater number of antibodies conferring a greater risk of developing T1D.[6]

T1D is thought to be a predominantly T cell–mediated process wherein there is an imbalance between T effector (Teff) and T regulatory (Treg) cell function.[7,8] Treg function is thought to be suppressed and, therefore, self-tolerance to β cells in the pancreas is lost, resulting in autoimmune destruction of the β cells.[8] Usually, by the time of diagnosis of clinically overt T1D, significant loss of β-cell function has occurred and only about 20% to 30% residual function is present and C-peptide levels continue to decline after diagnosis.[9,10]

Genetic susceptibility, especially certain HLA markers, is noted to be more prevalent in people that develop T1D. HLA DR4-DQ8 and HLA DR3-DQ2 haplotypes are thought to confer high risk for T1D.[11] There are certain other genetic loci that also play a role in pathogenesis of T1D, such as protein tyrosine phosphatase nonreceptor type 22 (PTPN22), preproinsulin, and interleukin 2 receptor subunit α (IL2RA).[11] Other environmental factors, such as viral infections, are also thought to play a role. Enteroviruses are strong contenders in this category, and research in this field is studying epitopes that might trigger the autoimmune process and vaccines that might prevent the process.[12]

In the first few months after initial diagnosis, there is usually a phase when the body seems to recover some β-cell function, called the honeymoon or partial remission (PR) phase. Although complete remission is rare, PR is more commonly observed and manifests with the reduced need for exogenous insulin while maintaining optimal blood glucose control. Although PR was initially described in 1940 by Jackson and colleagues,[13] the etiopathogenesis of this phase has not been fully described.

Several studies have shown that even a small amount of residual β-cell function leads to decreased incidence of microvascular complications, such as nephropathy and retinopathy.[14] There is also less risk for severe hypoglycemia.[15] Therefore, it is imperative to study and understand the honeymoon phenomenon so interventions can be devised that help preserve β-cell function or reverse autoimmunity.

HONEYMOON PHASE OR PARTIAL REMISSION PHASE

Initially, the predominant view was that after the diagnosis of T1D and commencement of insulin therapy came a phase of "β-cell rest" and a decrease in glucose toxicity that allowed some of the residual β cells in the pancreas to recover and generate insulin again. This view was supported by some studies in β-cell lines, wherein β cells cultured in a medium with elevated glucose concentrations showed decreased ability to secrete insulin, with recovery of insulin-secreting ability after glucose concentration in the medium was reduced. This reduction in secretion seemed to be proportionate to the duration of exposure; a longer duration of exposure was associated with a reduced ability to recover. Permanent loss of insulin-secreting ability was noted with chronic exposure.[16] This is an inadequate explanation because even with continued good control, β-cell dysfunction and reduced ability to make endogenous insulin returns, such that after a few weeks to months, exogenous insulin needs to be increased to control hyperglycemia.

The current prevailing view is that there is a relative quiescent phase in autoimmunity a few weeks to months after diagnosis that results in more functional β-cell mass in the pancreas.[17] Over the last couple of decades, T1D has been regarded as a remitting and relapsing disease with waxing and waning of the autoimmune process until, eventually, near total destruction of β cells occurs.[18]

DIAGNOSIS AND STAGES OF TYPE 1 DIABETES

T1D is diagnosed according to the classic criteria proposed by the American Diabetes Association (**Box 1**).[19] The TrialNet Pathway to Prevention study assessed the natural course of T1D development in at-risk individuals. It has been recognized that T1D starts months to years before overt diagnosis when patients present with classic symptoms of polyuria, polydipsia, nocturia, and weight loss. A long prodrome of a preclinical phase is recognized wherein autoantibodies are present without any dysglycemia. In stage 1, two or more antibodies are present but without any blood glucose abnormalities. In stage 2, dysglycemia is noted, although patients remain asymptomatic, usually until significant fasting hyperglycemia occurs. In stage 3, there is clinically apparent diabetes with classical symptoms of polyuria, polydipsia, and weight loss or when diagnostic criteria are met via oral glucose tolerance test (**Fig. 1**).[20] Although stage 1 may last several years, usually there is an acute decrease in C-peptide levels about 6 to 12 months before diagnosis of T1D. The peak incidence of the honeymoon phase is noted to be about 3 months after diagnosis with an average duration of about 9 months. By about 12 months after diagnosis only about 10% to 11% of new-onset diabetes patients are still in PR.[21]

DEFINITIONS OF THE HONEYMOON PHASE

International Society for Pediatric and Adolescent Diabetes guidelines from 2014 and 2018 defined the honeymoon phase as a period after T1D diagnosis when the insulin dose requirement is less than 0.5 U/kg/d with hemoglobin A_{1c} (HbA_{1c}) level less than 7%.[22,23] The Hvidoere study group proposed a different methodology back in 2008. They defined the honeymoon phase as the period when the calculated insulin dose adjusted HbA_{1c} ($IDAA_{1c}$) is below 9%, calculated based on the following formula:

$IDAA_{1c}$ = Actual A_{1c} + [4 x Total daily dose of insulin (units/kg/d)][24]

This measure was subsequently validated by Anderson and colleagues[25] in a Danish group of 126 children. It has also been used to assess prevalence of the honeymoon phase of T1D and factors associated with this prevalence in various populations.[26,27,28] Yet other studies have used differing definitions of PR, such as International Society for Pediatric and Adolescent Diabetes definition or insulin use of less than 0.3 U/kg body weight/d, or 0.4 U/kg/d with HbA_{1c} values of less than 7.5% or 7%.[29–31]

Box 1
American Diabetes Association criteria for the diagnosis of type 1 diabetes

1. Fasting blood sugar >126 mg/dL (after at least 8 hours of fasting).

2. Random blood sugar >200 mg/dL with overt symptoms, such as polyuria, polydipsia, or nocturia.

3. Fasting blood sugar >126 mg/dL or 2-hour blood sugar >200 mg/dL after a glucose tolerance test (1.75 g/kg up to a maximum dose of 75 g of glucose to be administered in a fasting state).

4. Hemoglobin A_{1c} >6.5% with any of the blood glucose abnormalities noted above.

Data from Chiang JL, Kirkman MS, Laffel LM, Peters AL; Type 1 Diabetes Sourcebook Authors. Type 1 diabetes through the life span: a position statement of the American Diabetes Association. Diabetes Care. 2014;37(7):2034-2054.

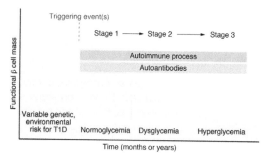

Fig. 1. Stages of T1D. The graph shows functional β-cell mass through the stages of T1D. The blue shaded area shows insulin secretory capacity with time on the x-axis reflecting a broad range ranging from months to years. (*Adapted from* Powers AC. Type 1 diabetes mellitus: much progress, many opportunities. *J Clin Invest.* 2021;131(8):e142242.)

The benefits of using the $IDAA_{1c}$ methodology are that it takes into consideration insulin doses and level of metabolic control, correlates well with C-peptide levels, and is a validated methodology. Although $IDAA_{1c}$ seems to be a useful tool, it is not always used in a busy clinic setting. It uses HbA_{1c} as a surrogate marker of residual C-peptide secretion and, because HbA_{1c} reflects T1D control over the preceding 3 months, it may not always give a true picture of the current situation. Also, this formula correlates with residual C-peptide secretion of about 300 pmol/L. Although this degree of C-peptide production is seen in older children, because of reduced body size and β-cell mass, this might underestimate the prevalence of PR in younger children who may have only lower levels of residual C-peptide production. In addition, this formula does not differentiate between β-cell failure leading to increased insulin use and increased insulin use because of obesity/overweight status that is causing insulin resistance. Therefore, it underestimates the prevalence of PR in obese children, which is especially observed in overweight females in Europe and minority populations in the United States, such as Hispanic and African American populations. Also, baseline HbA_{1c} levels are at least 0.4% higher in African American populations as compared with non-Hispanic White populations for the same mean blood glucose values, which again leads to underestimation of PR prevalence rates.[32] Therefore, further studies are needed to define the honeymoon phase in different racial/ethnic groups and age ranges.

Prevalence of the remission phase varies in different studies. In the Glucose Evaluation Trial for Remission (GETREM) in T1D study in 12 European centers, overall prevalence of clinical remission was noted to be about 22%.[33] Studies from Germany report close to 60% of children with T1D going into remission,[28] whereas studies from the United States show approximately 42% of children going into remission.[27] Other centers from Europe, such as Poland, report about 60% remission rates.[31] The previously mentioned rates are for PR; complete remission, where children are able to stop insulin therapy for at least 2 weeks with HbA_{1c} of less than 6.5%, is extremely rare and mostly limited to case reports. Although some variability in rates is caused by different definitions used in many of these studies, there is also individual variability in the autoimmune process.

FACTORS INFLUENCING THE HONEYMOON PHASE

Various factors have been shown to influence the honeymoon phase in children; **Table 1** describes the main factors. In some studies, older age at diagnosis, male

Table 1
Factors influencing remission rates

Factors	Influence on Remission Rate	Sources
Age at diagnosis	Reduced remission rate in children <5 y of age	26–28,34
Gender	Reduced remission rate in females	27,28,35
Diabetic ketoacidosis at diagnosis	Reduced remission rate in diabetic ketoacidosis: with bicarbonate <15	26–28,34
HbA$_{1c}$ at diagnosis	Uncertain influence	28,34,35
Antibodies	Reduced remission rate in multiple antibodies (>3–4 antibodies)	27,28,30 (no influence of antibodies)

gender, no diabetic ketoacidosis at diagnosis, and low number of autoantibodies have been positively associated with going into remission.

PATHOPHYSIOLOGY AND BIOMARKERS OF REMISSION

The pathophysiology of the remission phase is still being elucidated. Metabolic control and immunologic mechanisms seem to be important. After exogenous insulin initiation and reduction in hyperglycemia, there is some β-cell recovery and increased endogenous insulin production. Also, peripheral insulin resistance is decreased after control of hyperglycemia. It is purported that some degree of β-cell regeneration results from the development of immunologic tolerance. However, with new β-cell regeneration is increased antigen presentation, such that after a while there is renewed autoimmune destruction.[36] The balance eventually shifts to slow continuous β-cell loss and usually about a 40% further reduction of β-cell mass occurs in the first year after diagnosis.[37,38]

BIOMARKERS

Various biomarkers have been studied to assess if the honeymoon phase can be better characterized. Although T1D is predominantly thought to be a T cell–driven process, B lymphocytes and cells of the innate immune system, such as natural killer (NK) cells, are also implicated in the pathogenesis.[39] Several studies have tried to correlate serum levels of various T-lymphocyte subsets and cytokines, but results have been inconsistent. In addition, there has not been a good correlation made between serum levels of these markers and the autoimmune inflammatory process in the pancreas.[40] Although the number of antibodies predict the risk of nonremission with greater than three to four antibodies strongly associated with nonremission, antibody titers do not seem to correlate.

Various studies to assess T-cell characteristics have been performed. In a study by Gomez-Muñoz and colleagues,[41] patients in the PR phase showed increased percentages of effector memory T cells, terminally differentiated effector memory T cells, and neutrophils. Studies have also shown that patients with T1D with the highest frequency of CD4$^+$CD25$^+$CD127Hi Tregs at disease onset are associated with having a longer remission period.[42] Similarly, Fitas and colleagues[43] found decreases in neutrophils, NK cells, T helper 17 (Th17) cells, and T cytotoxic 17 (Tc17) cells at onset of

T1D. During remission, neutrophil counts gradually recovered and were normal when remission was over. NK cell counts continued to remain lower. Th17 and Tc17 followed the pattern of neutrophils. B cells were lowest during remission and Treg cells declined after remission. Low cytokine responders had higher C-peptide levels at onset and longer duration of remission.[43]

In another study, Musthaffa and colleagues[44] found CD4$^+$ T-cell proliferative responses to proinsulin autoantigens to be common before and immediately after T1D diagnosis but declined thereafter. They also noted that after T1D diagnosis, proinsulin$_{33-63}$ specific peripheral blood CD4$^+$ T-lymphocyte proliferation correlated with estimated C-peptide and predicted survival in PR. The association of these cells with future remission shows that they may have some regulatory function with potentially some capability to delay disease progression.[44]

In study by Li and colleagues,[45] programmed cell death-1 (PD-1) and its ligand (PD-L1) were noted to differ in various phases of T1D and were highest during mid-PR. PD-1 and PD-L1 are immunosuppressive molecules that are expressed in activated T and B cells. The authors also noted that PD-1 expression on CD 8$^+$ T cells in the mid-PR phase was positively correlated with remission duration. However, the percentages of circulating Tregs and IL-35$^+$ Tregs showed no relation to PR.[45]

Recently, the concept of T1D endotypes was introduced because of heterogeneity in the pathophysiology of T1D and the variability noted in responses to immunotherapies in clinical trials. This idea is primarily with the understanding that a one drug/therapy approach may not work for everyone and immunomodulatory therapy may need to be tailored to specific endotypes. For example, individuals that develop T1D at a young age seem to have more insulin-reactive B cell in islets. This is associated with rapid progression of T1D and aggressive course with a limited honeymoon phase.[46]

Histologic studies using human donor pancreatic tissue show that autoreactive CD8$^+$ and CD4$^+$ T cells are also in the pancreas of people without diabetes.[7] Intrinsic β-cell factors are thought to act in attracting these autoreactive cells, which were previously ignoring self-antigens, to activate and expand them, thus setting off an autoimmune process. It is not clearly known what cues drive this process, but cytokines, chemokines, oxidative stress, and altered antigen presentation are all thought to play a role.

Cytokines, such as CXCL10 interferons, have been shown in various studies to be recruiters of autoreactive T cells. IL-6 was noted to be expressed by β and α cells of the pancreas in healthy individuals and autoantibody-positive prediabetic individuals but was lower in the pancreas of T1D donors.[47] β-Cell intrinsic events include islet cell hyperexpression of MHC class 1 molecules.[48] Interferon-α induces MHC 1 hyperexpression resulting in activation of cytotoxic CD8$^+$ T cells.[49] Also, viral infections, such as coxsackievirus B and enteroviruses, can induce MHC class 1 hyperexpression.[50] CXCL10 is one of the most important cytokines in the pathogenesis of T1D.[51] CXCR3, the receptor for CXCL10, is observed on proinsulin-specific cells in patients with T1D. Islets of donors without diabetes are devoid of CXCL10 and CXCR3.[52,53]

TREG CELLS

CD4$^+$CD25$^+$FOXP3$^+$ Tregs are important in preventing autoimmunity.[54] In patients with IPEX syndrome, characterized by deficiency of FOXP3 expression, multiple autoimmune disorders are present, and T1D is a prominent feature. CD25 acts as IL-2 sink and deprives T cells of this important growth factor thereby decreasing Teff cell function. Suppression of autoimmunity can also stem from other factors, such as transforming growth factor-β, IL-10, IL-35, and adenosine and expression of molecules, such as lymphocyte activation gene 3 (LAG-3), cytotoxic T lymphocyte associated antigen 4 (CTLA-4), and granzyme B. However, there is a large degree of overlap of FOXP3 Treg function in people with T1D and non-T1D subjects. Only a subgroup of patients with T1D have suppression of Treg function.[55]

Another subset of Tregs, namely, CD4[+]FOXP3[-] cells, called T regulatory 1 (Tr1) cells, which secrete IL-10, are also thought to be important in decreasing islet autoimmunity. In people with T1D, Tregs have unstable FOXP3 expression and, thereby, are less able to control Teff cell proliferation and inflammatory cytokine production.[56] Similarly, IL-10-expressing T cells have been shown to suppress antigen-presenting cells that present self-antigens. In high-risk individuals who do not have T1D, IL-10-secreting T cells are noted to be enhanced.[57] It has been shown that patients with T1D who have higher pancreatic IL-10-expressing T cells have less aggressive autoimmunity, as evidenced by slow progression and fewer numbers of autoantibodies and have later age of onset and superior glycemic control.[58]

EFFORTS TO PRESERVE β-CELLS

Several immunotherapies have been tried to preserve β-cell function because even a small amount of residual function correlates with better clinical outcomes, including less hypoglycemia risk and fewer long-term microvascular complications. Selective immunomodulation has been tried with rituximab (anti-CD 20), teplizumab, abatacept, alefacept, high-dose ATG, and low-dose ATG. Because the autoimmune process is heterogenous, there is variable success with these therapies and, as of now, there is no specific therapy approved for clinical use to modulate autoimmunity and preserve β-cell function. There are also some studies focused on inducing tolerance via plasmid expressing preproinsulin 2 and a combination of immunomodulatory cytokines including transforming growth factor-β1, IL-10, and IL-2. This therapy is purported to induce antigen-specific tolerization without inducing global immune suppression.[59] These are discussed in detail elsewhere in this issue.

SUMMARY

Honeymoon phase or PR phase occurs through a combination of metabolic factors, such as reduction in glucotoxicity, β-cell rest, reduction in insulin resistance, and immunologic phenomena, such as development of immunologic tolerance, β-cell regeneration, and waxing and waning autoimmunity. Because autoimmune destruction of β cells is the fundamental pathophysiology behind development of T1D, the honeymoon phase provides a unique opportunity to study the autoimmune process in detail. Studies are underway to prolong the honeymoon phase and to reverse the autoimmune process.

CLINICS CARE POINTS

- The honeymoon phase is a period of improved β-cell function that is seen shortly after clinical diagnosis of T1D and the start of exogenous insulin therapy.
- During this phase there is reduced need for exogenous insulin while optimal blood glucose control is maintained.
- Many different factors contribute to this improved function. β-Cell rest and decreased insulin resistance after exogenous insulin initiation improves endogenous insulin secretion from residual β cells.

- The autoimmune process in T1D is waxing and waning. During the honeymoon phase, the autoimmune process is believed to be more quiescent leading also to some β-cell regeneration.
- Understanding the pathophysiology behind the honeymoon phase is important because even small amounts of residual β-cell function are noted to decrease risk for severe hypoglycemia and microvascular complications.
- Studies are underway to prolong the honeymoon phase and/or reverse the autoimmune process.

DISCLOSURE

A. Viswanathan: Nothing to disclose. J. Wood: Has research funding from Mannkind, Insulet, and BI. All unrelated to this topic. B. Hatipoglu: Nothing to disclose.

REFERENCES

1. Atkinson MA, Eisenbarth GS, Michels AW. Type 1 diabetes. Lancet 2014; 383(9911):69–82.
2. DiMeglio LA, Evans-Molina C, Oram RA. Type 1 diabetes. HHS public access. Lancet 2019;176(3):139–48.
3. Mayer-Davis EJ, Lawrence JM, Dabelea D, et al. Incidence trends of type 1 and type 2 diabetes among youths, 2002–2012. New England Journal of Medicine 2017;376(15):1419–29.
4. Ilonen J, Kiviniemi M, Lempainen J, et al. Genetic susceptibility to type 1 diabetes in childhood: estimation of HLA class II associated disease risk and class II effect in various phases of islet autoimmunity. Pediatric Diabetes 2016;17:8–16.
5. So M, Speake C, Steck AK, et al. Advances in type 1 diabetes prediction using islet autoantibodies: beyond a simple count. Endocrine Reviews 2021;42(5): 584–604.
6. So M, O'Rourke C, Bahnson HT, Greenbaum CJ, Speake C. Autoantibody reversion: changing risk categories in multiple-autoantibody–positive individuals. Diabetes Care 2020;43(4):913–7.
7. von Herrath M, Bonifacio E. How benign autoimmunity becomes detrimental in type 1 diabetes. Proc Natl Acad Sci U S A 2021;118(44):1–3.
8. Budd MA, Monajemi M, Colpitts SJ, et al. Interactions between islets and regulatory immune cells in health and type 1 diabetes. Diabetologia 2021. https://doi.org/10.1007/s00125-021-05565-6/.
9. Hao W, Gitelman S, di Meglio LA, Boulware D, Greenbaum CJ. Fall in C-peptide during first 4 years from diagnosis of type 1 diabetes: variable relation to age, HbA1c, and insulin dose. Diabetes Care 2016;39(10):1664–70.
10. Greenbaum CJ, Beam CA, Boulware D, et al. Fall in C-peptide during first 2 years from diagnosis: evidence of at least two distinct phases from composite type 1 diabetes TrialNet data. Diabetes 2012;61(8):2066–73.
11. Redondo MJ, Steck AK, Pugliese A. Genetics of type 1 diabetes. Pediatric Diabetes 2018;19(3):346–53.
12. Geravandi S, Liu H, Maedler K. Enteroviruses and T1D: is it the virus, the genes or both which cause T1D. Microorganisms 2020;8(7):1–20.
13. Jackson RL, Boyd JD, Smith TE. Stabilization of the diabetic child. Am J Dis Child 1940;59:332–41.

14. Lam A, Dayan C, Herold KC. A little help from residual β cells has long-lasting clinical benefits. J Clin Invest 2021;131(3):e143683.
15. Gubitosi-Klug RA, Braffett BH, Hitt S, et al. Residual β cell function in long-term type 1 diabetes associates with reduced incidence of hypoglycemia. Journal of Clinical Investigation 2021;131(3). https://doi.org/10.1172/JCI143011.
16. Gleason CE, Gonzalez M, Harmon JS, Robertson RP. Downloaded from Journals. Physiology.Org/Journal/Ajpendo at Cleveland Clinic 2000;279. Available at: http://www.ajpendo.org.
17. Aly HH, Gottlieb P. The honeymoon phase: intersection of metabolism and immunology. Current Opinion in Endocrinology, Diabetes and Obesity 2009;16(4): 286–92.
18. von Herrath M, Sanda S, Herold K. Type 1 diabetes as a relapsing-remitting disease? Nat Rev Immunol 2007;7(12):988–94.
19. Chiang JL, Kirkman MS, Laffel LM, Peters AL. Type 1 Diabetes Sourcebook Authors. Type 1 diabetes through the life span: a position statement of the American Diabetes Association. Diabetes Care 2014;37(7):2034–54.
20. Greenbaum CJ, Speake C, Krischer J, et al. Strength in numbers: opportunities for enhancing the development of effective treatments for type 1 diabetes: the TrialNet experience. Diabetes 2018;67(7):1216–25.
21. Zhong T, Tang R, Gong S, Li J, Li X, Zhou Z. The remission phase in type 1 diabetes: changing epidemiology, definitions, and emerging immuno-metabolic mechanisms. Diabetes Metab Res Rev 2020;36(2):e3207.
22. Cameron FJ, Amin R, de Beaufort C, et al, International Society for Pediatric and Adolescent Diabetes. ISPAD clinical practice consensus guidelines 2014. Diabetes in adolescence. Pediatr Diabetes 2014;15(Suppl 20):245–56.
23. Couper JJ, Haller MJ, Greenbaum CJ, et al. ISPAD clinical practice consensus guidelines 2018: stages of type 1 diabetes in children and adolescents. Pediatr Diabetes 2018;19(Suppl 27):20–7.
24. Mortensen HB, Hougaard P, Swift P, et al. New definition for the partial remission period in children and adolescents with type 1 diabetes. Diabetes Care 2009; 32(8):1384–90.
25. Andersen ML, Hougaard P, Pörksen S, et al. Partial remission definition: validation based on the insulin dose-adjusted HbA1c (IDAA1C) in 129 Danish children with new-onset type 1 diabetes. Pediatr Diabetes 2014;15(7):469–76.
26. Chiavaroli V, Derraik JGB, Jalaludin MY, et al. Partial remission in type 1 diabetes and associated factors: analysis based on the insulin dose-adjusted hemoglobin A1c in children and adolescents from a regional diabetes center, Auckland, New Zealand. Pediatr Diabetes 2019;20(7):892–900.
27. Marino KR, Lundberg RL, Jasrotia A, et al. A predictive model for lack of partial clinical remission in new-onset pediatric type 1 diabetes. PLoS One 2017;12(5): e0176860.
28. Nagl K, Hermann JM, Plamper M, et al. Factors contributing to partial remission in type 1 diabetes: analysis based on the insulin dose-adjusted HbA1c in 3657 children and adolescents from Germany and Austria. Pediatr Diabetes 2017;18(6): 428–34.
29. Lundberg RL, Marino KR, Jasrotia A, et al. Partial clinical remission in type 1 diabetes: a comparison of the accuracy of total daily dose of insulin of <0.3 units/kg/ day to the gold standard insulin-dose adjusted hemoglobin A1c of ≤9 for the detection of partial clinical remission. J Pediatr Endocrinol Metab 2017;30(8): 823–30.

30. Humphreys A, Bravis V, Kaur A, et al. Individual and diabetes presentation characteristics associated with partial remission status in children and adults evaluated up to 12 months following diagnosis of type 1 diabetes: an ADDRESS-2 (After Diagnosis Diabetes Research Support System-2) study analysis. Diabetes Res Clin Pract 2019;155:107789.

31. Chobot A, Stompór J, Szyda K, et al. Remission phase in children diagnosed with type 1 diabetes in years 2012 to 2013 in Silesia, Poland: an observational study. Pediatr Diabetes 2019;20(3):286–92.

32. Nwosu BU. Partial clinical remission of type 1 diabetes mellitus in children: clinical applications and challenges with its definitions. Eur Med J Diabetes 2019; 4(1):89–98.

33. Pozzilli P, Manfrini S, Buzzetti R, et al. Glucose evaluation trial for remission (GE-TREM) in type 1 diabetes: a European multicentre study. Diabetes Res Clin Pract 2005;68(3):258–64.

34. Bowden SA, Duck MM, Hoffman RP. Young children (<5 yr) and adolescents (>12 yr) with type 1 diabetes mellitus have low rate of partial remission: diabetic ketoacidosis is an important risk factor. Pediatr Diabetes 2008;9(3 Pt 1):197–201.

35. Wong TWC, Wong MYS, But WMB. Features of partial remission in children with type 1 diabetes using the insulin dose-adjusted A1c definition and risk factors associated with nonremission. Ann Pediatr Endocrinol Metab 2021;26(2):118–25.

36. Fonolleda M, Murillo M, Vázquez F, Bel J, Vives-Pi M. Remission phase in paediatric type 1 diabetes: new understanding and emerging biomarkers. Horm Res Paediatr 2017;88(5):307–15.

37. Bogun MM, Bundy BN, Goland RS, Greenbaum CJ. C-peptide levels in subjects followed longitudinally before and after type 1 diabetes diagnosis in TrialNet. Diabetes Care 2020;43(8):1836–42.

38. Shields BM, McDonald TJ, Oram R, et al. C-peptide decline in type 1 diabetes has two phases: an initial exponential fall and a subsequent stable phase. Diabetes Care 2018;41(7):1486–92.

39. Gomez-Muñoz L, Perna-Barrull D, Villalba A, et al. NK cell subsets changes in partial remission and early stages of pediatric type 1 diabetes. Front Immunol 2021;11:611522.

40. Wesley JD, Pfeiffer S, Schneider D, et al. Peripheral autoreactive CD8 T-cell frequencies are too variable to be a reliable predictor of disease progression of human type 1 diabetes. Clin Transl Immunology 2021;10(7):e1309.

41. Gomez-Muñoz L, Perna-Barrull D, Caroz-Armayones JM, et al. Candidate biomarkers for the prediction and monitoring of partial remission in pediatric type 1 diabetes. Front Immunol 2022;13:825426.

42. Narsale A, Lam B, Moya R, et al. CD4+CD25+CD127hi cell frequency predicts disease progression in type 1 diabetes. JCI Insight 2021;6(2):e136114.

43. Fitas AL, Martins C, Borrego LM, et al. Immune cell and cytokine patterns in children with type 1 diabetes mellitus undergoing a remission phase: a longitudinal study. Pediatr Diabetes 2018;19(5):963–71.

44. Musthaffa Y, Hamilton-Williams EE, Nel HJ, et al. Proinsulin-specific T-cell responses correlate with estimated C-peptide and predict partial remission duration in type 1 diabetes. Clin Transl Immunology 2021;10(7):e1315.

45. Li X, Zhong T, Tang R, et al. PD-1 and PD-L1 expression in peripheral CD4/CD8+ T cells is restored in the partial remission phase in type 1 diabetes. J Clin Endocrinol Metab 2020;105(6):dgaa130.

46. Smith MJ, Cambier JC, Gottlieb PA. Endotypes in T1D: B lymphocytes and early onset. Curr Opin Endocrinol Diabetes Obes 2020;27(4):225–30.

47. Rajendran S, Anquetil F, Quesada-Masachs E, et al. IL-6 is present in beta and alpha cells in human pancreatic islets: expression is reduced in subjects with type 1 diabetes. Clin Immunol 2020;211:108320.

48. Richardson SJ, Rodriguez-Calvo T, Gerling IC, et al. Islet cell hyperexpression of HLA class I antigens: a defining feature in type 1 diabetes. Diabetologia 2016; 59(11):2448–58.

49. Marroqui L, Dos Santos RS, Op de Beeck A, et al. Interferon-α mediates human beta cell HLA class I overexpression, endoplasmic reticulum stress and apoptosis, three hallmarks of early human type 1 diabetes. Diabetologia 2017; 60(4):656–67.

50. Schulte BM, Lanke KH, Piganelli JD, et al. Cytokine and chemokine production by human pancreatic islets upon enterovirus infection. Diabetes 2012;61(8):2030–6.

51. Roep BO, Kleijwegt FS, van Halteren AG, et al. Islet inflammation and CXCL10 in recent-onset type 1 diabetes. Clin Exp Immunol 2010;159(3):338–43.

52. Bender C, Rajendran S, von Herrath MG. New insights into the role of autoreactive CD8 T cells and cytokines in human type 1 diabetes. Front Endocrinol (Lausanne) 2021;11:606434.

53. Uno S, Imagawa A, Saisho K, et al. Expression of chemokines, CXC chemokine ligand 10 (CXCL10) and CXCR3 in the inflamed islets of patients with recent-onset autoimmune type 1 diabetes. Endocr J 2010;57(11):991–6.

54. Glisic-Milosavljevic S, Waukau J, Jailwala P, et al. At-risk and recent-onset type 1 diabetic subjects have increased apoptosis in the CD4+CD25+ T-cell fraction. PLoS One 2007;2(1):e146.

55. Hull CM, Peakman M, Tree TIM. Regulatory T cell dysfunction in type 1 diabetes: what's broken and how can we fix it? Diabetologia 2017;60(10):1839–50.

56. Schneider A, Rieck M, Sanda S, Pihoker C, Greenbaum C, Buckner JH. The effector T cells of diabetic subjects are resistant to regulation via CD4+ FOXP3+ regulatory T cells. J Immunol 2008;181(10):7350–5.

57. Arif S, Tree TI, Astill TP, et al. Autoreactive T cell responses show proinflammatory polarization in diabetes but a regulatory phenotype in health. J Clin Invest 2004; 113(3):451–63.

58. Arif S, Leete P, Nguyen V, et al. Blood and islet phenotypes indicate immunological heterogeneity in type 1 diabetes. Diabetes 2014;63(11):3835–45 [published correction appears in Diabetes. 2015 Sep;64(9):3334].

59. Pagni PP, Chaplin J, Wijaranakula M, et al. Multicomponent plasmid protects mice from spontaneous autoimmune diabetes. Diabetes 2021;db210327, published online ahead of print, 2021 Aug 13.

Islet Cell Therapy and Stem Cell Therapy for Type 1 Diabetes: There Will Always Be a Hope

Betul A. Hatipoglu, MD[a,b,]*, Julia Blanchette, PhD, RN[c]

KEYWORDS

• Beta cell • Type 1 diabetes • Diabetes • Transplant • Pancreas

KEY POINTS

• The cure for type 1 diabetes is getting closer as current work is focusing on renewable sources of β cells, transplantation methods without immunosuppressives, and methods to preserve β-cell function.
• Methods that may pave the way for the cure to type 1 diabetes include β-cell encapsulation, scaffolding, immune modulation, gene editing, and disease-modifying therapies.
• Barriers to making some of these therapies a reality include the lack of population screening to identify people at risk of developing type 1 diabetes or those who are early in disease progression, of insurance coverage and cost burden, and of engagement among marginalized populations borne from historical mistreatment.

INTRODUCTION

The dysfunctional pancreas theory by Mering and Minkowski in 1889 led to the discovery of the β cell. After the ability to isolate insulin by Banting and Best in 1921, the focus of diabetes research was to find ways to replace β cells and eliminate the need for people with type 1 diabetes (T1D) to depend on subcutaneous insulin. The ultimate goal of β-cell replacement therapy is to transplant and generate mature, fully functional β cells successfully. Fully functional β cells can secrete appropriate amounts of insulin in response to glucose.

Our previous article[1] described pancreas transplantation methods, autotransplantations and allotransplantations of islet cells, xenotransplantation, stem cell

[a] Department of Medicine, Case Western Reserve University School of Medicine, Cleveland, OH, USA; [b] Adult Endocrinology, Department of Medicine, University Hospitals Cleveland Medical Center, 11100 Euclid Avenue, Cleveland, OH 44106, USA; [c] Division of Endocrinology, University Hospitals Cleveland Medical Center, Center for Diabetes and Obesity, 11100 Euclid Avenue, Cleveland, OH 44106, USA
* Corresponding author. Department of Medicine, Adult Endocrinology, University Hospitals Cleveland Medical Center, 11100 Euclid Avenue, Cleveland, OH 44106.
E-mail address: bxh258@case.edu

Endocrinol Metab Clin N Am 52 (2023) 187–193
https://doi.org/10.1016/j.ecl.2022.07.001
0889-8529/23/© 2022 Elsevier Inc. All rights reserved.

transplantation, and mechanical replacement of β-cell function up to year 2018. We concluded that islet cell allotransplants are not a feasible cure for T1D without advancements in transplant sites or increasing volume of islet cells and that stem cell transplants for β replacement are promising. Although the lack of human donors is not a barrier to stem cell therapies, stem cell transplants do not reverse the autoimmune attack, require chronic immunosuppressant usage, and pose risks of immune rejection and tissue damage.[2] Broad immunosuppression therapy that reduces the risk of rejection and graft-versus-host disease comes with unwanted side effects, such as a heightened risk of opportunistic infections. In addition, there is a risk of β-cell hypoxia, poor revascularization, and inflammatory reactions. Therefore, we emphasized that technologies, such as the bionic pancreas, improves glycemic outcomes and quality of life in people with T1D as we wait for a cure. The purpose of this article is to review progress in β-cell therapies over the past 5 years.

To date, there is a focus on determining solutions so that stem cell transplants allowing for renewable sources of β cells become a reality. Current work focuses on evaluating renewable sources of β cells, transplantation methods for β cells that eliminate the need for immunosuppressives while keeping cells alive and functional, and methods to stop and reduce β-cell destruction as it occurs. These methods include β-cell encapsulation, scaffolds, immune modulation, gene editing, and disease-modifying therapies.

ENCAPSULATION

Encapsulation methods use a physical barrier to block an immune attack while ensuring the survival and function of β cells. The long-term goal of encapsulation is to allow for immunoprotection of transplanted islets or cells that mature into β cells and no need for lifelong immunosuppressant therapy. For successful encapsulation, there must be adequate transportation of nutrients, such as oxygen, glucose, and insulin, and hormone transport. Cells that are embedded in semipermeable structures made of biomaterials are protected from immune cells and have the ability for adequate nutrient and hormone transport.[3]

There are multiple kinds of encapsulation devices, including macroencapsulation, microencapsulation, and nanoencapsulation. Macroencapsulation devices are made of polymers, house a high volume of cells, and are most extensively studied thus far.[3] Macroencapsulation devices have been subcutaneously implanted containing PEC-01 cells that mature into a mixture of islet cells (pancreatic α, β, and δcells).[4] Macroencapsulation devices allow for direct vascularization of cells leading to cell engraftment and insulin production.[4] Macroencapsulation methods have not been studied long term, so the long-term survival of these stem cells is not yet determined in humans. Microencapsulation devices, however, are made of biomaterials and allow for more accessible nutrient and oxygen exchange, potentially allowing for better vascularization.[3] Gaps remain in understanding the long-term feasibility of encapsulation methods, further studying microencapsulation and nanoencapsulation methods, and developing even better biomaterials to prevent scar tissue formation.

SCAFFOLDS

Scaffolds are multiuse platforms that enable engineering of local environment to keep cells alive through porous structures that can deliver medications. The main benefit of scaffolds is the ability to deliver oxygen to support cell survival and medications to promote blood vessel growth. Their porous structures allow for the delivery of nutrients and glucose and insulin regulation. In a preliminary clinical trial, cell pouches were implanted in the abdominal wall to evaluate safety and efficacy. Therapy consists of initial device placement and follow-up islet cell transplants.[5] Thus far, the cell pouches are safe, well tolerated, demonstrate the growth of blood vessel networks, and have increased serum C-peptide in a small sample.[5] Requirement of immunosuppressant therapy after islet cell transplant remains a limitation. Further testing of cell pouches with scaffold technology needs to be further evaluated for optimizing clinical outcomes.[5]

IMMUNE MODULATION

Immune modulation alters the immune response to implanted cells at the local level, allowing the implanted cells to thrive. Biomaterials allow for controlled delivery of medications directly to the implantation site to suppress immune rejection. A recent study implanted unmodified islet cells using immune modulation technology in nonhuman primates. In this animal study, sustained glycemic control, C-peptide levels, and graft survival remained over 6 months, whereas the control group rejected islet cell grafts.[6] Although under early investigation, immune modulation therapies have translational potential for nonimmunosuppressants requiring β-cell replacement therapies in humans.

GENE EDITING

Gene editing to enhance survival and function of implanted β cells is currently being studied. Ideally, other cells will be converted into β cells through delivery signals. Evaluation of gene therapies to target specific genes and proteins involved in immune recognition, autoimmunity, and tolerance to make converted cells more robust and enhance their functionality is being studied. CRISPR is a technique that allows for precise, directed changes to DNA. Allogenic (donor-device) stem cells gene-edited using CRISPR are being studied to replace β cells. This therapy would allow for the regeneration of β cells while eliminating the need for immunosuppressant therapy. However, to date, this therapy is under early investigation.

DISEASE-MODIFYING THERAPIES

In addition to β-cell regeneration, there is a focus on delaying the onset of T1D in those at risk of development. Disease-modifying therapies aim to delay β-cell apoptosis through therapies that control autoimmunity and preserve or regenerate β cells. These therapies change the course of T1D and are aimed at populations within certain stages of T1D onset. Before stage 1 of T1D, there is recognition of self and activation of the immune system. During stage 1, there is glucose homeostasis, but 2 or more autoantibodies are present. During stage 2, glycemic excursions and dysregulation begin to present. Stage 3 is when some insulin secretion remains (honeymoon phase), but external insulin dependence presents. A clinical diagnosis of T1D is often made during stage 3. Stage 4 is when T1D is established. Most disease-modifying therapies are targeted at individuals with a family history of T1D who screen positive for multiple T1D autoantibodies or soon after clinical T1D diagnosis during stage 3.

Teplizumab

Teplizumab is a humanized anti-CD3 monoclonal antibody given via intravenous (IV) infusion, being evaluated for preventing or delaying the onset of T1D. In those at high risk of developing T1D or first-degree relatives, with at least 2 autoantibodies and an abnormal oral glucose tolerance test (OGTT), a single 2-week IV course of

Teplizumab was given.[7] The mean time to progression to T1D diagnosis was 48.4 months in the Teplizumab group versus 24.4 months in the placebo group ($P = .006$). In the extended follow-up study, the median times to diagnosis were 59.6 months in the Teplizumab group and 27.1 months in the placebo group ($P = .01$), indicating a course of Teplizumab delayed time to diagnosis of T1D.[7,8] In the extended follow-up study, Teplizumab improved β-cell function as evidenced by lower OGTT levels and higher C-peptide responses than in the placebo group.[8] These findings support that T1D is a chronic T-cell–mediated disease and that immunomodulation before development to clinical disease can help preserve β-cell function.[7] Furthermore, delay in time without daily management of T1D has a meaningful impact on quality of life. In addition, β-cell preservation to delay β-cell atrophy is beneficial in reducing incidences of T1D with diabetic ketoacidosis (DKA) at diagnosis.[7] Teplizumab is currently under review by the Food and Drug Administration (FDA) for treatment to delay T1D onset and is promising in delaying the onset of T1D in high-risk individuals. Gaps remain in identifying cost-effective methods and persuading insurance companies to cover T1D screening for the general population, as 90% of people who develop T1D do not have a family history.[9]

Verapamil

Verapamil is an FDA-approved antihypertensive medication that has been used for decades. Preclinical studies and mouse models showed Verapamil to reduce expression of TXNIP, prevent β-cell apoptosis, promote β-cell mass, and improve glycemic regulation.[10] Recently, it has been shown that oral Verapamil can promote endogenous β-cell function in adults with T1D onset within the previous 3 months. In a randomized, double-blind, placebo-controlled phase 2 clinical trial (N = 32), adults recently diagnosed with T1D who were given Verapamil required less exogenous insulin and were able to achieve better glycemic control than the placebo group at 3 months ($P<.05$) and 12 months ($P<.05$).[10] These effects were achieved without adverse events, such as hypotension or electrocardiographic changes.[10] To make this treatment a reality, large-scale limitations remain in identifying people with recently diagnosed T1D soon enough for effective therapy. Furthermore, the effectiveness of Verapamil needs to be further tested in more extensive trials.

Imatinib

Imatinib is a tyrosine kinase inhibitor used for chronic myelogenous leukemia that may impact immunologic and metabolic pathways, such as countering high levels of endoplasmic reticulum stress in β cells to preserve and reduce β-cell apoptosis.[11] Those with recently diagnosed T1D who were positive for at least 1 autoantibody and had peak stimulated C-peptide of greater than 0.2 during a mixed-meal tolerance test were enrolled in the imatinib study.[11] A 26-week treatment of imatinib slowed the decrease in β-cell function for up to 12 months, but not 24 months. The β-cell glucose sensitivity decreased when participants were off active treatment.[11] These results are promising, but gaps remain in identifying the ideal dose and duration of therapy, safety and efficacy in children, ability to delay or prevent progression of T1D, and potential combinations with other therapies.[11] Furthermore, real-world utilization would require intervention before progression to stage 4 of T1D, which may be difficult to catch in time for many individuals.

Anti-Interleukin-21 Antibody and Liraglutide

Another pathway to reduce β-cell stress and prevent apoptosis is the combination of anti–interleukin-21 (IL-21) and glucagon-like peptide-1 receptor agonists (GLP-1 RA).

The IL-21 medication is immunotherapy central to the role of the cytokine in promoting CD8[+] lymphocytes from lymph nodes and the exocrine pancreas islets.[12] Liraglutide, a GLP-1 RA, has been found to reduce β-cell stress and prevent apoptosis while protecting against cytokine-mediated effects on glucose-stimulated insulin secretion.[12] The combination of IL-21 and Liraglutide integrates immunomodulation and has shown promising results in mouse models. Adults recently diagnosed with T1D and residual C-peptide (≥0.2 nmol/L) (N = 308) who received a combination of anti-IL-21 and liraglutide had significantly reduced insulin requirements compared with the placebo groups (P<.001) without any adverse safety events.[12] However, these benefits diminished upon treatment cessation, and changes in immune cell subsets were mild over time.[12] Remaining gaps include understanding the ideal duration of time for liraglutide delivery, the current expensive cost and lack of insurance coverage for liraglutide, and the need to identify individuals with early-onset T1D before progression to stage 4.

BIONIC PANCREAS UPDATE

As we wait for functional and efficient β-cell regeneration and preservation therapies to become a reality, we can lean on diabetes technologies that improve glycemic outcomes and quality of life. The iLet bionic pancreas system mimics the function of the β and α cells to deliver insulin and glucagon based on glucose trends. The system consists of an insulin pump to deliver subcutaneous insulin and dasiglucagon, integration with a continuous glucose monitor to detect glucose levels, and an autonomous mechanical dosing algorithm to adjust insulin delivery.[13]

Glucose data from a continuous glucose monitor sensor are sent to the insulin pump, which contains an algorithm. The algorithm bases its initial decisions on the individual's body mass and uses the sensor glucose data to determine if more insulin delivery is required or if dasiglucagon is required to keep glucose in the target range. If warranted, insulin or dasiglucagon is delivered subcutaneously.[13] In addition to being one of the first systems to mimic both α- and β-cell function, it is user-friendly, practical in populations with lower literacy levels, requires minimal user input information (only body weight) to start up the system, and does not require the patient to precisely enter carbohydrates.[13] In an open-label, random-order, cross-over, home-use trial, the bihormonal system was used safely and resulted in 79% ± 9% time in range (70–180 mg/dL) and mean glucose of 139 ± 11 mg/dL.[13] This bihormonal system continues to be tested and remains a promising interim self-management solution for people living with T1D.

DISCUSSION

We have entered a time of multiple, promising β-cell therapies with the potential to cure T1D. However, as we enter this new era, we must acknowledge the remaining gaps. Specifically, we must acknowledge the historical mistreatment of marginalized populations, which has contributed to a lack of trust among these populations. It is critical to build trust with and ensure the inclusion of individuals with T1D from these populations in pharmacologic and device trials, continuing to evaluate these emerging therapies to ensure generalized efficacy. In addition, a considerable limitation of many emerging disease-modifying therapies is the timely identification of those at risk of T1D development and catching those who develop T1D during phase 3; otherwise, many of these therapies have little meaning. Clinicians, scientists, and industry leaders should advocate for insurance coverage and implementation of widespread screening of T1D to identify individuals during stage 3 and early stage 4 of T1D progression to benefit from these potential therapies. Large-scale screening for T1D is cost-effective in communities with high DKA incidences[14] and may continue to have benefits if the disease-modifying therapies come to market. Last, we must keep in mind that although the potential and current therapies described are promising, we need to advocate to insurance companies regarding the cost-benefit and importance of coverage for all people living with T1D, specifically those on public health insurance.

SUMMARY

Cures for T1D are finally on the horizon, and the advances addressed above result from tremendous efforts to change the lives of people living with T1D. However, we still wait for the day we can administer therapies to those early on in T1D progression or who have recently been diagnosed with T1D to improve the course of their disease management significantly. For now, technologies, such as the bionic pancreas, are exciting and give us promise to improve the lives of people with T1D.

DISCLOSURE

Dr B. Hatipoglu reports no conflicts of interest related to the content of the work. Dr J. Blanchette is on the advisory board of Cardinal Health-Edgepark, Proventin Bio, and Lifescan, a consultant for WellDoc, and an independent contractor for Tandem Diabetes, and Insulet Corporation.

The work was partially funded by the Mary B. Lee Chair in Adult Endocrinology (Dr. Hatipoglu

REFERENCES

1. Rodeman KB, Hatipoglu B. Beta-cell therapies for type 1 diabetes: transplants and bionics. Cleve Clin J Med 2018;85(12):931–7.
2. Deb L, Jenkins M, Meredith M, et al. The role of stem cells in the treatment of type 1 diabetes mellitus and associated complications. Georgetown Med Rev 2021; 5(1). https://doi.org/10.52504/001c.29777.
3. Bourgeois S, Sawatani T, Van Mulders A, et al. Towards a functional cure for diabetes using stem cell-derived beta cells: are we there yet? Cells 2021;10(1):191.
4. Shapiro AMJ, Thompson D, Donner TW, et al. Insulin expression and C-peptide in type 1 diabetes subjects implanted with stem cell-derived pancreatic endoderm cells in an encapsulation device. Cell Rep Med 2021;2(12):100466.
5. Bachul PJ, Perez-Gutierrez A, Juengel B, et al. 306-OR: modified approach for improved islet allotransplantation into prevascularized sernova cell pouch device: preliminary results of the phase i/ii clinical trial at University of Chicago. Diabetes 2022;71(Supplement_1):30CR.
6. Lei J, Coronel MM, Yolcu ES, et al. FasL microgels induce immune acceptance of islet allografts in nonhuman primates. Sci Adv 2022;8(19):eabm9881.
7. Herold KC, Bundy BN, Long SA, et al. An anti-CD3 antibody, teplizumab, in relatives at risk for type 1 diabetes. N Engl J Med 2019;381(7):603–13.
8. Sims EK, Bundy BN, Stier K, et al. Teplizumab improves and stabilizes beta cell function in antibody-positive high-risk individuals. Sci Transl Med 2021;13(583): eabc8980.
9. Greenbaum CJ. A Key to T1D prevention: screening and monitoring relatives as part of clinical care. Diabetes 2021;70(5):1029–37.
10. Ovalle F, Grimes T, Xu G, et al. Verapamil and beta cell function in adults with recent-onset type 1 diabetes. Nat Med 2018;24(8):1108–12.

11. Gitelman SE, Bundy BN, Ferrannini E, et al. Imatinib therapy for patients with recent-onset type 1 diabetes: a multicentre, randomised, double-blind, placebo-controlled, phase 2 trial. Lancet Diabetes Endocrinol 2021;9(8):502–14.
12. Von Herrath M, Bain SC, Bode B, et al. Anti-interleukin-21 antibody and liraglutide for the preservation of β-cell function in adults with recent-onset type 1 diabetes: a randomised, double-blind, placebo-controlled, phase 2 trial. Lancet Diabetes Endocrinol 2021;9(4):212–24.
13. Castellanos LE, Balliro CA, Sherwood JS, et al. Performance of the insulin-only ilet bionic pancreas and the bihormonal ilet using dasiglucagon in adults with type 1 diabetes in a home-use setting. Diabetes Care 2021;44(6):e118–20.
14. McQueen RB, Geno Rasmussen C, Waugh K, et al. Cost and cost-effectiveness of large-scale screening for type 1 diabetes in Colorado. Diabetes Care 2020; 43(7):1496–503.

Moving?

Make sure your subscription moves with you!

To notify us of your new address, find your **Clinics Account Number** (located on your mailing label above your name), and contact customer service at:

Email: **journalscustomerservice-usa@elsevier.com**

800-654-2452 (subscribers in the U.S. & Canada)
314-447-8871 (subscribers outside of the U.S. & Canada)

Fax number: **314-447-8029**

**Elsevier Health Sciences Division
Subscription Customer Service
3251 Riverport Lane
Maryland Heights, MO 63043**

*To ensure uninterrupted delivery of your subscription, please notify us at least 4 weeks in advance of move.

Printed and bound by CPI Group (UK) Ltd, Croydon, CR0 4YY

08/05/2025

01864719-0001